Harper College Library

3 2158 00479 9985

OCT 2

P9-DHT-890

DATE DUE

GAYLORD | | | PRINTED IN U.S.A.

Early Diagnosis and Treatment of Cancer: Head and Neck Cancer

Early Diagnosis and Treatment of Cancer

Series Editor: Stephen C. Yang, MD

Breast Cancer
Edited by Lisa Jacobs and Christina A. Finlayson

Colorectal Cancer
Edited by Susan Lyn Gearhart and Nita Ahuja

Head and Neck Cancer
Edited by Wayne M. Koch

Ovarian Cancer
Edited by Robert E. Bristow and
Deborah K. Armstrong

Prostate Cancer
Edited by Li-Ming Su

EARLY DIAGNOSIS AND TREATMENT OF CANCER

Series Editor: Stephen C. Yang, MD

Head and Neck Cancer

Edited by

Wayne M. Koch, MD

Professor
Department of Otolaryngology–Head and Neck Surgery
The Johns Hopkins Hospital
Baltimore, Maryland

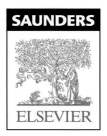

SAUNDERS

ELSEVIER

SAUNDERS
ELSEVIER

1600 John F. Kennedy Blvd.
Ste 1800
Philadelphia, PA 19103-2899

EARLY DIAGNOSIS AND TREATMENT OF CANCER: ISBN-13: 978-1-4160-5202-9
HEAD AND NECK CANCER

Copyright © 2010 by Saunders, an imprint of Elsevier Inc. All rights reserved.

No part of this publication may be reproduced or transmitted in any form or by any means, electronic
or mechanical, including photocopying, recording, or any information storage and retrieval system,
without permission in writing from the publisher. Details on how to seek permission, further
information about the Publisher's permissions policies and our arrangements with organizations such as
the Copyright Clearance Center and the Copyright Licensing Agency, can be found at our website:
www.elsevier.com/permissions.

This book and the individual contributions contained in it are protected under copyright by the Publisher
(other than as may be noted herein).

Notices

Knowledge and best practice in this field are constantly changing. As new research and experience
broaden our understanding, changes in research methods, professional practices, or medical
treatment may become necessary.

Practitioners and researchers must always rely on their own experience and knowledge in
evaluating and using any information, methods, compounds, or experiments described herein.
In using such information or methods they should be mindful of their own safety and the safety
of others, including parties for whom they have a professional responsibility.

With respect to any drug or pharmaceutical products identified, readers are advised to check
the most current information provided (i) on procedures featured or (ii) by the manufacturer of
each product to be administered, to verify the recommended dose or formula, the method and
duration of administration, and contraindications. It is the responsibility of practitioners, relying on
their own experience and knowledge of their patients, to make diagnoses, to determine dosages and
the best treatment for each individual patient, and to take all appropriate safety precautions.

To the fullest extent of the law, neither the Publisher nor the authors, contributors, or editors,
assume any liability for any injury and/or damage to persons or property as a matter of products
liability, negligence or otherwise, or from any use or operation of any methods, products,
instructions, or ideas contained in the material herein.

Library of Congress Cataloging-in-Publication Data

Early diagnosis and treatment of cancer : head and neck cancer / edited by Wayne M. Koch.
     p. ; cm.—(Early diagnosis and treatment of cancer series)
  ISBN 978-1-4160-5202-9
  1. Head—Cancer. 2. Neck—Cancer. I. Koch, Wayne M. II. Title: Head and neck
cancer. III. Series: Early diagnosis and treatment of cancer series.
  [DNLM: 1. Head and Neck Neoplasms—diagnosis. 2. Early Diagnosis. 3. Head and Neck
Neoplasms—therapy. WE 707 E12 2010]
  RC280.H4E27   2010
  616.99′491—dc22

                                                        2009028019

Acquisitions Editor: Dolores Meloni
Design Direction: Steven Stave

Printed in China.

Last digit is the print number: 9 8 7 6 5 4 3 2 1

Working together to grow
libraries in developing countries

www.elsevier.com | www.bookaid.org | www.sabre.org

ELSEVIER   BOOK AID
            International   Sabre Foundation

HARPER COLLEGE LIBRARY
PALATINE, ILLINOIS 60067

Contents

Series Preface

Seen on a graph, the survival rate for many cancers resembles a precipice. Discovered at an early stage, most cancers are quickly treatable, and the prognosis is excellent. In late stages, however, the typical treatment protocol becomes longer, more intense, and more harrowing for the patient, and the survival rate declines steeply. No wonder, then, that one of the most important means in fighting cancer is to prevent or screen for earlier stage tumors.

Within each oncologic specialty, there is a strong push to identify new, more useful tools for early diagnosis and treatment, with an emphasis on methods amenable to an office-based or clinical setting. These efforts have brought impressive results. Advances in imaging technology, as well as the development of sophisticated molecular and biochemical tools, have led to effective, minimally invasive approaches to cancer in its early stages.

This series, *Early Diagnosis and Treatment of Cancer*, gathers state-of-the-art research and recommendations into compact, easy-to-use volumes. For each particular type of cancer, the books cover the full range of diagnostic and treatment procedures, including pathologic, radiologic, chemotherapeutic, and surgical methods, focusing on questions like these:

- What do practitioners need to know about the epidemiology of the disease and its risk factors?
- How do patients and their families wade through and interpret the many tests they face?
- What is the safest, quickest, least invasive way to reach an accurate diagnosis?
- How can the stage of the disease be determined?
- What are the best initial treatments for early-stage disease, and how should the practitioner and the patient choose among them?
- What lifestyle factors might affect the outcome of treatment?

Each volume in the series is edited by an authority within the subfield, and the contributors have been chosen for their practical skills as well as their research credentials. Key Points at the beginning of each chapter help the reader grasp the main ideas at once. Frequent illustrations make the techniques vivid and easy to visualize. Boxes and tables summarize recommended strategies, protocols, indications and contraindications, important statistics, and other essential information. Overall, the attempt is to make expert advice as accessible as possible to a wide variety of health care professionals.

For the first time since the inception of the National Cancer Institute's annual status reports, the 2008 "Annual Report to the Nation on the Status of Cancer," published in the December 3 issue of the *Journal of the National Cancer Institute*, noted a statistically significant decline in "both incidence and death rates from all cancers combined." This mark of progress encourages all of us to press forward with our efforts. I hope that the volumes in *Early Diagnosis and*

Treatment of Cancer will make health care professionals and patients more familiar with the latest developments in the field, as well as more confident in appling them, so that early detection and swift, effective treatment become a reality for all our patients.

Stephen C. Yang, MD
The Arthur B. and Patricia B. Modell
Professor of Thoracic Surgery
Chief of Thoracic Surgery
The Johns Hopkins Medical Institutions
Baltimore, Maryland

Preface

Early detection of cancer is one of the "Holy Grails" of management of that disease, made all the more urgent by the recent announcement that cancer is expected to supersede heart disease as the number one cause of death in the United States by 2010. The fundamental concept is based on the time-honored observation that treatment is most successful with earliest staged lesions. Together with the concept that tumors grow and increase in stage in a generally uniform manner over time, clinical experience of improved outcome when cancer is detected early provides enormous intuitive benefit to early detection. Whether this logic follows the observations is arguable, but the rationale is strong enough to drive many clinical and laboratory endeavors, which we outline in the chapters that follow.

Endeavors to improve early detection of head and neck cancer face some challenges common to all types of cancer and some that are particular to upper aerodigestive malignancy. From a population and demographic vantage point, head and neck cancer is much less common than the most common adult malignancies—lung, prostate, breast, and colon—but it ranks in the top ten in the United States, about as common as lymphoma or melanoma. Elsewhere, head and neck cancer is a bigger public health problem. Long the most common adult cancer in India, the emerging economy in China has opened that population to the risk of smoking-related cancers including HNSCC. It is too common a cancer to ignore with no effort at public health endeavors for detection and prevention, but uncommon enough to raise problems with who to screen and how to raise and maintain health provider skill and awareness for the task. The dental community has embraced head and neck cancer screening through useful efforts of the American Dental Association and the National Institute of Dental and Craniofacial Research, and, indeed, for those Americans who visit the dentist regularly, dental screening of soft tissues makes sense. Dental providers look at the mouth routinely, gaining a familiarity with normal and diseased states, and they see their clients frequently enough to maintain a regular program of screening. However, those most at risk for traditional forms of head and neck cancer are heavy smokers and drinkers, a group that often does not visit the dentist regularly. Furthermore, dental screening ends at the tonsil arch, where a new epidemic of cancer affecting nonsmokers and attributed to the human papillomavirus begins. Therefore, despite the advent of several new products marketed to help dental professionals with oral screening (which can be billed to the cash-paying client at a markup), dental screening alone will not adequately address all early detection concerns for head and neck cancer.

Primary care providers can visualize the tissues of the oral cavity and can palpate the neck for metastatic nodes, but all other regions of the upper aerodigestive tract are inaccessible for screening by visualization or palpation except by expert clinicians, chiefly otolaryngologists. Hence, like colon cancer, head and neck cancer screening is relegated to a specialist-referral arrangement outside the routine of health maintenance paradigms. Unlike prostate cancer, there is no blood test that adequately screens for head and neck cancer, and individuals cannot perform effective self-exams as they can for breast cancer. Even for the specialist, small cancers deep within crypts of the lympho-epithelium of the oropharyngeal tonsillar tissue (palatine and lingual tonsils) or within hidden folds in the hypopharynx or laryngeal ventricle may remain elusive for years before suspected and detected.

Turning to technology, hope for an effective screening tool for head and neck cancer has been the impetus for a great deal of research during the past decade, much of which is outlined in this volume. The challenge to identify markers for cancer that can be detected quickly, noninvasively, and cheaply with high specificity and sensitivity is daunting. Even if such a test were available, individuals at risk would still need to be reached by the health care establishment in order to receive the test, and then a clinically detectable lesion would need to be identified prior to initiating intervention. Still, efforts to apply radiographic studies, molecular detection of tumor-specific proteins, or nucleic acid alterations examining various specimens, including both blood and saliva, are underway across the country and around the world.

Much of this volume is dedicated to treatment of early cancers of the head and neck, where the goal is to effectively eradicate cancer while preserving both function and form of vital tissues and organs. Each region within the upper aerodigestive tract is unique in its challenges in this regard. Small lesions within the larynx are amenable to laser excision with great precision, avoiding collateral damage to remaining portions and preserving laryngeal function. Oral cavity lesions, likewise, are accessible to simple surgical extirpation, often with acceptable functional result. However, in both these regions, occult changes within cells surrounding the clinical lesion lead to a high rate of recurrence of cancer over time, particularly in the smoking population. Cancers of the nasopharynx and oropharynx are more sensitive to radiation, making this the treatment of choice after early detection. However, radiation delivered to these areas is a one-time tactic, making management of those cases that are not controlled a much greater strategic problem. Salvage surgery in these areas is hampered by the need to detect persistence early in a treatment-altered field even more limited in its access to physical and radiographic screening.

This timely volume seeks to address these issues in a comprehensive manner, pointing out the need, the challenges, and the prospects for future innovation. With cancer on the ascent in public concern in the United States, and increasing in frequency along with tobacco use in major population centers worldwide, it is difficult to overestimate the importance of early detection. It is our hope that the thoughtful submissions that follow will contribute in coming years to endeavors to improve the plight of many individuals who contract this most debilitating and deadly disease.

Wayne M. Koch, MD

Contributors

Anthony Alberg, Ph.D.
Division of Head and Neck Oncologic Surgery,
Medical University of South Carolina, Charleston,
South Carolina

Gopal Bajaj, M.D.
Radiation Oncologist, Radiation Oncology Department,
Inova Fairfax Hospital, Falls Church, Virginia

Anthony Bared, M.D.
Head and Neck Surgery, University of Miami Leonard M.
Miller School of Medicine, Miami, Florida

Joseph A. Califano III, M.D.
Professor, Department of Otolaryngology, Johns Hopkins
Head and Neck Surgery, The Milton J. Dance, Jr., Head
and Neck Center, Greater Baltimore Medical Center,
Baltimore, Maryland

Gabrielle Cannick, D.M.D.
Division of Head and Neck Oncologic Surgery, Medical
University of South Carolina, Charleston, South Carolina

Matthew Carpenter, M.D.
Division of Head and Neck Oncologic Surgery, Medical
University of South Carolina, Charleston, South Carolina

Angela Chi, D.M.D.
Assistant Professor, Division of Head and Neck Oncologic
Surgery, Medical University of South Carolina,
Charleston, South Carolina

Francisco J. Civantos, M.D.
Associate Professor, Head and Neck Surgery, University of
Miami Leonard M. Miller School of Medicine, Miami,
Florida

Terry Day, M.D.
Director, Head and Neck Tumor Program, Hollings
Cancer Center; Director, Division of Head and Neck
Oncologic Surgery, Medical University of South Carolina,
Charleston, South Carolina

Richard R. Drake, Ph.D.
Professor, Department of Microbiology and Molecular Cell
Biology, Eastern Virginia Medical School, Norfolk, Virginia

Joel B. Epstein, D.M.D., M.S.D.
Professor, Department of Oral Medicine and Diagnostic
Sciences; Department of Otolaryngology and Head and
Neck Surgery, College of Medicine, University of Illinois,
Chicago, Illinois

Tarik Y. Farrag, M.D.
Post-Doctoral Fellow, Department of Otolaryngology,
Johns Hopkins University School of Medicine, Baltimore,
Maryland

Marvella Ford, Ph.D.
Division of Head and Neck Oncologic Surgery, Medical
University of South Carolina, Charleston, South Carolina

Michael K. Gibson, M.D.
Associate Professor, Division of Hematology/Oncology,
University of Pittsburgh Medical Center, Pittsburgh,
Pennsylvania

David Goldenberg, M.D.
Associate Professor, Division of Otolaryngology—Head
and Neck Surgery, The Pennsylvania State University, The
Milton S. Hershey Medical Center, Hershey, Pennsylvania

Patrick K. Ha, M.D.
Assistant Professor, Department of Otolaryngology, Johns
Hopkins Head and Neck Surgery, The Milton J. Dance,
Jr., Head and Neck Center, Greater Baltimore Medical
Center, Baltimore, Maryland

Boris Hristov, M.D.
Chief Resident, Department of Radiation Oncology and
Molecular Radiation Sciences, The Johns Hopkins
University School of Medicine, Baltimore, Maryland

Heather A. Jacene, M.D.
Assistant Professor, Russell H. Morgan Department of
Radiology and Radiological Science, Division of Nuclear
Medicine, The Johns Hopkins University School of
Medicine, Baltimore, Maryland

Emad H. Kandil, M.D.
Assistant Professor of Surgery, Clinical Assistant Professor
of Medicine, Chief of Endocrine Surgery Section, Tulane
University School of Medicine, New Orleans, Louisiana

Rachel A. Koch, B.A.
Administrative Intern, Lawndale Community Health
Center, Chicago, Illinois

Wayne M. Koch, M.D.
Professor, Department of Otolaryngology—Head and
Neck Surgery, The Johns Hopkins Hospital, Baltimore,
Maryland

Oleg Militsakh, M.D.
Division of Head and Neck Oncologic Surgery, Medical
University of South Carolina, Charleston, South Carolina

Peter Miller, M.D.
Division of Head and Neck Oncologic Surgery, Medical
University of South Carolina, Charleston, South Carolina

Kavita Malhotra Pattani, M.D.
Instructor/Fellow, Department of Otolaryngology, The
Johns Hopkins Medical Institutions, Baltimore, Maryland

Britt C. Reid, D.D.S., Ph.D.
Assistant Professor, University of Maryland School of
Dentistry, University of Maryland, Baltimore, Maryland

James J. Sciubba, D.M.D., Ph.D.
Professor, The Johns Hopkins University School of
Medicine (Ret.); Consultant, The Milton J. Dance, Jr.,
Head and Neck Center, Greater Baltimore Medical
Center, Baltimore, Maryland

Ian M. Smith, M.D.
Resident, Department of Otolaryngology—Head and
Neck Surgery, The Johns Hopkins Medical Institutions,
Baltimore, Maryland

Edward M. Stafford, M.D.
Department of Otolaryngology, The Johns Hopkins
Hospital, Baltimore, Maryland

Natalie Sutkowski, Ph.D.
Division of Head and Neck Oncologic Surgery, Medical
University of South Carolina, Charleston, South Carolina

Ralph P. Tufano, M.D.
Associate Professor of Otolaryngology—Head and Neck
Surgery, The Johns Hopkins Medical Institutions,
Baltimore, Maryland

J. Trad Wadsworth, M.D.
Vice Chairman, Clinical Affairs; Associate Professor,
Department of Otolaryngology—Head and Neck Surgery,
Emory University School of Medicine, Atlanta, Georgia

Martha A. Zeiger, M.D.
Professor of Surgery, Chief of Endocrine Surgery Section,
The Johns Hopkins Medical Institutions, Baltimore,
Maryland

Robert Zitsch, M.D.
Head and Neck Surgery, University of Miami Leonard M.
Miller School of Medicine, Miami, Florida

1

Molecular Gene Alterations as Early-Detection Markers

Ian M. Smith, Joseph A. Califano III, and Patrick K. Ha

KEY POINTS

- Early diagnosis of head and neck squamous cell carcinoma (HNSCC) is the most significant factor in predicting survival for each tumor site.
- HNSCC has many promising molecular markers including human papilloma virus (HPV), p53, cyclin D1, p16, cyclooxygenase-2 (COX-2), epidermal growth factor (EGF), and vascular endothelial growth factor (VEGF).
- Molecular markers have been applied in several ways: early detection of cancer or screening and disease follow-up and progression.
- Population-based screening tests are extremely difficult to successfully undertake, owing to the low overall incidence and the associated rates of false-positive results in this sample set.
- Alternative efforts for molecular detection that do not require as much specificity for clinical use include molecular surgical margin analysis, lymph node analysis, disease surveillance after treatment, molecular staging, and/or molecularly tailored therapies.
- To date, few of the approaches for molecular screening and diagnosis have been taken to clinical trials. Notable exceptions are tests for loss of heterozygosity (for prognosis of premalignant lesions) and toluidine blue (for early detection).
- Many detection sources have been studied including saliva, salivary rinses, mouth scrapings, and blood serum or plasma.
- Major developmental efforts have been conducted on specific alterations including p53 mutation detection, mitochondrial mutations, promoter hypermethylation, loss of heterozygosity, and HPV detection.

Introduction

Early diagnosis is the most significant factor in predicting survival for each tumor site (Table 1-1). With the advent of newer biomedical technologies, there has been an increased interest in the development of early screening tests and noninvasive diagnostic tests for head and neck squamous cell carcinoma (HNSCC). Basic science understanding of the genetic and epigenetic alterations in the pathogenesis of cancer has yielded new molecular diagnostic approaches. Our understanding of tumor molecular biology has led to translating these advances into relevant clinical situations and applied pathology. Many promising molecular markers have been found including human papilloma virus (HPV), p53, cyclin D1, p16, cyclooxygenase-2 (COX-2), epidermal growth factor (EGF), and vascular endothelial growth factor (VEGF). This chapter discusses HNSCC molecular biomarkers—their benefits and limitations.

Molecular markers have been applied in several ways: early detection of cancer, disease follow-up and progression, specialized applications such as molecular surgical margin and lymph node analysis, molecular staging, and selection of tailored therapies. Each use of molecular markers is intended to improve patient survival, but these markers do so in different ways.

Table 1-1. Five-year Survival of Head and Neck Squamous Cell Carcinoma by Site and Extent of Disease at Presentation

Tumor Site	Extent of Disease		
	Local	Regional	Distant
Lip	91.4	82.6	52.2
Oral cavity	71.4	45.8	21.8
Salivary gland	85.5	56.7	23.4
Oropharynx	58.4	41.2	20.3
Nasopharynx	65.3	50.9	28.8
Hypopharynx	46.8	29.7	15.7
Larynx	79.2	54.8	35.4
Other	61.8	38.4	11.6

Adapted from Carvalho AL, Nishimoto IN, Califano JA, Kowalski LP: Trends in incidence and prognosis for head and neck cancer in the United States: a site-specific analysis of the SEER database. Int J Cancer 114(5):806–816, 2005.

This chapter discusses applications for molecular markers, premalignant disease and cancer progression model, body fluids, and mechanisms for detection, and it gives a background of genetic alterations used for detection. Several underlying assumptions should be mentioned at the outset. Tumor development is now widely recognized as a process involving multiple alterations affecting the genetic code that accumulate over time. Key molecular pathways may be affected by alterations in one of several targets, which may accrue over time in an order that may vary from case to case. There are several recognized clinical subsets of head and neck cancer, such as HPV-related oropharyngeal cancer, typical smoker-drinker cancers of the oral cavity or larynx, nonsmoker, nondrinker cancers of the lateral tongue, and so on. Each of these subsets may have somewhat distinctive molecular profiles.

The use of molecular markers for early detection therefore depends on the relative prevalence of specific alterations in the population to be tested and on the relative position of each alteration in the tumor progression pathway. Interpretation of collected molecular data must take into consideration several issues. First, is the molecular target truly indicative of the fully transformed malignant state, or by itself is it indicative only of risk or probability of cancer? Some markers may be present to a greater degree in cancer but still present in benign states. If so, how distinct is the breakpoint between benign and malignant state?

Molecular Marker Applications

Early Detection (Screening)

Head and neck squamous cell tumors have a tendency toward late-stage presentation because these growing neoplasms are often asymptomatic and taken as a whole. The noted exception is laryngeal lesions, which can often arise on the vocal folds and cause hoarseness, leading to an earlier medical presentation as well as anterior oral cavity lesions that may be easily visualized by the patient or the primary care or dental professional. Other head and neck cancers manifest as dysphagia, odynophagia, or a mass—symptoms associated with late-stage presentation. This chapter covers areas of investigation in molecular diagnostics, which include tests that may be adapted to screen high-risk populations without previous symptoms or findings, and the development of tests that may be used for detection of occult, persistent, or recurrent disease in patients who have already been diagnosed with HNSCC.

Within the realm of early detection, population-based screening tests are extremely difficult to successfully develop and deploy, owing to the low overall incidence and the associated rates of false-positives in this sample set. Population-based screening tests do benefit from well-outlined risk factors including tobacco and alcohol use. Even so, they suffer because of the difficulty of producing tests with adequate sensitivity to be useful in detection and with adequate specificity to not generate large numbers of false-positive results in the setting of low incidence. Furthermore, it is known that many of the common genetic alterations in HNSCC can be detected in patients who smoke but who do not have evidence of overt carcinoma. Other molecular detection applications, such as molecular margin detection, detection of nodal metastasis, and disease surveillance after treatment, simply do not require this level of testing specificity because the pertinent markers can be identified from the analysis of existing tumor tissue.

Tests developed in the laboratory for molecular diagnosis must be validated in clinical trials. To date, few of the approaches for molecular screening and diagnosis have been taken to clinical trials. Notable exceptions are tests for loss of heterozygosity (LOH) used for prognosis and toluidine blue staining of oral lesions as a means of enhancing detection.

Disease Surveillance: Follow-up and Progression

Routinely, patients who are postoperative or post-chemotherapy or radiation therapy are monitored by interval physical examination and radiologic imaging. Identifying early recurrence would be expected to have survival benefit or at least a benefit in reduced morbidity and tumor burden in patients with recurrences. Many of the molecular techniques discussed here lack the requisite sensitivity and specificity for population-based screening. However, because primary tumors can be studied directly in the setting of disease surveillance for recurrence, molecular alterations can be directly tailored to the patient. These efforts show remarkable promise in monitoring recurrence and treatment outcomes. Prominent examples of techniques include toluidine blue and LOH.[1]

Molecular Margin or Lymph Node Analysis

Traditional intraoperative frozen section and paraffin sections have been used to detect the presence of negative surgical margins and lymph node metastasis. However, intraoperative frozen sections are expensive, time-consuming, and effort-intensive and may not be as accurate as nonfrozen histopathology. Therefore, some surgeons rely on postoperative reports of margin detection based on hematoxylin-and-eosin (H&E)–stained slides to guide therapy. If margins are positive, patients may be subjected to repeat operations. Quick, reliable, and sensitive molecular detection techniques would augment surgical management. Published studies have used p53 mutation detection, p53 expression, and methylation markers to assess the presence of positive margins with varying success.[2,3]

Nodal status has a significant impact on overall survival in HNSCC, underscoring the importance of accurate staging of cervical lymph nodes. The traditional diagnostic approach relies on H&E staining; however standard methods of pathologic examination can yield false-negative results. Often, isolated neoplastic cells or micrometastases can be missed.[4] Investigators have attempted to use techniques such as quantitative reverse transcription-polymerase chain reaction (qRT-PCR), to detect cancer-specific antigens fast enough for use with pathologic frozen-section analysis. No studies have shown adequate usefulness for wide-scale adoption in detecting tumor spread to lymph nodes. Yet, pilot scale studies have shown promise in improving nodal staging. Molecules used successfully for detection include pemphigus vulgaris antigen[5] and squamous cell carcinoma antigen.[6] These studies offer promise that molecular detection will be translated into the clinic. One significant caveat remains that the clinical significance of molecular-positive cervical metastasis has not been demonstrated to date. The identification of tumor in a pathologically N0 neck, resulting in upstaging to N+ would be expected to have a greater impact than identification of additional nodes in cases already pathologically N+. Carefully designed prospective trials are a must to prove the efficacy of these applications.

Molecular Staging and Molecularly Designed Therapies

Efforts to coordinate clinical trial treatment arms to molecular diagnostic criteria have been made in the last 10 years. Adequate predictors of response have been elusive, but some promising targets have been found. One group has found that cyclin D1 overexpression correlates with cisplatin sensitivity in cell lines.[7] Overexpression of epidermal growth factor receptor (EGFR) has also been implicated in cisplatin resistance.[8]

Cancer Progression Model

Approaches to molecular diagnosis rely on heritable, documented changes involved in the pathogenesis of cancer. The head and neck cancer progression model was initially derived from Vogelstein's description of colon cancer progression.[9] This theory states that cancer results from multiple accumulated, progressively transforming genetic alterations in clonal population cells. This hypothesis is based on several principles, including the following: (1) neoplasms are caused by tumor suppressor gene inactivation and/or proto-oncogene activation; (2) an accumulation of genetic and epigenetic events causes the development of a tumor phenotype; and (3) net accumulation of alterations rather than a specific order of events determines the malignant phenotype.[10,11] In oral cancer, a similar stepwise progression model has also been described.

HNSCC is highly correlated with environmental exposures such as cigarette smoke, smokeless tobacco, and alcohol. Most theories concerning the etiology of HNSCC derive from accumulated molecular changes that are inflicted by DNA-damaging, carcinogenic exposures. Through comparison of the spectrum of alterations in premalignant and invasive cancers, genetic and epigenetic alterations can be classified as early or late.

Several common clinical lesions that may represent the premalignant state leading to HNSCC are leukoplakia, erythroplakia, oral lichen planus, and submucous fibrosis. Clearly an elevated cancer risk is associated with these lesions, but controversy remains regarding whether cancers develop from these lesions directly or are merely heralded by their appearance with invasive tumor and eventually appear elsewhere in the upper aerodigestive tract. Predicting which lesions progress and also being able to detect these lesions early can help in early disease eradication. Several published reports indicate that dysplastic leukoplakic lesions can be stratified for their ability to develop into cancer, based on allelic LOH.[12,13] Molecular analysis may indicate the likelihood of progression of both free-standing dysplastic lesions and those that remain after previous treatment of invasive cancer. Reliable prediction of cancer development in these lesions is discussed in several sections of this chapter.

Mechanisms of Detection

Sample Collection

To date, samples for molecular detection have primarily come from oral fluids (brushings, washings, or saliva) or blood (plasma or serum). Unlike with cervical cancer,

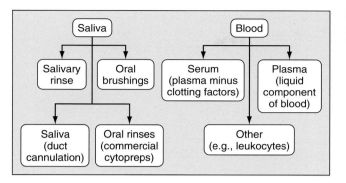

Figure 1-1. Body fluid compartment sources for diagnostic and screening studies in head and neck squamous cell carcinoma (HNSCC).

traditional pathologic approaches (e.g., cytology) have failed to yield adequate test sensitivity and specificity for clinical usefulness. Figure 1-1 shows different methods of sample collection.

Blood

Blood is a convenient source of DNA for molecular diagnostic efforts to find genetic and epigenetic alterations that are cancer-specific. Studies use either the *blood plasma*—the liquid component of blood, or the *serum*—blood plasma in which clotting factors (e.g., fibrin) have been removed. Other studies have considered changes in *blood leukocytes*, such as oxidative 8-oxoguanine DNA damage to predict cancer risk and treatment response.[14]

Oral Cavity

Several collection methods exist for surveying tumor-associated molecular changes from the oral cavity. *Salivary rinses* refer to sample collection in which a patient rinses the mouth with saline or other liquid and simply expels it into a specimen cup. Saliva can be collected by repeated expectoration over time, from the gingival pocket, or from salivary duct cannulation. Usually, centrifugation is used to produce fluid devoid of cells and debris. Finally, commercially available cytology kits harvest cells using *oral brushings*. Brushes used in suspicious areas to scrape oral mucosa yield markedly more cells than do rinses.

Assays

DNA Techniques

Molecular assays depend on the specific requirements of the cellular molecule to be detected: DNA, RNA, or protein. Classic techniques for DNA detection include big dye termination sequencing, polymerase chain reaction (PCR), quantitative real-time PCR (qPCS), and in situ hybridizations. In addition, epigenetic alterations (e.g., promoter methylation) can be detected by bisulfite sequencing, methylation-specific PCR (MSP), or in a quantitative fashion by quantitative methylation-specific PCR (qMSP).

RNA Techniques

RNA detection can be accomplished by RT-PCR or by quantitative RT-PCR, or the entire mRNA complement can be detected with an expression microarray. Expression microarrays use small silicon chips or glass slides with embedded short segments of DNA (termed *oligos*) to detect and quantitate the presence of specific sequences. The advantage of expression microarrays is the large scale of screening afforded. Chips are devised that can accurately measure the expression of all 40,000 plus genes in the genome. The disadvantage is the statistical and logistic management of such a large quantity of data.

Protein Techniques

Proteins have been detected by traditional assays such as Western blot, ELISA (enzyme-linked immunosorbent assay), and immunohistochemistry. Novel proteomic techniques have the ability to assay expression in a high-throughput fashion across the entire human genome. New discovery techniques include two-dimensional SDS-PAGE gels (separates proteins based on size, charge, and isoelectric point) along with innovations in mass spectography, SELDI-TOF (surface-enhanced laser desorption and ionization time-of-flight mass spectrometry), and MALDI-TOF (matrix-assisted laser desorption ionization time-of-flight mass spectrometry). These proteomic techniques can assay expression of a large number of different proteins, and efforts are being made to apply these to samples such as saliva and blood for molecular cancer detection.

Specific Genetic Alterations

Cytogenetic Alterations: CGH/FISH/SKY

HNSCC displays many cytogenetic alterations including aneuploidy, chromosomal gain, chromosomal loss, and translocations. Several techniques exist to assess the presence of cytogenetic alterations: spectral karyotyping (SKY), which is a chromosomal staining technique that is helpful in finding translocations, and fluorescence in situ hybridization (FISH), which uses probes designed to detect specific copy number changes in chromosomes. These techniques allow for the detection of large-scale genetic alterations or rearrangements that may not be detected using other molecular assays. Figure 1-2 shows one type of well-studied cytogenetic alteration in head and neck cancer: LOH, in which there is cytogenetic or genetic loss of one allele.

Others have considered whole-chromosomal alterations, specifically aneuploidy. Sudbo and colleagues[15] in 2001 showed that chromosomal copy changes (aneuploidy) could have prognostic significance in HNSCC. Sudbo's group found a significant association between cancer progression in premalignant lesions and chromosomal aneuploidy. This work[15] has been retracted because of data inconsistencies. At this

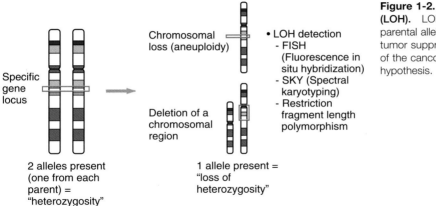

Figure 1-2. Loss of heterozygosity (LOH). LOH refers to loss of one parental allele that usually harbors a tumor suppressor gene. This forms half of the canconical Knudson two-hit hypothesis.

time, further work is being conducted to investigate whether there is any valid effect of chromosomal aneuploidy on the progression of premalignant lesions.

PCR–Based Detection: Loss of Heterozygosity/Microsatellite Instability

Microsatellite instability (MSI) refers to alterations in copy number of small repeats of a short nucleotide motif (usually one to five nucleotides long) in the genetic sequence of a cell. It was discovered initially in colon cancer,[16] but also has been found to be a feature of head and neck cancer.[17] Figure 1-3 demonstrates how MSI is detected. The most common microsatellite in humans is a dinucleotide repeat of cytosine and adenine, which occurs in tens of thousands of locations in our genome. When MSI is present, these areas are aberrantly replicated, leading to expansion or contraction of the locus. MSI has been found to be associated with errors in DNA replication and DNA repair enzymes.[18] After the discovery of MSI, efforts were made to use these microsatellite alterations to detect cancer cells in a background of normal tissue. Microsatellite analysis by PCR can reveal either MSI or LOH (loss of one portion of a parental chromosomal). LOH is one possible mechanism of tumor suppressor gene inactivation fulfilling Knudson's two-hit hypothesis.

According to Knudson, complete silencing of a suppressor gene occurs by inactivation of each allele through a variety of mechanisms. Researchers have used these tumor-specific alterations for cancer detection using saliva or plasma of HSNCC patients. A group of MSI alterations was initially reported in the serum of 29% of patients with HNSCC.[19] These alterations were then used to assay saliva samples of patients with HNSCC in a pilot study to detect tumor-specific genetic alterations in exfoliated oral mucosal cell samples. Spafford and colleagues[20] studied samples from 44 HNSCC patients and 43 healthy control subjects. They showed LOH or MSI in at least one marker in 38 (86%) of 44 primary tumors with identical alterations found in the saliva samples in 35 of the 38 cases (92% of those with markers; 79% overall). MSI was detectable in the saliva in 24 of 25 cases (96%) in which it was present in the tumor; LOH was identified in the test sample in 19 of 31 cases (61%) in which it was found in the primary tumor. No microsatellite alterations were detected in any of the samples from the healthy control subjects.[20]

Microsatellite testing is now clinically available. However, other studies have found greater rates of background MSI in normal samples, which has mitigated the sensitivity in widespread application of these tests.[21]

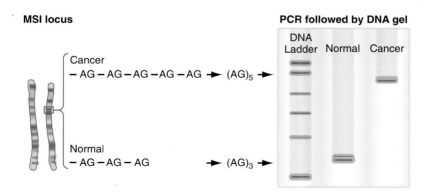

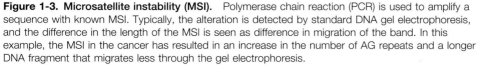

Figure 1-3. Microsatellite instability (MSI).   Polymerase chain reaction (PCR) is used to amplify a sequence with known MSI. Typically, the alteration is detected by standard DNA gel electrophoresis, and the difference in the length of the MSI is seen as difference in migration of the band. In this example, the MSI in the cancer has resulted in an increase in the number of AG repeats and a longer DNA fragment that migrates less through the gel electrophoresis.

Another application for LOH testing is the diagnosis and prognostic estimation of oral premalignant lesions and squamous cell carcinoma. Early changes in HNSCC include LOH of two specific chromosome sites (sites 3p14 and 9p21).[22] Groups have found that these areas of LOH have a correlation with clinical outcome. In a study of 48 oral squamous cell carcinomas, allelic imbalance at 3p24-26, 3p13, and 9p21 had a 25-fold increase in mortality rate.[23] Increased frequency of allelic imbalance at more loci ($P = .002$) was found in any area of dysplasia that developed into cancer ($n = 39$ cases) compared with case-matched dysplastic lesions that did not progress into cancer. Many of these subsequent developing cancers occurred in a different site, in accord with the theory of field cancerization (genetic changes caused by mutagens that produce a field effect).[24] Rosin and associates[25] studied 116 premalignant cases for LOH at 19 microsatellite loci on 7 chromosome arms (3p, 4q, 8p, 9p, 11q, 13q, and 17p) and found that those with LOH at 3p and/or 9p and additional losses (on 4q, 8p, 11q, or 17p) showed a 33-fold increase in relative cancer progression risk. Rosin and associates also found that this technique of LOH detection had significant promise for monitoring oral lesions via assay of the cell cytology because they frequently showed the same LOH that was found in the primary tumors.

Sequence Alterations

p53

p53 is one of the most well-known and frequently altered tumor suppressor genes in human cancers. It functions primarily as a transcription factor with many tumor-suppressive downstream targets activated. It was initially found underlying the inherited syndrome of cancer susceptibility, Li-Fraumeni. This transcription factor binds to the promoter sequence of many downstream targets and causes activation of mRNA transcription. *p53* is activated and expressed in normal cells under a variety of circumstances, most commonly after DNA damage. It induces cell-cycle arrest in response to DNA damage as well as either DNA repair activation or activation of apoptosis, depending on the context of the DNA injury (Fig. 1-4).

Over 50% of head and neck cancers harbor mutations (typically missense) of the *p53* tumor suppressor gene.[25a] Detecting these mutations in body fluids of HNSCC patients has been the subject of many studies. Early efforts used plaque hybridization

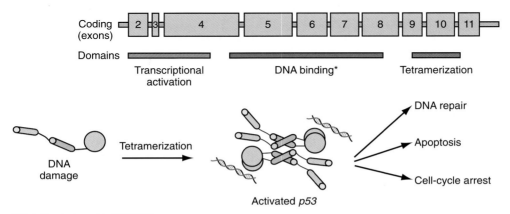

*Mutation hot spot in HNSCC

Figure 1-4. *p53* tumor-suppressor gene. DNA damage causes activation via tetramerization, resulting in transcriptional activation of a number of targets and resulting in increase of DNA repair, arrest of the cell cycle, and activation of apoptosis. In head and neck cancers, missense mutations can occur at almost any point in the coding sequence, but most are in the DNA-binding domain. HNSCC, head and neck squamous cell cancer.

to identify known *p53* mutations that had already been identified in the primary tumor. The salivary rinse had the same *p53* mutation in 5 of 7 patients.[26,27]

One other approach to *p53* mutation detection has been to measure *p53* antibodies in the serum of cancer patients. One group found that 27% (7 of 26) of patients with oral squamous cell carcinomas had circulating antibodies against *p53* (ELISA).[28] Others considered a group of 126 patients with oral squamous cell carcinomas compared with 80 control patients, assaying with ELISA for *p53* autoantibodies in the serum collected during a post-treatment surveillance period of 5 years. None of the control patients had these antibodies, but 18.6% of the primary cancer patients and 50% of the recurrent patients had *p53* autoantibodies detected. In addition, the *p53* antibody-positive patients had noticeably poorer prognosis ($P < .005$), and overall survival rate at 5 years for the *p53*-positive group was 24% (half that of the *p53*-negative group).[29]

Mitochondria

Studies over the last decade have pointed increasingly to the role of mitochondrial alterations in human cancers and HNSCC in particular. Mitochondria are involved in many cell pathways implicated in carcinogenesis. They are central to the apoptosis pathway (programmed cell death), the site of oxidative phosphorylation, the generator of free radicals, as well as the source of cellular energy (respiration) in cells. Their role in the tumorigenesis of head and neck cancer has been slowly coming to light.

Zhou and colleagues[30] found that 41 of 83 (49%) HNSCC tumors contained mtDNA mutations. Mutations occurred within noncoding (D-loop) and coding regions. Mitochondria have their own genome (Fig. 1-5) that includes genes encoding for the electron transport chain (NADH, cytochrome *c*, and cytochrome c oxidase), ATP synthase, and protein synthesis genes. Mitochondrial DNA also is present at higher concentrations facilitating detection studies. As a screening tool, Fliss and associates[31] found detectable mitochondrial mutations by PCR in 67% (6 of 9) of salivary rinse samples from head and neck cancer patients that corresponded to mutations found in tumors.

A change has been noted in the overall content of mitochondrial DNA that increases as a proposed compensation for general mitochondrial dysfunction. Mitochondrial DNA content has been conclusively demonstrated to increase with progressive degrees of mild, moderate, to severe dysplasia and finally carcinoma.[32] This

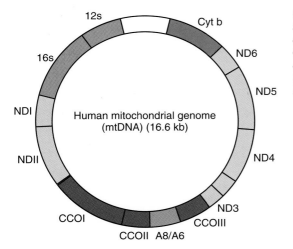

Figure 1-5. Map of the human mitochondrial genome. Shown are the seven subunits of NADH dehydrogenase-coenzyme Q oxidoreductase (ND), one unit of the coenzyme Q-cytochrome *c* oxidoreductase (Cyt *b*), three subunits of cytochrome *c* oxidase (CCO), two subunits of ATP synthase (A), and the protein synthesis genes (12S and 16S). Not shown are the genes for the 22 tRNAs.

change was used for a salivary detection strategy by Jiang and associates.[33] In the saliva, multivariate analysis showed a significant and independent association of high levels with diagnosis of HNSCC by measuring salivary mtDNA/nuclear DNA using two mitochondrial genes: COX 1 and COX 2.

Epigenetic Changes

Somatic genetic and epigenetic alterations have been the focus of studies of HNSCC pathogenesis. Epigenetics changes are heritable DNA alterations that do not affect the coding sequence but do affect the regulation of genes. Examples of these changes are promoter hypermethylation, acetylation, and histone modifications.

Methylation

By far the most useful and best studied of these in HSNCC has been gene promoter hypermethylation. This functional alteration takes place in the regulatory units of the genome (the promoters) in areas termed CpG islands. Molecularly, CpG (cytosine-guanine dinucleotides) can be modified at the 5′ carbon of the carbon ring of cytosine (Fig. 1-6) by the addition of a methyl group from S-adenyl methionine (SAM) by the DNA methyltransferase enzyme family (DNMT). Although this phenomenon was initially shown to be the cause of X-chromosome inactivation and genetic imprinting, inactivation of tumor suppressor genes in this manner has been increasingly shown to play a role in tumorigenesis. This adheres to the canconical Knudson two-hit hypothesis, which suggests that tumor suppressor genes are inactivated by two separate silencing events. Methylation has been shown to be sufficient to cause a "hit" to one allele in multiple genes. After both alleles have been silenced, the cell may undergo changes to its phenotype that contribute to malignancy (e.g., cell-cycle alterations, inhibition of apoptosis, and so on).

One advantage of methylation as a tumor marker is its ready use for screening. DNA is stable in the blood or saliva, and very small levels of methylation can be detected in a background of other DNA products by sophisticated means, including bisulfite sequencing and quantitative or standard methylation-specific PCR (Fig. 1-7).

Early methylation studies of HNSCC examined a panel of four putative tumor suppressor genes whose inactivation was associated with a cancer phenotype. At least one of these four genes—p16, MGMT, GST, and DAPK—exhibited significant promoter hypermethylation in 42% of primary tumors.[34] Other genes epigenetically

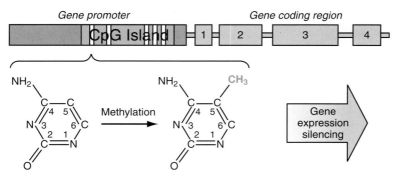

Figure 1-6. Cytosine-guanine dinucleotide (CpG) methylation. Individual Cpg shown within the context of a CpG island, which is found in the promoter segment of a gene upstream from the transcription start site. Methylation performs a gene-silencing function through alterations in tertiary structure, direct binding of methylation-sensitive promoters and repressors, and activation of the deacetylation complexes.

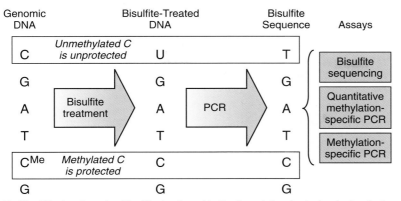

Figure 1-7. Bisulfite treatment. Bisulfite treatment is the foundation for technologies that assess promoter and CpG island methylation status. Methylated cytosine residues are protected from the bisulfite reaction, and changes from cytosine to thymine can be seen in unmethylated bases. Methylated cytosines can be differentiated from unmethylated cytosines in this manner. After bisulfite treatment, methylation can be studied by bisulfite sequencing, methylation-specific polymerase chain reaction (PCR; MSP), which uses primers specific to methylated versus unmethylated CpGs, and quantitative MSP (qMSP), which does the same with real-time PCR.

silenced in HNSCC include *RASSF1A*,[35] *hMLH1* (DNA mismatch repair gene),[36] *E-cadherin*,[37] and *STAT1*.[38]

Once these molecular changes were identified, efforts were undertaken to use them for molecular diagnosis. Recent studies have shown correlation in the presence of methylation of *p16* between tumors, saliva, and serum via MSP. Normal controls showed no *p16* methylation.[39] Another group found methylation in the oral rinses of patients with premalignant lesions corresponding to that of reported oral rinse methylation rates for invasive cancer. In fact, *p16* and *MGMT* were observed to be methylated by MSP in 44% and 56%, respectively, of the premalignant oral rinse samples.[40] However, to date it has been difficult to develop assays with sufficient sensitivity (HNSCC tumors are heterogeneous in their genetic changes) and specificity (normal cells may have methylated alleles) for clinical application for early detection.

Expression Array

An emerging technology that offers unparalleled assessment of the expression of many genes simultaneously is expression microarray. Small silicon chips or glass slides are embedded with thousands of gene-specific oligonucleotides to study the simultaneous mRNA expression of many genes within a sample. This technology has the ability to compare gene expressions of the human genome in many samples to explore significant differences in gene expression patterns between tumor tissues and normal tissues, or to compare aggressive tumors with indolent tumors. From the standpoint of molecular diagnostics, it is hoped that this technology will reveal a gene expression signature that can differentiate normal aerodigestive mucosa from that of HNSCC. Gene expression microarray has already been used clinically in breast cancer to produce a tool with demonstrable efficacy for predicting treatment effects and prognosis in clinical trials. In head and neck cancer, this approach has been used for screening and diagnosis. Using saliva and blood serum to look for early detection markers, premalignant oral lesions have been shown to have marked differences in expression patterns compared with tumors and normal mucosa.[11]

mRNA expression differences have been studied in the saliva of patients with HNSCC. A group at University of California—Los Angeles found 1679 genes (*P* < .05) with differing expression levels in the saliva of HNSCC compared with those of controls. The most promising salivary RNA biomarkers were IL8, IL1B, DUSP1, HA3, OAZ1, S100P, and SAT. Combination of the biomarkers resulted in a 91% sensitivity accompanied by a 91% specificity to distinguish HNSCC patients.[41] These findings have yet to be validated in an independent set. Recently, researchers have questioned the efficacy of RNA detection in the saliva. A feasibility study concluded:

> the combination of (a) a minimal microarray signal, which was unaffected by RNase treatment, (b) the presence of a conventional RT-PCR housekeeper product in both RNase-treated and no-RT saliva samples, (c) the absence of a conventional RT-PCR housekeeper product in DNase-treated conditions, and (d) the absence of an RNA-specific RT-PCR product shows that any microarray or RT-PCR signal in the saliva must arise from genomic DNA, not RNA. Thus, saliva extracts do not support mRNA expression studies.[42]

Viral Detection

Human Papilloma Virus

A popular area of research in recent years has interrogated the role of HPV in the carcinogenesis of HNSCC. HPV, specifically high-risk types (16, 18, and so on), is a well-characterized primary cause of cervical cancer. Especially enticing is the fact that its recognition in cervical cancer has yielded one of the most effective forms of cancer screening, early detection, and increased cure rates in cancer to date. HPV is now recognized as a likely cause of a subset of head and neck cancer,[43] particularly in oropharyngeal and tonsillar lesions. There are numerous subtypes of this virus (more than 20), but most have not been shown to be carcinogenic. HPV subtypes 16 and 18 are the most-studied high-risk subtypes, but the majority of evidence in head and neck cancer has implicated HPV subtype 16 as an etiologic agent in more than 90% of HPV-related head and neck cancers.

HPV produces two key proteins, E6 and E7, which have the potential to transform human cells. These viral oncogenes have been shown to inactivate two crucial human tumor suppressor genes: *p53* (E6) and *pRb* (E7). This inactivation results in loss of cell-cycle control, impaired cell differentiation, increased mutations, and chromosomal instability.[44]

Overall in HNSCC, HPV genomic DNA can be detected by real-time PCR-based methods in 26% of all cancers.[45] However, in head and neck cancer, this virus has a predilection for the lingual and palatine tonsils of the oropharynx. Data looking at only the subset of the oropharynx suggest that 50% or more of these tumors are HPV-positive.

It is interesting that HPV-associated cancers have tended to have increased survival and better outcomes. Schwartz and colleagues[46] found that HPV-16–positive patients had significantly reduced overall and disease-specific mortality rates compared with other patients after adjustment for age, stage, treatment, smoking, alcohol, education, and comorbid disease.

New studies show promising molecular screening approaches that have increased sensitivity for detection. Real-time PCR of HPV-associated DNA is now the standard for detection at low thresholds. However, use of these technologies as screening tests suffers from low sensitivity.[47] Saliva screening for the HPV virus by Zhao and associates[48] found a 45.6% incidence of tumor HPV positivity in HNSCC patients, of whom 57% had detectable salivary rinse HPV-16. Salivary rinse for HPV DNA detection had a sensitivity of 32.6%. Depending on the threshold for HPV-16 positivity in the assay, specificity increased only slightly—from 97.2% to 98.7% at the higher cutoff, and the authors suggest that more than 99% specificity would be required for population-based screening.

HPV seropositivity has also been an intriguing risk factor for the development of head and neck cancer. The largest study examining HPV-16 seropositivity found an odds ratio of 2.2 for developing head and neck cancer in a cohort of 292 patients who were followed up in a screening study and who had eventually developed HNSCC. Fifty percent of the oropharyngeal and 14% of tongue cancers contained HPV-16 DNA, according to PCR analysis.[49] The diagnostic utility is again limited by the number of HPV-seropositive patients who will not develop head and neck cancer or have seropositivity from any number of other sources. Technologies such as competitive PCR combined with mass spectrometry have promise for yielding more specificity with positive results of one one-copy number of DNA over real-time PCR, but the issue of false-positive nonpathologic detection of HPV remains.[50] In a case-control study examining HPV-16 in the saliva, 19% of head and neck cancer patients ($n = 201$) were saliva-positive, and 10% of control subjects ($n = 333$) were positive, yielding an odds ratio of 2.6.[51] HPV likely has low utility for population-based screening. HPV positivity, though, may eventually play a role in disease monitoring, surveillance, and clinical decision making.

Epstein-Barr Virus for Nasopharyngeal Carcinoma

The association between the Epstein-Barr virus (EBV) and nasopharyngeal carcinoma (NPC) has long been known. NPC is a common epithelial neoplasm among the Chinese populations in southern China and Southeast Asia. EBV gene products are frequently detected in NPC tissues along with elevated serum viral load and antibodies against viral proteins (VCA and EA). Elevated plasma EBV DNA load is an important marker for disease presence and for monitoring disease progression. Tan and colleagues[52] looked at 78 untreated NPC patients, and plasma EBV DNA was quantified using qRT-PCR. They found a significant decrease in EBV DNA plasma load after treatment (1669 ± 637 copies/mL → 57 ± 37 copies/mL; $P < .05$). In addition, plasma EBV DNA load was shown to be a good prognosticator of disease progression and clinical outcome.

EBV antibodies have been used to predict development of disease. It has been noted that a serologic window of elevated titers of the EBV antibody can be detected in patients who go on to develop NPC. Ji and associates[53] found EBV antibody levels to be an early marker of NPC with considerable positive predictive value in a study of 39 NPC patients followed up for 15 years. Serologic screening at enrollment identified patients who already had elevated titers and had clinical manifestations earlier (median = 28 months) than those who developed higher levels after enrollment (median = 90 months).

Viral load has also been considered as a molecular staging means. In one study, circulating EBV DNA load data were combined with TNM staging to determine the efficacy of molecular staging in 376 patients with NPC. Pretherapy circulating EBV DNA load was an independent prognostic factor for overall survival in NPC patients.[54]

Serum Protein Markers

CD44

The soluble adhesion molecule CD44 has gained recent attention in the HNSCC literature. Prince and associates[55] used this marker for cell sorting by flow cytometry to define a malignant subpopulation of potential cancer stem cells in HNSCC. CD44 has previously been implicated in HNSCC pathogenesis. One of its advantages is its cell surface location and its availability for detection by routine clinical approaches such as ELISA. In one study, the levels of sCD44st, sCD44v5, sCD44v6, sICAM-1, and sVCAM-1 were considered in 81 patients with HNSCC versus 20 controls, before and after treatment. The levels of all five of these markers were significantly higher in the HNSCC group than in those of the control group. In addition, sCD44st, sCD44v5, and sCD44v6 median serum levels were significantly reduced after treatment.[56] However, a separate group considering CD44 isoforms in the serum used ELISA to show that there was no significant difference between the serum levels of sCD44v6 in HNSCC individuals and those in healthy smokers. Moreover, there was no correlation between the serum level of sCD44v6 and UICC (International Union Against Cancer) stage, TNM stage, or histologic grade.[57]

Epithelial Growth Factor Receptors

HNSCCs commonly have upregulation of epithelial growth factor (EGF) pathways. The epithelial growth factor receptor (EGFR) is in the molecular tyrosine kinase family of cell surface receptors that are implicated in the pathogenesis of many forms of cancer. EGFR overexpression is observed in 42% to 80% of head and neck cancers.[58] A meta-analysis showed worse outcomes for patients with EGFR overexpression in seven of eight studies.[59] Recently, overexpression of EGFR has been targeted with immunomagnetic cell enrichment and RT-PCR to detect circulating head and neck tumor cells. This technique was successful in finding 1 cancer cell per 10^5 total leukocytes 77.8% of the time.[60]

Vascular Endothelial Growth Factor (VEGF)

VEGF is also a tyrosine kinase receptor and a promising serum biomarker. One study found that serum VEGF levels (by ELISA) was higher in patients with larynx cancer (317.22 ± 25.46 pg/mL) compared with a group of control patients (47.83 ± 0.13 pg/mL). This increase was significant ($P < .001$). In univariate analysis, elevated s-VEGF correlated with poor Karnofsky performance status for all patients with advanced laryngeal carcinoma ($P < .08$).[61]

Proteomic Approaches

Novel proteomic techniques provide the ability to assay protein expression in samples in a high-throughput manner across the translated human genome. These technologies may enable researchers to identify unique protein expression, or expression patterns, in cancer compared with normal tissues. In conjunction with screening approaches seeking blood or saliva markers, new clinical tests may be found for screening, premalignant progression, or tissue diagnosis. Traditional techniques include two-dimensional SDS-PAGE gels that separate proteins based on size, charge, and isoelectric point. Improvements of mass spectography and SELDI-TOF (surface-enhanced laser desorption and ionization time-of-flight mass spectrometry) as well as MALDI-TOF (matrix-assisted laser desorption ionization time-of-flight mass spectrometry) techniques can assay expression of a large number of different proteins in a given sample. Protein-based microarray technologies with chips embedded with a library of known antibodies (more than 10,000 are now possible) are also available to look at genome-wide protein expression in a sample.

These proteomic techniques have recently been used for HNSCC molecular research. Soltys and colleagues[62] used SELDI-TOF to assay protein expression in the plasma of 56 patients with head and neck cancer, with 52 controls, and compiled

37,356 data points representing a particular protein's expression for each sample. From these two groups, significant differences in expression were isolated to 65 specific SELDI-TOF peaks. This study also included a completely separate "validation set" of 57 cancer patients and 52 normal controls. The goal was to demonstrate the predictive ability of these markers in the plasma. Results were promising showing correct identification of 39 of 57 HNSCC patients and 40 of 52 noncancer controls, for a sensitivity of 68% and a specificity of 73%. It is interesting to note that their model tended to overpredict cancer in control smokers, which is often a problem in cancer marker studies. A group from Pittsburgh recently used a multiplexed immunobead-based panel to assay in the serum 60 biomarkers in 116 HNSCC patients before treatment, 103 patients successfully treated, and 117 smoker controls. The highest diagnostic power was found in a panel comprising 25 biomarkers, including EGF, EGFR, interleukin 8 (IL8), tissue plasminogen activator inhibitor-1 (TPA inhibitor-1), α-fetoprotein, matrix metallopeptidase 2 (MMP2), matrix metallopeptidase 3 (MMP3), interferon-alpha (IFN-α), interferon-gamma (IFN-γ), interferon inducible protein-10 (IFN-inducible protein-10), regulated on activation, normal T cell expressed and secreted (RANTES), macrophage inflammatory protein-1α, IL-7, IL-17, IL-1 receptor-α, IL-2 receptor, granulocyte colony-stimulating factor, mesothelin, insulin-like growth factor-binding protein 1, E-selectin, cytokeratin-19, vascular cell adhesion molecule, and cancer antigen-125. This study had impressive sensitivity (84.5%) and specificity (98%). Ninety-two percent of patients in the active disease group were correctly classified from a cross-validation serum set. These extremely promising data suggest that use of many markers in tandem may enable adequate sensitivity and specificity for reliable molecular detection.[63]

Other Applications

Molecular markers can be used to probe surgical margin and lymph nodes for the detection of minimal residual disease and micrometastases. Traditional pathologic review can easily miss individual tumor cells or small nests of metastases. Molecular detection methods can lead to improved staging and better outcomes by reducing local and regional recurrence rates. p53 was an early target used for the study of surgical margins and lymph nodes.

Surgical Margins

Tissues that were deemed histologically free of cancer were found to contain tumor-specific TP53 mutations in 13 of 25 cases, and negative lymph nodes actually harbored a mutation in 6 of 28 cases.[64] Five cases with molecular evidence of involved margins experienced local recurrence of disease within the first 3 years after treatment. The need to distinguish positive surgical margins from dysplasia indicative of local field effects (genetic changes affecting a large area of tissue caused by tobacco smoke, for example) has complicated this field significantly. Precancerous cells around the index tumor may share only some tumor-specific molecular alterations, and so may elude detection, or be counted as minimal residual fully transformed tumor cells. One study considered primary tumors, surgical margins, and local recurrences using a panel of LOH markers. Based on variations in the spectrum of molecular alterations in the index tumor and surrounding mucosal cells, they showed that 61% (8 of 13) of locally recurrent lesions studied actually had not come from the primary tumor, but rather from field effect cancerization. These results demonstrate the difficulty in relying on molecular marker analysis at the margin of a resection.[65]

In a pilot study considering the feasibility of early detection using methylation markers, QMSP (quantitative tumor suppressor gene hypermethylation assay) was used to assay operative margins intraoperatively. Methylated DNA was present in the margins in 50% of patients in whom the primary tumor was also methylated.[66] Another effort considered immunohistochemical expression of p53 and eIF4E (4E) and found significant differences in disease-free interval between patients with 4E-positive and 4E-negative margins ($P = .003$), but no significant association with p53, which remained after multivariate analysis.[2] These results suggest that molecular detection at the margin will eventually prove to have prognostic significance and possibly guide surgical management.

Lymph Nodes

Because lymph nodes do not contain normal epithelium, detection of subclinical deposits of metastatic HNSCC in nodes does not present as great a problem with false-positive results as does margin analysis. This improves detection specificity using tumor-specific markers and suggests that nodal detection is likely to be used clinically before margin analysis. However, survival benefit from the detection of microscopic foci of disease in lymph nodes has not been clinically documented.

Detection of nodal disease may have a direct effect on postoperative treatment selection in that radiation is typically used whenever nodes are involved. Therefore, molecular detection converting a case from N0 to N+ would result in appropriate escalation of treatment.

The first attempt to detect nodal micrometastasis with molecular markers targeted TP53 mutations. The investigators found that 5 of 33 nodes examined (15%) showed metastases by light microscopy, but 11 of 33 (33%) were found to be tumor-positive with molecular diagnosis.[67] The *p53* tumor suppressor gene is mutated in more than 50% of HNSCC tumors, but the large variety of mutations limits its applicability as a quick and reliable method of detection.

Others have looked at squamous cell carcinoma antigen (SCAA) mRNA expression by nested PCR. They found that in 198 histologically negative nodes SCCA was expressed in 37 (18.7%). A micrometastatic focus was found in nine of these lymph nodes (4.6%) by additional sectioning.[6] Other studies have considered the *MUC1* gene, *E48*, cytokeratin 14 (CK14), CK20 primarily using RT-PCR. Ferris and associates[5] published promising reports of four qRT-PCR markers for intraoperative nodal diagnosis. This feasibility study assessed 40 previously reported markers in 19 histologically positive nodes and 21 negative nodes. Using qRT-PCR they found four markers that discriminated between positive and benign nodes with accuracy greater than 97%. These were pemphigus vulgaris antigen, SCCA1/2, parathyroid hormone-related protein (PTHrP), and tumor-associated calcium signal transducer 1 (TACSTD1).

Each study has been shown to successfully uncover subclinically node-positive patients. However, although the clinical management of head and neck cancer dictates that patients with even a slight risk of nodal metastasis based on tumor site and staging receive therapy that treats the nodal basins of the neck with either radiation therapy or surgical node dissection, this increased fidelity in finding regional lymph node disease has not translated to improved regional control or survival.

Conclusion

Additional basic science effort is needed to identify and validate markers to bring molecular detection to the clinic. The technologies discussed in this chapter are in the preclinical research stage. At present, there are many novel markers and techniques that are promising. Many new technologies are revolutionizing this field: expression arrays (mRNA expression arrays), proteomic approaches (protein microarrays, SELDI/MALDI-TOF), and molecular imaging techniques (positron emission tomography [PET]). Older technologies remain critical: RT-PCR, quantitative DNA PCR, QMSP, ELISA. Many areas of potential clinical utility exist: screening high-risk patients for disease, predicting malignant progression, improvements in staging and prediction, therapy selection, adequate margin assessment, and diagnosis of lymph node disease.

As translational research moves forward, rigid statistical analysis is required, particularly with adequate multivariate analyses. Multiple markers may need to be combined to produce clinical useful assays. Promising diagnostic markers require independent validation cohorts. Intelligent design of prospective clinical studies is critical to validate and prove efficacy. There is considerable reason for optimism that novel molecular markers will change the way patients are diagnosed, surgically staged, and followed up after treatment.

References

1. Zhang L, Williams M, Poh CF, et al: Toluidine blue staining identifies high-risk primary oral premalignant lesions with poor outcome. Cancer Res 65(17):8017–8021, 2005.
2. Nathan CA, Amirghahri N, Rice C, et al: Molecular analysis of surgical margins in head and neck squamous cell carcinoma patients. Laryngoscope 112(12):2129–2140, 2002.
3. van Houten VM, Leemans CR, Kummer JA, et al: Molecular diagnosis of surgical margins and local recurrence in head and neck cancer patients: a prospective study. Clin Cancer Res 10(11):3614–3620, 2004.
4. Jose J, Coatesworth AP, MacLennan K: Cervical metastases in upper aerodigestive tract squamous cell carcinoma: histopathologic analysis and reporting. Head Neck 25(3):194–197, 2003.
5. Ferris RL, Xi L, Raja S, et al: Molecular staging of cervical lymph nodes in squamous cell carcinoma of the head and neck. Cancer Res 65(6):2147–2156, 2005.
6. Hamakawa H, Fukizumi M, Bao Y, et al: Genetic diagnosis of micrometastasis based on SCC antigen mRNA in cervical lymph nodes of head and neck cancer. Clin Exp Metastasis 17(7):593–599, 1999.
7. Akervall J, Kurnit DM, Adams M, et al: Overexpression of cyclin D1 correlates with sensitivity to cisplatin in squamous cell carcinoma cell lines of the head and neck. Acta Otolaryngol 124(7):851–857, 2004.
8. Nozawa H, Tadakuma T, Ono T, et al: Small interfering RNA targeting epidermal growth factor receptor enhances chemosensitivity to cisplatin, 5-fluorouracil and docetaxel in head and neck squamous cell carcinoma. Cancer Sci 97(10):1115–1124, 2006.
9. Fearon ER, Vogelstein B: A genetic model for colorectal tumorigenesis. Cell 61(5):759–767, 1990.
10. Califano J, van der Riet P, Westra W, et al: Genetic progression model for head and neck cancer: implications for field cancerization. Cancer Res 56(11):2488–2492, 1996.
11. Ha PK, Benoit NE, Yochem R, et al: A transcriptional progression model for head and neck cancer. Clin Cancer Res 9(8):3058–3064, 2003.
12. Rosin MP, Cheng X, Poh C, et al: Use of allelic loss to predict malignant risk for low-grade oral epithelial dysplasia. Clin Cancer Res 6(2):357–362, 2000.
13. Zhang L, Cheung KJ, Jr, Lam WL, et al: Increased genetic damage in oral leukoplakia from high risk sites: potential impact on staging and clinical management. Cancer 91(11):2148–2155, 2001.
14. Paz-Elizur T, Ben-Yosef R, Elinger D, et al: Reduced repair of the oxidative 8-oxoguanine DNA damage and risk of head and neck cancer. Cancer Res 66(24):11683–11689, 2006.
15. Sudbo J, Kildal W, Risberg B, et al: DNA content as a prognostic marker in patients with oral leukoplakia. N Engl J Med 344(17):1270–1278, 2001.
16. Ionov Y, Peinado MA, Malkhosyan S, et al: Ubiquitous somatic mutations in simple repeated sequences reveal a new mechanism for colonic carcinogenesis. Nature 363(6429):558–561, 1993.
17. El-Naggar AK, Hurr K, Huff V, et al: Microsatellite instability in preinvasive and invasive head and neck squamous carcinoma. Am J Pathol 148(6):2067–2072, 1996.
18. de la Chapelle A: Microsatellite instability. N Engl J Med 349(3):209–210, 2003.
19. Nawroz H, Koch W, Anker P, et al: Microsatellite alterations in serum DNA of head and neck cancer patients. Nat Med 2(9):1035–1037, 1996.
20. Spafford MF, Koch WM, Reed AL, et al: Detection of head and neck squamous cell carcinoma among exfoliated oral mucosal cells by microsatellite analysis. Clin Cancer Res 7(3):607–612, 2001.
21. Coulet F, Blons H, Cabelguenne A, et al: Detection of plasma tumor DNA in head and neck squamous cell carcinoma by microsatellite typing and p53 mutation analysis. Cancer Res 60(3):707–711, 2000.
22. Mao L, Lee JS, Fan YH, et al: Frequent microsatellite alterations at chromosomes 9p21 and 3p14 in oral premalignant lesions and their value in cancer risk assessment. Nat Med 2(6):682–685, 1996.
23. Partridge M, Emilion G, Pateromichelakis S, et al: The prognostic significance of allelic imbalance at key chromosomal loci in oral cancer. Br J Cancer 79(11–12):1821–1827, 1999.
24. Partridge M, Pateromichelakis S, Phillips E, et al: A case-control study confirms that microsatellite assay can identify patients at risk of developing oral squamous cell carcinoma within a field of cancerization. Cancer Res 60(14):3893–3898, 2000.
25. Rosin MP, Epstein JB, Berean K, et al The use of exfoliative cell samples to map clonal genetic alterations in the oral epithelium of high-risk patients. Cancer Res 57(23):5258–5260, 1997.
25a. Poeta ML, Manola J, Goldwasser MA, et al: TP53 mutations and survival in squamous-cell carcinoma of the head and neck. N Engl J Med 357(25):2552–2561, 2007.
26. Boyle JO, Mao L, Brennan JA, et al: Gene mutations in saliva as molecular markers for head and neck squamous cell carcinomas. Am J Surg 168(5):429–432, 1994.
27. Koch WM, Boyle JO, Mao L, et al: p53 gene mutations as markers of tumor spread in synchronous oral cancers. Arch Otolaryngol Head Neck Surg 120(9):943–947, 1994.
28. Warnakulasuriya S, Soussi T, Maher R, et al: Expression of p53 in oral squamous cell carcinoma is associated with the presence of IgG and IgA p53 autoantibodies in sera and saliva of the patients. J Pathol 192(1):52–57, 2000.
29. Hofele C, Schwager-Schmitt M, Volkmann M: [Prognostic value of antibodies against p53 in patients with oral squamous cell carcinoma—five years survival rate]. Laryngorhinootologie 81(5):342–345, 2002.
30. Zhou S, Kachhap S, Sun W, et al: Frequency and phenotypic implications of mitochondrial DNA mutations in human squamous cell cancers of the head and neck. Proc Natl Acad Sci U S A 104(18):7540–7545, 2007.
31. Fliss MS, Usadel H, Caballero OL, et al: Facile detection of mitochondrial DNA mutations in tumors and bodily fluids. Science 287(5460):2017–2019, 2000.

32. Kim MM, Clinger JD, Masayesva BG, et al: Mitochondrial DNA quantity increases with histopathologic grade in premalignant and malignant head and neck lesions. Clin Cancer Res 10(24): 8512–8515, 2004.

33. Jiang WW, Masayesva B, Zahurak M, et al: Increased mitochondrial DNA content in saliva associated with head and neck cancer. Clin Cancer Res 11(7):2486–2491, 2005.

34. Sanchez-Cespedes M, Esteller M, Wu L, et al: Gene promoter hypermethylation in tumors and serum of head and neck cancer patients. Cancer Res 60(4):892–895, 2000.

35. Dong SM, Sun DI, Benoit NE, et al: Epigenetic inactivation of RASSF1A in head and neck cancer. Clin Cancer Res 9(10 Pt 1):3635–3640, 2003.

36. Liu K, Zuo C, Luo QK, et al: Promoter hypermethylation and inactivation of hMLH1, a DNA mismatch repair gene, in head and neck squamous cell carcinoma. Diagn Mol Pathol 12(1):50–56, 2003.

37. Hasegawa M, Nelson HH, Peters E, et al: Patterns of gene promoter methylation in squamous cell cancer of the head and neck. Oncogene 21(27):4231–4236, 2002.

38. Xi S, Dyer KF, Kimak M, et al: Decreased STAT1 expression by promoter methylation in squamous cell carcinogenesis. J Natl Cancer Inst 98(3):181–189, 2006.

39. Nakahara Y, Shintani S, Mihara M, et al: Detection of p16 promoter methylation in the serum of oral cancer patients. Int J Oral Maxillofac Surg 35(4):362–365, 2006.

40. Lopez M, Aguirre JM, Cuevas N, et al: Gene promoter hypermethylation in oral rinses of leukoplakia patients—a diagnostic and/or prognostic tool? Eur J Cancer 39(16):2306–2309, 2003.

41. Li Y, St John MA, Zhou X, et al: Salivary transcriptome diagnostics for oral cancer detection. Clin Cancer Res 10(24):8442–8450, 2004.

42. Kumar SV, Hurteau GJ, Spivack SD: Validity of messenger RNA expression analyses of human saliva. Clin Cancer Res 12(17):5033–5039, 2006.

43. Schwartz SM, Daling JR, Doody DR, et al: Oral cancer risk in relation to sexual history and evidence of human papillomavirus infection. J Natl Cancer Inst 90(21):1626–1636, 1998.

44. Munger K, Howley PM: Human papillomavirus immortalization and transformation functions. Virus Res 89(2):213–228, 2002.

45. Kreimer AR, Clifford GM, Boyle P, et al: Human papillomavirus types in head and neck squamous cell carcinomas worldwide: a systematic review. Cancer Epidemiol Biomarkers Prev 14(2): 467–475, 2005.

46. Schwartz SR, Yueh B, McDougall JK, et al: Human papillomavirus infection and survival in oral squamous cell cancer: a population-based study. Otolaryngol Head Neck Surg 125(1):1–9, 2001.

47. Ha PK, Pai SI, Westra WH, et al: Real-time quantitative PCR demonstrates low prevalence of human papillomavirus type 16 in premalignant and malignant lesions of the oral cavity. Clin Cancer Res 8(5):1203–1209, 2002.

48. Zhao M, Rosenbaum E, Carvalho AL, et al: Feasibility of quantitative PCR-based saliva rinse screening of HPV for head and neck cancer. Int J Cancer 117(4):605–610, 2005.

49. Mork J, Lie AK, Glattre E, et al: Human papillomavirus infection as a risk factor for squamous-cell carcinoma of the head and neck. N Engl J Med 344(15):1125–1131, 2001.

50. Yang H, Yang K, Khafagi A, et al: Sensitive detection of human papillomavirus in cervical, head/neck, and schistosomiasis-associated bladder malignancies. Proc Natl Acad Sci U S A 102(21):7683–7688, 2005.

51. Smith EM, Ritchie JM, Summersgill KF, et al: Human papillomavirus in oral exfoliated cells and risk of head and neck cancer. J Natl Cancer Inst 96(6):449–455, 2004.

52. Tan EL, Selvaratnam G, Kananathan R, et al: Quantification of Epstein-Barr virus DNA load, interleukin-6, interleukin-10, transforming growth factor-beta1 and stem cell factor in plasma of patients with nasopharyngeal carcinoma. BMC Cancer 6:227, 2006.

53. Ji MF, Wang DK, Yu YL, et al: Sustained elevation of Epstein-Barr virus antibody levels preceding clinical onset of nasopharyngeal carcinoma. Br J Cancer 96(4):623–630, 2007.

54. Leung SF, Zee B, Ma BB, et al: Plasma Epstein-Barr viral deoxyribonucleic acid quantitation complements tumor-node-metastasis staging prognostication in nasopharyngeal carcinoma. J Clin Oncol 24(34):5414–5418, 2006.

55. Prince ME, Sivanandan R, Kaczorowski A, et al: Identification of a subpopulation of cells with cancer stem cell properties in head and neck squamous cell carcinoma. Proc Natl Acad Sci U S A 104(3):973–978, 2007.

56. Kawano T, Yanoma S, Nakamura Y, et al: Evaluation of soluble adhesion molecules CD44 (CD44st, CD44v5, CD44v6), ICAM-1, and VCAM-1 as tumor markers in head and neck cancer. Am J Otolaryngol 26(5):308–313, 2005.

57. Andratschke M, Chaubal S, Pauli C, et al: Soluble CD44v6 is not a sensitive tumor marker in patients with head and neck squamous cell cancer. Anticancer Res 25(4):2821–2826, 2005.

58. Ford AC, Grandis JR: Targeting epidermal growth factor receptor in head and neck cancer. Head Neck 25(1):67–73, 2003.

59. Lothaire P, de Azambuja E, Dequanter D, et al: Molecular markers of head and neck squamous cell carcinoma: promising signs in need of prospective evaluation. Head Neck 28(3):256–269, 2006.

60. Tong X, Yang L, Lang JC, et al: Application of immunomagnetic cell enrichment in combination with RT-PCR for the detection of rare circulating head and neck tumor cells in human peripheral blood. Cytometry B Clin Cytom 72:310–323, 2007.

61. Teknos TN, Cox C, Yoo S, et al: Elevated serum vascular endothelial growth factor and decreased survival in advanced laryngeal carcinoma. Head Neck 24(11):1004–1011, 2002.

62. Soltys SG, Le QT, Shi G, et al: The use of plasma surface-enhanced laser desorption/ionization time-of-flight mass spectrometry proteomic patterns for detection of head and neck squamous cell cancers. Clin Cancer Res 10(14):4806–4812, 2004.

63. Linkov F, Lisovich A, Yurkovetsky Z, et al: Early detection of head and neck cancer: development of a novel screening tool using multiplexed immunobead-based biomarker profiling. Cancer Epidemiol Biomarkers Prev 16(1):102–107, 2007.

64. Brennan JA, Mao L, Hruban RH, et al: Molecular assessment of histopathological staging in squamous-cell carcinoma of the head and neck. N Engl J Med 332(7):429–435, 1995.

65. Tabor MP, Brakenhoff RH, Ruijter-Schippers HJ, et al: Genetically altered fields as origin of locally recurrent head and neck cancer: a retrospective study. Clin Cancer Res 10(11):3607–3613, 2004.

66. Goldenberg D, Harden S, Masayesva BG, et al: Intraoperative molecular margin analysis in head and neck cancer. Arch Otolaryngol Head Neck Surg 130(1):39–44, 2004.

67. Partridge M, Li SR, Pateromichelakis S, et al: Detection of minimal residual cancer to investigate why oral tumors recur despite seemingly adequate treatment. Clin Cancer Res 6(7): 2718–2725, 2000.

2

Molecular Proteomics in Early Detection of Head and Neck Cancer

J. Trad Wadsworth and
Richard R. Drake

KEY POINTS

- The human proteome is defined as the full set of proteins encoded by the genome.
- Proteomics, or protein pattern analysis, is the characterization and quantification of proteins in tissues and body fluids.
- SELDI (surface-enhanced laser desorption/ionization) analysis and classification algorithms have been established by several groups to have both high throughput and robust sensitivity and specificity in differentiating serum samples between head and neck squamous cell carcinoma (HNSCC) patients and control patients.
- Using MALDI-TOF (matrix-assisted laser desorption/ionization-time of flight) technology as a discovery platform may allow generating biomarker panels for use in more accurate prediction of prognosis and treatment efficacies for HNSCC.
- These proteomic technologies hold tremendous promise for providing clinicians with tools that may allow screening of high-risk populations, such as tobacco users and those with known human papilloma virus, for HNSCC.
- Detection of HNSCC cancers in earlier stages may finally provide our patients with the improved disease-specific survival that both researchers and clinicians have long hoped for.

Introduction

Head and neck squamous cell carcinoma (HNSCC) remains a significant disease, making up over 5% of all cancers in the United States and an even larger proportion of cancers worldwide.[1] Along with squamous cell carcinoma of the lung, it is one of the few human cancers that appears to be primarily due to environmental causes. These causes are generally identifiable. Tobacco use, excess alcohol consumption, and human papilloma virus (HPV) are well-established risk factors for HNSCC.

Over the last 30 years, there have been many changes in the way HNSCC is diagnosed, treated, and even studied. Imaging technologies including computed tomography, magnetic resonance imaging, and positron emission tomography allow physicians much improved adjuncts to standard physical examination for both diagnosis and surveillance. Organ preservation via combined chemotherapy and radiation therapy has become a standard of care for many subsites of HNSCC, including many laryngeal, oropharyngeal, and sinonasal tumors. New and improved surgical extirpative techniques, complex reconstruction utilizing free tissue transfer, and improved speech and swallowing rehabilitation, have maximized both functional and cosmetic outcomes. All these advances have allowed a perceived improvement in the quality of life for HNSCC patients. Yet, little progress has been documented regarding improved survival rates, begging the obvious question: why not?

There may be many answers to this question. One intuitive answer is that given the usual location of these tumors within the upper aerodigestive tract, tumor symptoms mimic those of common ailments. Tumors are therefore often discovered in advanced stages. Because the American Joint Committee on Cancer (AJCC) staging system is specifically tied to survival by design, advanced-stage illness equates to poorer survival.[2] Despite increased awareness and education about the potential effects of tobacco and alcohol use, the incidence of HNSCC in the United States has changed very little, since elimination of the known environmental causes seems impractical. Indeed, prevention and early diagnosis are therefore accepted as main-stays of successful HNSCC treatment. Nevertheless, no accepted screening test exists for this cancer type. In fact, screening for HNSCC is not mentioned in recent screening guidelines of the American Cancer Society[3] presumably because of the lack of sufficient screening tools available to physicians. Aside from a complete head and neck history and physical examination with imaging studies in patients with suspicious clinical findings or symptoms, there are no accepted methods for screening for the appearance and recurrence of these cancers. To remedy this situation, many researchers have dedicated much of their work to facilitate early detection of HNSCC, the importance of which is exemplified by this textbook series.

The search for biomarkers and biomarker patterns predictive of HNSCC has focused largely on the detection of genetic abnormalities that lead to the development of HNSCC.[4,5] This topic is specifically covered in depth in Chapter 1. Despite the identification and characterization of multiple genetic aberrations in HNSCC, none has yet been determined to enhance early detection of HNSCC. Recently, attention has therefore focused on deciphering the HNSCC proteome in search of diagnostic biomarkers.

The human proteome is defined as the full set of proteins encoded by the genome. Proteomics, or protein pattern analysis, is the characterization and quantification of proteins in tissues and body fluids. Proteomic methods can be used to compare protein expression patterns in normal versus cancer patients or to compare samples at different times from the same patient. Proteomic research has traditionally involved two-dimensional gel electrophoresis (2D-PAGE) to detect differences in protein expression in tissue and body fluid specimens between the healthy (control) group and the disease group.[6,7] In 2D-PAGE, proteins are separated on the basis of size and charge. Although 2D-PAGE has been the primary historical technique in conventional proteomic analyses, it has limitations in detection, particularly for proteins of low abundance and molecular mass less than 10,000 Da, is labor-intensive, has low throughput, and is not easily applied in the clinical setting.

Mass spectrometry analysis of proteins and peptides has evolved rapidly over the last decade. A mass spectrometer instrument consists of at least three common features: an ionization source, a mass analyzer, and a detector. For analysis of proteins, particularly from clinical samples, the two most common types of mass spectrometers involve an electrospray-ionization source coupled to an ion-trap mass analyzer (ESI-MS) or a matrix-assisted laser desorption/ionization (MALDI) source with a time of flight (TOF) mass analyzer. Because ESI-MS involves the generation of multiply charged ions in solution prior to mass analysis, interpretation of the data can be complicated in protein-dense clinical samples (such as serum) since extensive upfront purification and protease digestions are required, resulting in less sample throughput. The MALDI-TOF process involves the laser desorption of sample spotted on a metal plate, resulting in primarily single ion species. This allows for the profiling of multiple desorbed protein species and is more amenable to a higher throughput analysis required for many clinical specimens. Surface-enhanced laser desorption/ionization-time of flight (SELDI-TOF) mass spectrometry is an affinity surface, chip-array variant of MALDI-TOF. Although ESI-MS is a critical and useful tool in the analysis of proteins from clinical samples, it has not been extensively applied to HNSCC serum samples. Thus, in this review focus is on the applications of the MALDI-TOF and related SELDI-TOF approaches for assessing early detection assays for head and neck cancers.

Surface-Enhanced Laser Desorption/Ionization

One of the initial technologic advances in proteomics for the analysis of complex biologic mixtures is surface-enhanced laser desorption/ionization time of flight mass spectrometry (SELDI-TOF-MS).[8,9] As summarized in Figure 2-1, this modification of MALDI technology uses ProteinChip arrays that are coated with variable chemical surfaces (e.g., ionic, hydrophobic, or metallic) to affinity-capture protein molecules from patient samples (e.g., serum, tissue, and saliva). The chip is then irradiated with a laser, which causes the adherent proteins to "fly off" as charged ions. The ions travel through a vacuum tube, and the mass-to-charge (m/z) ratios are calculated based on their time of flight (TOF) through the ion chamber (reviewed in references 10 and 11).

In the early part of this decade, applications of this technology had shown great potential for early detection of prostate, breast, ovarian, and bladder cancers.[12–15] Interest in applying this technique to HNSCC soon followed, although there remains a relative paucity of published work on SELDI and HNSCC, with less than 10 studies currently in the literature. The first study combining HNSCC and SELDI was by Wu and associates[16] in 2002 in which the authors used SELDI techniques to augment their 2D-PAGE experiment investigating protein differences between two cell lines from a primary and metastatic tumor from a single HNSCC patient. The different protein bands determined by the 2D-PAGE analysis were cut out and processed via SELDI to arrive at m/z data that was then used to query a database to facilitate identification of the protein species. The researchers concluded that the proteins enolase-alpha, annexin-I, and annexin-II could be important in head and neck cancer metastasis. This study bridged the divide between the gold standard method of 2D-PAGE analysis and the newer SELDI techniques, and it furthered interest in applying SELDI in HNSCC analysis.

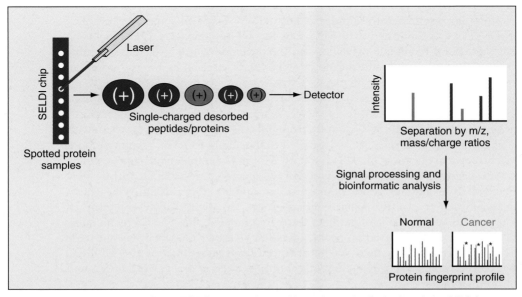

Figure 2-1. Schematic summary of SELDI-TOF (surface-enhanced laser desorption/ionization–time of flight) mass spectrometry profiling.

The use of SELDI for large-scale analysis of multiple HNSCC patient samples was not reported until 2004 by researchers at the Eastern Virginia Medical School.[17] In this study, SELDI was used to analyze serum from 99 HNSCC patients and 102 healthy nonsmoking control subjects. The serum protein expression profiles were then used to develop and train a classification and regression tree algorithm. This algorithm, or decision tree, when tested reliably achieved a sensitivity of 83.3% and a specificity of 100% in discriminating HNSCC from normal control serum samples. These results generated much excitement in the hope that the SELDI technique had potential for the development of a screening test for the detection of HNSCC. Soon after, Soltys and associates[18] published their work analyzing the proteomic spectra of 113 HNSCC cancer patients and 104 control subjects. In this work, half of the study group was used in training sets while the other half was used for testing their decision algorithm using a Lasso technique for data analysis. The results yielded a sensitivity of 68% and a specificity of 73%. Although the study showed lower accuracy in correctly classifying samples, the significance of this work was to show that with a heterogeneous control group that includes tobacco and alcohol users, one could expect higher misclassification rates. Both of these studies reflected the shift in paradigm from focusing on specific or novel tumor biomarker discovery to the use of this technology to assay the patterns of protein expression, regardless of whether the individual protein species for all peaks were known. However, it was clear that many samples of both HNSCC patients and controls of varying demographics would be needed to minimize confounding factors for this data analysis technique.

This issue was partially addressed later in 2004.[19] In this study, we analyzed 99 HNSCC, 102 healthy nonsmoker, and 25 healthy smoker serum samples. The serum protein expression profiles were used to develop a classification tree algorithm, which achieved a sensitivity of 83.3% and a specificity of 90% in discriminating HNSCC from normal and healthy smoker controls. The positive and negative predictive values were 80% and 92%, respectively. This showed that training the decision algorithm with a group of samples from tobacco users could enhance the accuracy of the analysis. Furthermore, this work was the first to show that this same SELDI method could allow for a known tumor marker, metallopanstimulin-1 (MPS-1), to be detected in sera from HNSCC patients based on its mass alone. The peak relative intensity of the 10,068-Da MPS-1 protein correlated consistently with MPS-1 levels detected by radioimmunoassay in serum samples of both HNSCC patients and controls. The 10,068-Da peak was confirmed to be MPS-1 by SELDI immunoassay. Our conclusion was that the SELDI technique may allow for the development of a reliable screening test for the early detection and diagnosis of HNSCC, as well as for the potential identification of specific tumor biomarkers.

One limitation of the studies discussed thus far is that the HNSCC populations were heterogeneous in both subsite and stage. A small study by Xiao and associates[20] specifically examined 33 HNSCC samples from only the larynx, comparing them with 31 matched healthy control samples using SELDI techniques. The results demonstrated correct classification of 97% for both HNSCC samples and controls. The results also suggested that the accuracy of SELDI-generated decision algorithms may be enhanced by examining more homogeneous samples. Gourin and colleagues[21] further attempted to stratify analysis by subgroups. In their study, sera from 78 HNSCC and 68 healthy control patients were compared. Using SELDI techniques, classification tree analysis based on peak expression yielded 82% sensitivity and 76% specificity. The researchers then specifically addressed subgroups of the HNSCC samples, correctly classifying 88% of laryngeal tumors, 83% of oral cavity tumors, and 81% of oropharyngeal tumors.

Another study specifically addressed the identification of a certain protein species using SELDI techniques. Le and associates[22] induced hypoxia in vitro in the cell line

FaDu, originally a hypopharyngeal HNSCC primary tumor, and used SELDI analysis to identify an upregulated protein species at 15 kDa. The researchers then identified this protein as galectin-1. After staining 101 HNSCC tissue samples for galectin-1, they used the immunohistochemical data to compare with historical patient data. They concluded that galectin-1 was a significant predictor of overall survival on multivariate analysis of the retrospective data. Roesch-Ely and colleagues[23] combined genomic and SELDI proteomic approaches. In their first study, the authors confirmed calgranulins A and B and annexins 1 and 2 to be downregulated in HNSCC at the genomic level, in contrast to cutaneous squamous cell carcinoma. This, too, proved true on SELDI protein profile analysis. They then showed novel expression patterns of calgranulins A and B in normal mucosa as well as in HNSCC mucosa. A second study by the same researchers examined 113 HNSCC tissue samples and 73 healthy samples.[24] They also tested mucosa distant from the primary tumor in 99 samples and adjacent to the tumor in 18 samples by SELDI-TOF-MS on IMAC30 (the most frequently used in HNSCC research) ProteinChip Arrays. It is interesting that the authors' prediction algorithm correctly classified normal mucosa and tumor samples with 94.5% and 92.9% accuracy, respectively. More important, when they applied the classification algorithm to the distant and adjacent mucosa, the distant tissue was accurately classified in only 59.6% of samples, and 27.3% of these histologically benign samples were classified as aberrant or HNSCC. Similarly, 72% of the adjacent tissue was predicted as aberrant. These data suggest that SELDI proteomic analysis can identify potential changes in the continuum from HNSCC to histologically benign tissue that otherwise would not be apparent on standard histology. When Roesch-Ely and colleagues[24] compared the protein profiles in the distant samples with clinical outcome of 32 patients, they noted that the association between aberrant profiles and tumor relapse was statistically significant ($P = .018$), concluding that SELDI proteomic profiling could be a significant adjunct to standard histopathologic diagnosis and may be useful in predicting clinical outcome.

SELDI analysis and classification algorithms have therefore been established by several groups to allow high throughput with robust sensitivity and specificity in differentiating serum samples between HNSCC patients and control patients. However, to be used in a screening method for a cancer that is as rare as HNSCC in the general population, the sensitivity and specificity need to be dramatically improved. Multi-institutional trials with shared samples, as carried out with other cancer types such as prostate cancer[25,26] are necessary to determine if SELDI protein expression pattern analysis can achieve its potential for HNSCC.

MALDI-TOF and MALDI-TOF/TOF

The demonstrated high-throughput capabilities and surface capture utility of SELDI-TOF have spurred the development and use of more sensitive MALDI-TOF instrumentation coupled with derivatized-magnetic beads or other nanoparticle surfaces as front-end protein capture strategies.[27–29] A summary schematic diagram is shown in Figure 2-2. From an instrumentation perspective, more sensitive MALDI-TOF/TOF tandem mass spectrometers continue to be developed. The first TOF analysis provides the protein profile scan, as has been described, and selected proteins of interest are further analyzed at the amino acid/peptide level in the second TOF to provide direct protein sequences and therefore protein identities. The magnetic beads allow robotic processing and automation of the samples onto the MALDI spot plates. MALDI spot plates differ from SELDI chips in that they generally contain 384 spots per steel plate; however, they are similar in that dimensions are similar to a standard 96-well plate. The other difference is that the beads provide the surface capture component and are separate from the spot plate that is inserted into the instrument.

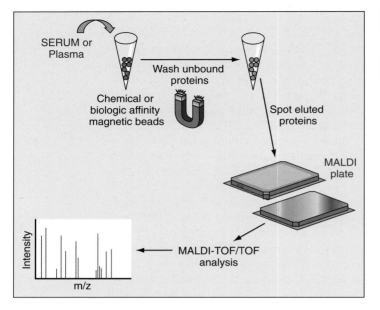

Figure 2-2. Schematic summary of bead-based fractionation combined with MALDI-TOF mass spectrometry profiling.   MALDI-TOF/TOF, matrix-assisted laser desorption/ionization-time of flight/time of flight.

The beads provide a scalability function to allow more sample to be interrogated than the defined SELDI chip surface area. Like the SELDI chip surface, these beads can be "derivatized" with multiple chemical or biologic affinity components. Eluted samples from the beads are mixed with matrix, spotted on the plate, and laser desorbed for mass analysis by TOF, as described for the SELDI process. The peak spectra generated are analyzed with the same types of algorithms that have been applied to SELDI data.

In one of the first published MALDI profiling studies of clinical serum sets, Sidransky and associates[30] evaluated sera from 99 patients with HNSCC, 92 patients with non-small cell lung carcinoma (NSCLC) and 143 control subjects. In this study, no enrichment by affinity capture surfaces was used as sera samples were diluted 1 : 100 in water and nondenaturing detergent, mixed with matrix and spotted directly onto a MALDI sample plate. The resulting spectra were evaluated using a t test feature-selection procedure and linear discriminant analysis (LDA) to determine whether the cancer patient profiles could individually be classified separately from the controls as well as to determine differences between the NSCLC and HNSCC cohorts. Using 45 features from each spectra, receiver operating characteristic (ROC) curves were derived, yielding an optimal cancer model cutoff of 73% sensitivity and 90% specificity. This cancer model could distinguish the NSCLC samples from healthy controls, and gave distinctly lower sensitivities relative to the HNSCC samples. Ten m/z peaks in the 5 to 111 kDa range were predominantly found to be overexpressed in HNSCC subjects compared with controls. The results from this initial study implied that distinct protein differences were present and reflective of HNSCC and NSCLC disease states, but no further protein identification or follow-up has been reported.

To compare results from our previous SELDI studies with newer proteomic expression profiling strategies, a subset of the same samples was used with an automated chemical affinity magnetic bead fractionation strategy for MALDI-TOF mass spectrometry analysis.[31] New cohorts of healthy smoker serum samples and a series of paired pretreatment and post-treatment HNSCC sera were also assessed. The TOF/TOF tandem mass spectrometry feature of the MALDI instrument used was applied to the identification of many low-molecular-weight peptides differentially expressed in the different serum cohorts.

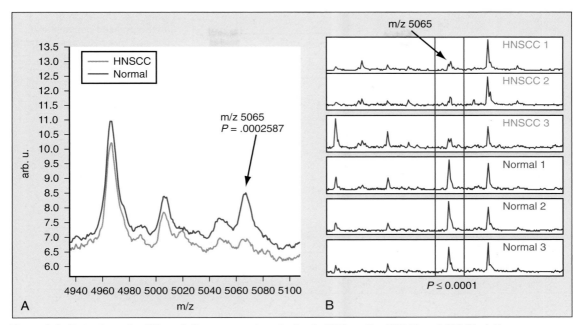

Figure 2-3. Detection of a differentially expressed peak at m/z 5065 on the MALDI and SELDI platforms.
A, A peak at m/z 5065 detected on the MALDI platform is underexpressed in HNSCC when compared with normal sera. **B,** A peak of m/z 5065 is found to be underexpressed in HNSCC sera on the SELDI platform. HNSCC, head and neck squamous cell carcinoma; MALDI, matrix-assisted laser desorption/ionization; SELDI, surface-enhanced laser desorption/ionization.

We designed a MALDI-TOF bead-based analysis for comparison with one of our previous SELDI-TOF studies of normal ($n = 27$), healthy smoker ($n = 25$), and HNSCC ($n = 24$) serum samples. An HNSCC cohort of 48 serum samples from 24 patients consisting of matched pretreatment and 6- to 12-month post-treatment samples was also used. An immobilized metal ion affinity chromatography-copper (IMAC-Cu) derivatized magnetic bead was used to bind low mass serum peptides, the same affinity surface used with the SELDI-TOF approach. Also, the magnetic beads allowed a 20 times higher amount of serum to be used in the initial binding reaction. All processing steps were automated with a Bruker Daltonics ClinProt robotic system, software (FlexAnalysis), and UltraFlex III MALDI-TOF/TOF mass spectrometer. As expected, there were shared peak features for both SELDI and MALDI analyses. As shown in Figure 2-3, the discriminatory peak at 5065 m/z was found to be underexpressed in HNSCC sera on both platforms. A separate profile of the spectra in this region obtained with MALDI-TOF is shown in Figure 2-4 for each of the three sample sets. Another underexpressed in HNSCC peak at 5132 m/z was also detected.

Visualization options of the resulting MALDI-TOF data have also improved. An example of a screenshot for the MALDI-TOF data generated is shown in Figure 2-5, and different views include heat maps, average peak intensities, principal component analysis, and three-dimensional spectral overlays. In the working mass range of 1000 to 10,000 m/z, about 200 peaks were resolved and used with a k-nearest neighbor genetic algorithm in FlexAnalysis to generate cross-validated classification models. The best model resulted in the correct classification of 89% normal, 93% benign, and 98% HNSCC samples compared with the SELDI-TOF study classification rates or 100% normal, 80% benign, and 83% HNSCC. An example of the differential spectra obtained for one of the peaks identified in the analysis at 1469 m/z, which was later

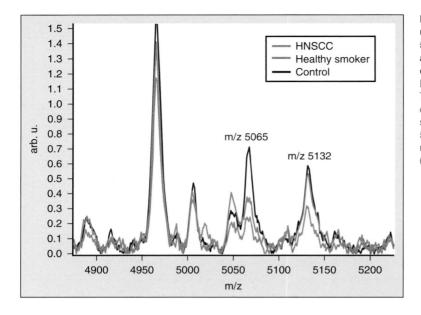

Figure 2-4. Detection of underexpressed peaks at m/z 5065 and m/z 5132 peak in head and neck squamous cell carcinoma (HNSCC) sera. Expanded view of averaged MALDI-TOF (matrix-assisted laser desorption/ionization-time of flight) spectra for peak profiles at m/z 5064 and m/z 5132 in healthy normal (*blue*), healthy smoker (*green*), and HNSCC (*red*) sera.

identified as fibrin A, is shown in Figure 2-6. A more specific principal component analysis of the intensities of two peaks at 1469 m/z and 4173 m/z is shown in Figure 2-7, which highlights the overexpression of 1469 m/z in cancer samples relative to underexpression of 4173 m/z in cancer samples.

Using weak cation exchange derivatized magnetic beads for serum protein capture, a two-way comparison of all pretreatment versus post-treatment samples was carried out. The *k*-nearest neighbor algorithm generated a cross-validated model that correctly predicted 79% classification of pretreatment HNSCC and 88% post-treatment samples. The low mass proteins and serum peptides were then analyzed by MALDI-TOF/TOF MS for sequence identification directly from the same magnetic bead-captured samples. The proteins identified that were differentially expressed represented fragments of kininogen-1 and fibrin peptide A. One conclusion from this aspect of the study was that further analysis of these low mass peptides is warranted, since it is still difficult to differentiate disease-specific differences from potential serum sample processing artifacts, reflected in the detection of the fibrin A clotting-associated peptides.

This initial study using newer high-resolution MALDI-TOF/TOF mass spectrometry combined with bead fractionation proved suitable for automated protein profiling. It also has the capability to simultaneously identify potential biomarker proteins for HNSCC. Furthermore, we were able to show some modest improvement with the MALDI-TOF in identifying groups with HNSCC when compared with our prior data using SELDI-TOF. Using this MALDI-TOF technology as a discovery platform may allow generation of biomarker panels for use in more accurate prediction of prognosis and treatment efficacies for HNSCC.

Future Applications

MALDI-TOF Imaging in Tissue

Proteomic analysis of cells derived directly from HNSCC tissues represents an increasingly attractive target as methods of isolation improve and sensitivities of mass

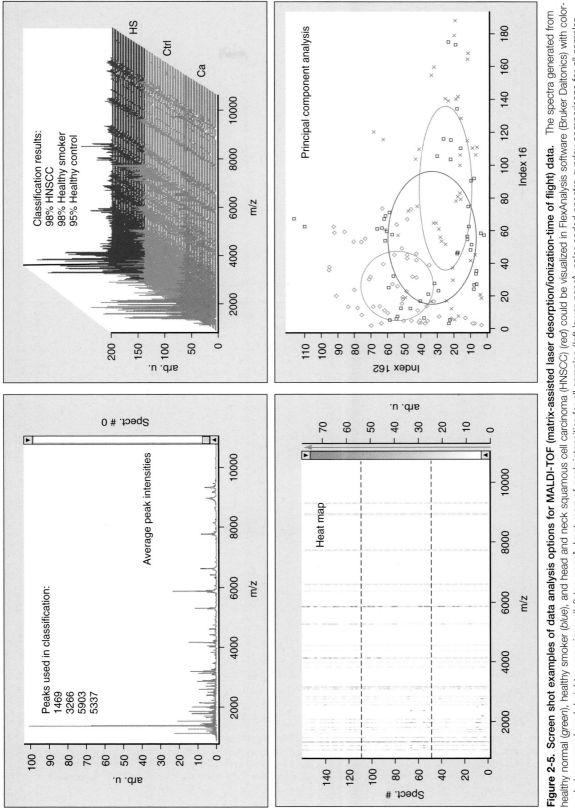

Figure 2-5. Screen shot examples of data analysis options for MALDI-TOF (matrix-assisted laser desorption/ionization-time of flight) data. The spectra generated from healthy normal (*green*), healthy smoker (*blue*), and head and neck squamous cell carcinoma (HNSCC) (*red*) could be visualized in FlexAnalysis software (Bruker Daltonics) with color-coded averaged peak height comparisons (*left top panel*), heat map of peak intensities for all samples (*left lower panel*), color-coded spectra overlay comparisons for all samples (*right top panel*), and principal component analysis distribution for two discriminating peaks in all samples (*right lower panel*).

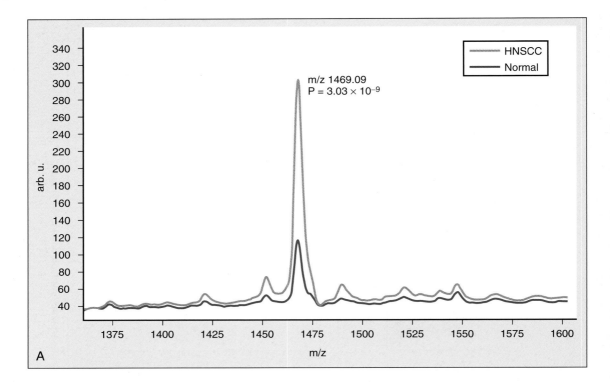

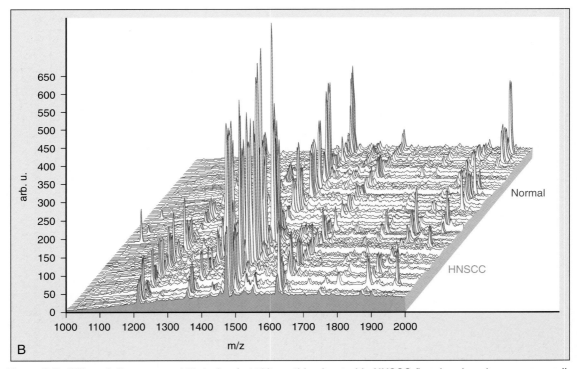

Figure 2-6. Differentially expressed fibrin A m/z 1469 peptide elevated in HNSCC (head and neck squamous cell carcinoma) sera. **A,** The upper spectra panel shows the averaged intensities of MALDI-TOF (matrix-assisted laser desorption/ionization-time of flight) peaks of fibrin A for ions at m/z 1469 in healthy normal (*blue*) and HNSCC (*red*). **B,** The stacked spectra overlay illustrates the m/z 1469 peak intensities for every sample analyzed: healthy normal versus HNSCC.

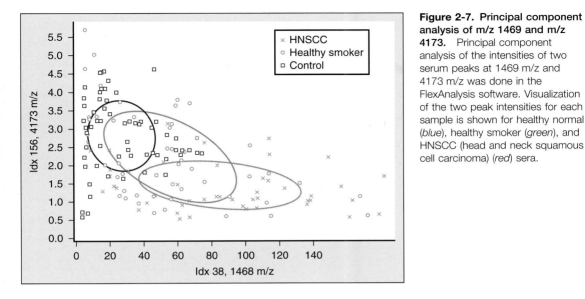

Figure 2-7. Principal component analysis of m/z 1469 and m/z 4173. Principal component analysis of the intensities of two serum peaks at 1469 m/z and 4173 m/z was done in the FlexAnalysis software. Visualization of the two peak intensities for each sample is shown for healthy normal (*blue*), healthy smoker (*green*), and HNSCC (head and neck squamous cell carcinoma) (*red*) sera.

spectrometers increase. One newly emerging application is that of MALDI-TOF imaging of frozen tissue samples prepped directly on MALDI plates.[32] Rather than being represented as peak heights, an individual protein or peptide is assigned a pixel intensity and color. Therefore, the larger the peak intensity at a given mass, the brighter the pixel color of that protein in the image of the tissue at that location. This allows simultaneous protein profiling analysis of all the cell types in a heterogeneous tumor tissue, and all these data are linked to pathology and cytology results. For HNSCC, this MALDI-TOF imaging approach has the potential to better define molecular tumor margins and aid in multiple prognostic and treatment decision-making processes.

Conclusion

Mass spectrometry techniques, such as MALDI-TOF and SELDI-TOF, allow for differentiation and classification of samples for a given disease state. The expression profiling studies described herein for HNSCC biomarkers have largely been pilot-sized and geared toward discovery applications. Based on what has been learned from larger-scale SELDI studies of serum from prostate cancer,[13,25,26] moving these studies toward clinical validation will require larger sample collections, standardization of the sample processing and storage conditions, calibration of instrumentation between institutions, and continued development of software to store and analyze complex datasets. This will obviously require a large investment in money and coordination of clinical resources.

The proteomic technologies nonetheless hold tremendous promise to provide clinicians with tools that may eventually allow screening of high-risk populations, such as tobacco users and those with known human papilloma virus, for HNSCC. Furthermore, detection of these cancers in earlier stages may finally provide our patients with the improved disease-specific survival that both researchers and clinicians have long hoped for. Finally, for patients who suffer with higher-staged disease, closer observation may become possible with proteome analysis, thereby detecting the presence of molecular disease before the detection of clinically evident disease.

References

1. Jemal A, Murray T, Samuels A, et al: Cancer Statistics, 2003. CA Cancer J Clin 53:5–26, 2003.
2. Greene FL, Fritz AG, Balch CM, et al (eds): AJCC Cancer Staging Handbook, 6th ed. New York: Springer, 2002.
3. Smith RA, Cokkinides V, Eyre HJ: American Cancer Society Guidelines for the Early Detection of Cancer, 2003. CA Cancer J Clin 53:27–43, 2003.
4. Gleich LL, Salamone FN: Molecular genetics of head and neck cancer. Cancer Control, 9:369–378, 2002.
5. Patel V, Leethanakul C, Gutkind JS: New approaches to the understanding of the molecular basis of oral cancer. Crit Rev Oral Biol Med 12:55–63, 2001.
6. Srinivas PR, Srivastava S, Hanash S, Wright GL, Jr: Proteomics in early detection of cancer. Clin Chem 47:1901–1911, 2001.
7. Adam BL, Vlahou A, Semmes OJ, Wright GL, Jr: Proteomic approaches to biomarker discovery in prostate and bladder cancers. Proteomics 1:1264–1270, 2001.
8. Kuwata H, Yip TT, Yip CL, et al: Bactericidal domain of lactoferrin: detection, quantitation, and characterization of lactoferricin in serum by SELDI affinity mass spectrometry. Biochem Biophys Res Commun 245:764–773, 1998.
9. Merchant M, Weinberger SR: Recent advancements in surface-enhanced laser desorption/ionization-time of flight-mass spectrometry. Electrophoresis 21:1164–1177, 2000.
10. Wright GL, Jr: SELDI protein chip MS: a platform for biomarker discovery and cancer diagnosis. Expert Rev Mol Diagn 2:549–563, 2002.
11. Wulfkuhle JD, Liotta LA, Petricoin EF: Proteomic applications for early detection of cancer. Nature Rev Cancer 3:267–275, 2003.
12. Li J, Zhang Z, Rosenzweig J, et al: Proteomics and bioinformatics approaches for identification of serum biomarkers to detect breast cancer. Clin Chem 48:1296–1304, 2002.
13. Adam BL, Qu Y, Davis JW, et al: Serum protein fingerprinting coupled with a pattern-matching algorithm distinguishes prostate cancer from benign prostate hyperplasia and healthy men. Cancer Res 62:3609–3614, 2002.
14. Cazares LH, Adam BL, Ward MD, et al: Normal, benign, preneoplastic, and malignant prostate cells have distinct protein expression profiles resolved by surface enhanced laser desorption/ionization mass spectrometry. Clin Cancer Res 8:2541–2552, 2002.
15. Petricoin EF, Ardekani AM, Hitt BA, et al: Use of proteomic patterns in serum to identify ovarian cancer. Lancet 359:572–577, 2002.
16. Wu W, Tang X, Hu W, et al: Identification and validation of metastasis-associated proteins in head and neck cancer cell lines by two-dimensional electrophoresis and mass spectrometry. Clin Exp Metastasis 19:319–326, 2002.
17. Wadsworth JT, Somers KD, Cazares LH, et al: Serum protein profiles to identify head and neck cancer. Clin Cancer Res 10(5):1625–1632, 2004.
18. Soltys SG, Le QT, Shi G, et al: The use of plasma surface-enhanced laser desorption/ionization time-of-flight mass spectrometry proteomic patterns for detection of head and neck squamous cell cancers. Clin Cancer Res 10(14):4806–4812, 2004.
19. Wadsworth JT, Somers KD, Stack BC, Jr, et al: Identification of patients with head and neck cancer using serum protein profiles. Arch Otolaryngol Head Neck Surg 130(1):98–104, 2004.
20. Xiao X, Zhao X, Liu J, et al: Discovery of laryngeal carcinoma by serum proteomic pattern analysis. Sci China C Life Sci 47:219–223, 2004.
21. Gourin CG, Xia ZS, Han Y, et al: Serum protein profile analysis in patients with head and neck squamous cell carcinoma. Arch Otolaryngol Head Neck Surg 132(4):390–397, 2006.
22. Le QT, Shi G, Cao H, et al: Galectin-1: a link between tumor hypoxia and tumor immune privilege. J Clin Oncol 23(35):8932–8941.
23. Roesch-Ely M, Nees M, Karsai S, et al: Transcript and proteome analysis reveals reduced expression of calgranulins in head and neck squamous cell carcinoma. Eur J Cell Biol 84(2–3):431–444, 2005.
24. Roesch-Ely M., Nees M, Karsai S, et al: Proteomic analysis reveals successive aberrations in protein expression from healthy mucosa to invasive head and neck cancer. Oncogene 26(1):54–64, 2007.
25. McLerran D, Grizzle WE, Feng Z, et al: Analytical validation of serum proteomic profiling for diagnosis of prostate cancer: sources of sample bias. Clin Chem 54:44–52, 2008.
26. McLerran D, Grizzle WE, Feng Z, et al: SELDI-TOF MS whole serum proteomic profiling with IMAC surface does not reliably detect prostate cancer. Clin Chem 54:53–60, 2008.
27. Drake RR, Cazares LH, Semmes OJ: Mining the low molecular weight proteome of blood. Proteomics. Clinical Applications 1:758–768, 2007.
28. Orvisky E, Drake SK, Martin BM, et al: Enrichment of low molecular weight fraction of serum for MS analysis of peptides associated with hepatocellular carcinoma. Proteomics 6:2895–2902, 2006.
29. Drake RR, Schwegler EE, Malik G, et al: Lectin capture strategies combined with mass spectrometry for the discovery of serum glycoprotein biomarkers. Mol Cell Proteomics 5:1957–1967, 2006.
30. Sidransky D, Irizarry R, Califano JA, et al: Serum protein MALDI profiling to distinguish upper aerodigestive tract cancer patients from control subjects. J Natl Cancer Inst 95:1711–1717, 2003.
31. Freed GL, Cazares LH, Fichandler CE, et al: Differential capture of serum proteins for expression profiling and biomarker discovery in pre- and posttreatment head and neck cancer samples. Laryngoscope 118:61–68, 2008.
32. Cornett DS, Mobley JA, Dias EC, et al: A novel histology-directed strategy for MALDI-MS tissue profiling that improves throughput and cellular specificity in human breast cancer. Mol Cell Proteomics 5:1975–1983, 2006.

3 Screening for Head and Neck Cancer: Health Services Perspective

Britt C. Reid

KEY POINTS

- Currently, there is insufficient evidence to support or refute the use of a visual or palpation examination or any other method of screening for oral cancer in the general population.
- A successful head and neck cancer screening program requires both supply and demand for services.
- Public awareness campaigns have sought to increase demand by promoting care-seeking and increased knowledge of head and neck cancers.
- Contact with health care providers represents a potential opportunity for increasing the supply of cancer screening. Adults visit a physician 3 to 10 times per person per year and visit a dentist 1 to 3 times per year.
- Organizational level factors mainly affect the supply side of the cancer screening equation. Applying information technology and aligning payment policy are two critical areas for organizational level interventions to improve head and neck cancer screening programs.
- Organizational level changes are likely to produce more substantial improvements in head and neck cancer screening outcomes than patient or provider level interventions.
- New head and neck cancer research is required to trigger relevant organizational changes at a national level as has happened for cancers of some other anatomic sites.

Overview of Screening

Evidence generated from randomized controlled trials takes an average of 17 years to be incorporated into clinical practice.[1] Add to this the years it may take to propose, acquire funding for, and conduct such trials, and a generation may easily pass between concept and practice. Meanwhile, head and neck cancers continue to arise, patients continue to need care for these cancers, and clinicians continue to be called on to provide that care. (U.S. incidence and survival rates are shown in Figures 3-1 and 3-2.) Clearly, we must assess and make the best use of the evidence we have at hand while allowing that new evidence may alter our practices. This chapter takes a public health viewpoint on the screening of head and neck cancer. From this vantage point, not only are tumor and patient level characteristics relevant, but so too are provider and organizational level factors. The effectiveness of a given screening test is determined by factors from all these levels, including such varied issues as the anatomic site of the tumor, patient beliefs, provider training, and system-wide access to care.

There is very little published evidence that is specific for health services issues regarding cancer screening and even less that is specific for head and neck cancer screening. In the discussion that follows, evidence specific to head and neck cancer is used when available and supplemented with relevant evidence from more general cancer screening studies.

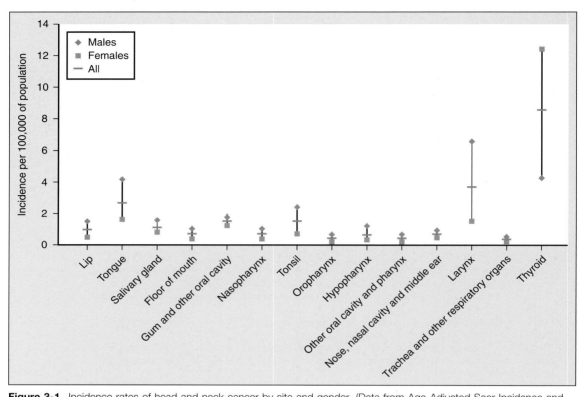

Figure 3-1. Incidence rates of head and neck cancer by site and gender. (Data from Age-Adjusted Seer Incidence and U.S. Death Rates and 5-Year Relative Survival Rates (2000–2004). http://seer.cancer.gov/csr/1975_2004/results_single/sect_01_table.04_2pgs.pdf)

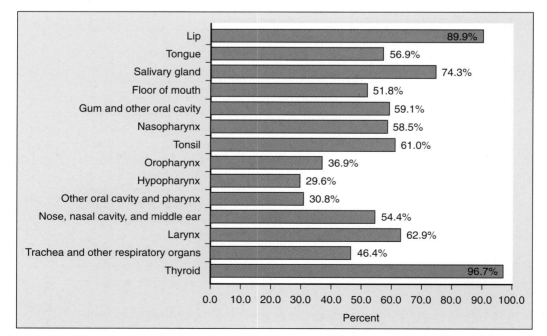

Figure 3-2. Five-year relative survival rates for head and neck cancers. (Data from Age-Adjusted Seer Incidence and U.S. Death Rates and 5-Year Relative Survival Rates. http://seer.cancer.gov/csr/1975_2004/results_single/sect_01_table.04_2pgs.pdf)

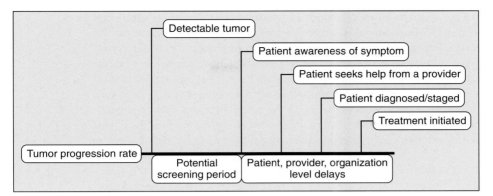

Figure 3-3. Head and neck cancer screening event timeline.

Screening versus Diagnosis

The purpose of population screening for head and neck cancers is to classify asymptomatic persons into those likely or unlikely to have the disease. Population screening assumes that head and neck cancer has a substantial detectable preclinical stage and that early treatment offers benefits that exceed the burdens and costs of screening. Those screened and found likely to have the disease get follow-up with more extensive testing using the current gold standard tests to form a final diagnosis. Figure 3-3 depicts the event timeline for head and neck cancer, with tumor progression rate largely determining the speed with which a given tumor moves along the timeline. Development of screening tests focuses on advancing the time point for detection to as early in the presymptomatic period as possible.

In current practice, visualization and palpation form a commonly used test for the screening of many head and neck cancers, whereas biopsy with pathology report form the gold standard for a final diagnosis. The costs and burdens of screening should include all considerations of finances, time, discomfort, acceptability, and morbidity resulting from screening.

By its very nature, screening for head and neck cancers should have costs and burdens that are substantially lower than those of the gold standard tests used for a final diagnosis. Unlike the tests used to make a final diagnosis, screening results in some false-negatives and false-positives. These false initial screening results are the trade-off for using a test with lower costs and burdens than those of the gold standard tests.

The development of new methods and tests for the screening of populations is guided by the desire to minimize the resulting burdens, costs, and false diagnoses, and to maximize the benefits—largely through the early identification of head and neck cancers.

Anatomic Sites Amenable to Screening

Direct Visualization and Intraoral and Extraoral Palpation

Not all anatomic sites are equally amenable to the screening of asymptomatic people using current methodology. In addition, the range of anatomic sites amenable to screening depends on the degree of specialized training and experience of the provider performing the screening. However, for most primary care providers, direct visualization and/or palpation are most easily accomplished for lip, oral cavity, salivary gland, and a few pharyngeal tumors and nearly impossible for many other head and neck tumors. Laryngeal tumors are rarely detected before symptoms are noted, although it is fortunate that the most prevalent symptom—hoarseness—is often displayed early. The most commonly used screening method takes advantage of the ability to directly visualize and palpate the anatomic sites of the lip, oral cavity, and some portions of the pharynx. An oral cancer examination involves three components: (1) an extraoral palpation, (2) an intraoral palpation, and (3) an intraoral visual inspection). Each step of an oral cancer examination with accompanying photos was provided to all American Dental Association (ADA) members in a recent supplemental publication in the *Journal of the American Dental Association* (Fig. 3-4). The ADA summary of important points to remember when screening for oral cancer is given in Box 3-1.

Clinicians need certain instruments and supplies to conduct a thorough and time-efficient examination. Suggested tools for the oral head and neck cancer examination include an adequate light source, mirrors (laryngeal and nasopharyngeal), gloves, tongue blades, and 2 × 2 gauze pads. For providers appropriately trained in their use, anesthetic nasal spray, a flexible nasopharyngolaryngoscope, an otoscope, and a nasal speculum are additional instruments that allow for visualization of an expanded range of anatomic sites (Fig. 3-5).

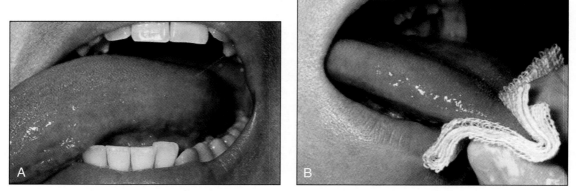

Figure 3-4. Step 6 (tongue) of the American Dental Association (ADA) 8-step, 90-second oral cancer examination.   The ADA recommends that all adult patients receive this screening on a routine basis as part of a regular oral examination. (From Perform a death-defying act. The 90-second oral cancer examination. J Am Dent Assoc 132:36S–40S, 2001.)

Box 3-1. Points to Remember When Screening for Oral Cancer

Most oral cancers are located on the lateral borders of the tongue, floor of the mouth and lips—special attention should be focused in these areas.

Tell your patient what you are doing with each procedure and why.

Always note any changes in color and texture of all soft tissues or any swelling. If you detect an abnormality, determine the history of the lesion; if the abnormality has been of more than two weeks' duration, take appropriate action to obtain a biopsy.[2]

Follow up to ensure a definitive diagnosis of an abnormality.

Teach your patients about the signs and symptoms of oral cancer.

If a patient uses tobacco products, provide appropriate counseling or refer patient for counseling.[2]

Remove all removable prostheses before starting the examination.

From Perform a death-defying act: the 90-second oral cancer examination. J Am Dent Assoc 132: 36S–40S, 2001.

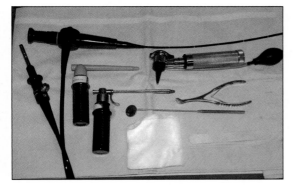

Figure 3-5. Instruments and supplies for conducting an examination for oral cancer.

Sensitivity, Specificity, and Positive Predictive Values of Visualization and Palpation

Direct visualization and/or palpation entail very low patient costs and burdens and require minimal training, suggesting that a wide range of types of providers could accomplish these screenings.[3,4] Visualization and palpation have reported ranges of 70% to 80% sensitivity, 70% to 99% specificity, and 40% to 60% positive predictive value.[5-11]

Evidence for Screening Benefits

Since the 1970s, the survival rates for oral and pharyngeal cancer have improved, but those for cancer of the larynx have declined (Fig. 3-6A and B). To reduce overall morbidity and mortality from head and neck cancer, Healthy People 2010 set goals to increase the number of adults with annual oral cancer screenings and the proportion of oral cancer diagnosed at local stage.[12] However, there is currently no evidence-based consensus regarding who should undergo oral cancer screenings and how often. The American Cancer Society recommends oral cancer screenings for all adults as part of a regular overall cancer screening.[13] Both the Canadian Task Force on Clinical Preventive Services and the U.S. Task Force on Clinical Preventive Services (USTFCPS) report that there is insufficient evidence to recommend routine population screening for oral cancer by health care professionals, but they do recommend an annual examination by a physician or dentist for high-risk patients (those over 60 with heavy alcohol and tobacco use).[14-15] Task Force statements reflect a lack of evidence to support population screening from randomized controlled trials. Such trials are unlikely to be conducted in the United States for reasons of practicality (low prevalence) and ethics (i.e., assigning subjects to not receive screening for head and neck cancer would fall below the current standard of care). Therefore, it is unlikely that an evidence-based guideline will be forthcoming in the United States in the near future.

Despite evidence of a protective effect of screening against advanced-stage disease, no reduction in mortality rate was recorded over a 10-year period from a national oral cancer control program in Cuba.[16] Only one randomized controlled trial of an oral cancer screening program has published results.[8] This study, conducted in India, shows no clear mortality reduction with screening, although several potential methodologic weaknesses may play a role in explaining this result. Nonetheless, at this point there is insufficient evidence to support or refute the use of a visual examination as a method of screening for oral cancer in the general population. In addition, "No robust evidence exists to suggest that other methods of screening, toluidine blue, fluorescence imaging or brush biopsy, are either beneficial or harmful."[17]

There are, however, advocated oral cancer guidelines that do not rise to the level of an evidence-based guideline but that may function as one. The Canadian Dental

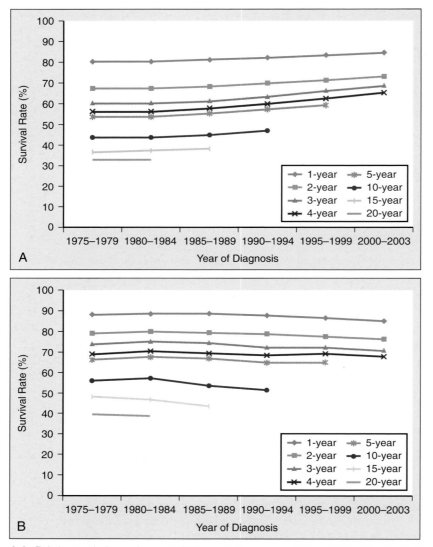

Figure 3-6. Relative survival rates by year of diagnosis of oral and pharyngeal cancer (**A**) and cancer of the larynx (**B**). (A, Data from SEER, at http://seer.cancer.gov/csr/1975_2004/results_single/sect_20_table.06A.pdf. B, Data from SEER, at http://seer.cancer.gov/csr/1975_2004/results_single/sect_12_table.06.pdf.)

Association recommends that all adults get an oral cancer examination as part of a regular examination on a 6-month time interval, and the British Dental Association recommends the same examination but with an annual time interval. The ADA advises patients to seek regular oral cancer screening as part of regular care without stating a specific time interval. Nonetheless, the ADA has initiated an oral cancer awareness campaign through its journal and the media, which includes instruction on how to perform all three components of an oral cancer examination for all adults "on a regular basis." Despite these recommendations, only 15.0% of adults 40 years of age and older report receiving an oral cancer examination in their lifetime[18]; the number rises to 25% when limited to adults with a recent dental visit. These screening rates are extremely low and probably reflect a combination of poor patient ability to recall events as well as providers not performing the screenings. Patient report of a screening varies little by smoking status,[19] a highly relevant risk factor for cancer.[20]

This finding seems to indicate that there is little targeting of high-risk patients by providers for screening. The most common reason given by dentists for not performing an oral cancer examination for patients 40 years of age and older on their initial visit was that acute problems or emergencies prevented it,[21] a statement that offers little in explaining the dramatically low rates reported by patients.

Tumor Factors in Cancer Screening

Tumor level factors play an important role in shaping screening efforts and are mentioned here to provide perspective on the discussion of the different levels of factors that follow. Anatomic site, stage at diagnosis, tissue type, and histologic grade all help to determine patient survival and morbidity directly or indirectly. Tumor progression rates vary widely and may be largely determined by the genetic profiles of the tumor and the patient. Variation in progression rates complicate attempts to demonstrate benefits from a screening program. For example, a rapidly progressing tumor may be diagnosed at an advanced stage and result in poor survival time despite being detected early by screening. Knowledge of molecular and genetic predictors of progression rates would go a long way toward understanding and improving screening efforts, but no consensus on markers has yet been achieved. Oral squamous cell carcinogenesis is associated with a wide range of genetic abnormalities, so much so that simple DNA ploidy may represent a valuable approach to population screening.[22]

The Supply-and-Demand Equation for Successful Cancer Screening

A successful head and neck cancer screening program requires both a supply and demand for the services. Demand generally arises from patient level factors, whereas supply is largely determined by provider and organizational level factors. A number of factors involving characteristics of the individual patient and the providers they contact are associated with whether or not a person receives timely cancer screening. It is obvious that a person must actually be "at risk of being screened" to have any hope of benefiting from the screening effort. For an individual to be at risk of cancer screening, a successful program must overcome factors that derive from three different levels—patient, provider, and organizational—that together form the supply-demand equation. Each of these levels of factors interacts with the other to determine whether an individual will receive timely screening for head and neck cancers. A summary of some of the factors reported to affect cancer screening rates can be found in Box 3-2. Many of these factors have not only direct effects on cancer screening but also indirect effects by interacting with the factors of other levels.

The Demand Side of the Equation

The first part of this successful screening equation is to have the patient perceive the process as being acceptable and potentially beneficial. Barriers to obtaining cancer screening in general are listed in Box 3-3.[23-25] It has been demonstrated among head and neck cancer patients that low levels of care-seeking behavior contribute to the risk of an advanced-stage diagnosis.[26,27] Patients fail to seek health care for a number of reasons, including attitudes about self-efficacy, fatalism, and self-esteem. Unfortunately, persons with the highest risk for developing head and neck cancers because of high exposures to tobacco and alcohol often display low care-seeking behaviors. For example, although dentists provide the majority of asymptomatic head and neck cancer diagnoses, there is strong evidence that smokers are less likely to visit a dentist for nonemergency care than are nonsmokers.[28] In addition, both general educational levels and specific cancer knowledge levels are associated with cancer stage at diag-

Box 3-2. Some Patient, Provider, and Organizational Level Factors
Reported to Affect Head and Neck Cancer Screening

Patient	Provider	Organizational
Age	Age	Reminder systems
Race	Gender	Science-based policy
Gender	Training	High-risk profiling
Income	Liability	Health care delivery system
Education	Distribution	Payment plan
Fatalism	Reimbursement	Legislative mandate
Comorbidity		Centralized administrations
Usual source of care		Economies of scale
Insurance coverage		Goal setting
Place of residence		Audits and formal feedback
Care-seeking behavior		Scope-of-practice laws
Knowledge of head and neck cancer		

Box 3-3. Barriers to Obtaining Cancer Screening

Lack of a usual source of care

Inadequate insurance coverage

Low educational attainment

Older age

Nonwhite race

Low income

Rural or inner city residence

nosis. In several studies, it was found that the public's poor knowledge of the risk factors and signs and symptoms of oral cancer may have led them to believe that an examination was unnecessary.[29–33] As a result, public awareness campaigns have sought to improve the situation and promote care-seeking and increased knowledge of head and neck cancers.[34,35] However, it is important to note that addressing the "demand side" only through patient level factors is not likely to result in a successful screening program.

Improving the demand side of the screening equation through various health promotion and education interventions is ultimately a necessary but insufficient approach to successful cancer screening. A patient who is educated to be health-seeking, who accepts the screening process and perceives its potential benefits, is still not a patient screened for head and neck cancer unless the "supply side," or provider and organizational level issues, are also adequately addressed.

The Supply Side of the Equation

What are some of the provider level factors involved in cancer screening? Note that some of the barriers to obtaining cancer screening in general that were previously listed as patient level factors also have provider level implications. For example, lack of a usual source of care and rural or inner-city residence may simply reflect a dearth of appropriate providers available to the patient as opposed to any individual patient level issues.[23-25] However, even when adequate numbers of providers are available, other issues may conspire against a successful screening program. More frequent and regular contact with the health care system, especially when the same provider is involved, has been found to increase the likelihood of being screened for several types of cancer.[36-38] However, among a population with no substantial barriers to access to health care, those with regular physician contact did not necessarily display fewer advanced-stage diagnoses among head and neck cancer patients.[39] Unlike cancer screening for other sites, head and neck cancer screening may not have been offered by the providers that these patients were visiting, at least not at rates sufficient to demonstrate any substantial advantages.[40] Studies of primary care physicians have found gaps in oral cancer knowledge, low rates of oral cancer screening, and high interest in obtaining continuing education to enhance their knowledge.[41,42] For example, individual physician characteristics that have been reported to be associated with higher breast cancer screening rates include younger age, being an internist, and being female.[43,44] Being an internist was also associated with earlier stage at diagnosis for head and neck cancer among their patients.[40]

National data suggest that, on average, adults visit a physician from 3 to 10 times per year and visit a dentist from 1 to 3 times per year.[45,46] Therefore, among the population visiting either of these provider types in a given year for nonemergent care, many potential opportunities arise for performing head and neck cancer screening. Currently, dentists provide most oral cancer examinations,[47] are more likely to detect asymptomatic lesions, and do more routine screening for oral cancer than physicians.[48] Dentists are also more likely to consider oral cancer screening within their scope of practice and to have the appropriate training to perform an examination.[47] Yet, only 15.0% of adults 40 years of age or older report undergoing an oral cancer examination in their lifetime,[49] and report of an examination varies little by smoking status.[19] Even if these patients are substantially underreporting oral cancer screening because of an inability to recall past efforts, there appears to be many missed opportunities for screening of head and neck cancers. These reports indicate that substantial problems exist with performing head and neck cancer screening on asymptomatic patients regardless of the patient's risk for cancer or the provider's training. In other words, improved provider training for screening patients may result in improvements in screening rates, but even among well-trained providers rates are low. This suggests that we should expect limited screening rate improvements from efforts focused only on provider training/education.

Interaction of Patient and Provider Factor Levels

It is interesting that not only do the different factor levels have their direct effects on cancer screening but patient and provider level factors also interact with each other. For example, Allison and colleagues[50] recently found that provider level delays in head and neck cancer diagnoses were associated with patient level factors such as comorbidity, age, and education in a multivariate analysis. Such interactions can suggest high leverage points for interventions. In many cases, an interaction of a number of difficult-to-address issues may be eliminated when the most easily modifiable among them is identified and addressed.

Organizational Factors in Cancer Screening

Organizational level factors tend most directly, but not exclusively, to affect the supply side of the screening equation. These factors generally manifest as policies and regulatory law driven by a combination of social contract and economic forces. Based on observed screening improvements for cancers at other anatomic sites, organizational level factors likely represent the most powerful areas for interventions among all the levels discussed in this chapter. Organizational factors may be usefully separated into two categories for exploring their potential impact on head and neck cancer screening.

Use of Information Technology

Opportunities for taking advantage of advances in information technology include both simple and complex approaches. At the simple end of the spectrum are prompts and reminder systems that could be implemented via stand-alone computers, internet or Web-based systems in a wide range of settings including single offices of solo practitioners to large networks of providers.[51,52] In fact, reminder systems consistently display two- and threefold improvements in cancer screening rates and represent one of the simplest and most effective interventions for accomplishing this.[53] At the more complex end of the spectrum are computing methodologies to model screening programs that maximize various health outcomes against limited resources. For example, when applying an artificial neural network using the known prevalence of risk factors for oral cancers in a given community and applying the sensitivity and specificity of visual and palpation screening methods, it was determined that 80% of all tumors would be discovered by screening only 25% of the population.[54,55] This result would be accomplished theoretically by identifying and screening only persons with a high risk for developing oral cancers.

Aligning Payment Policy with Screening

Financing of health care is fragmented in the United States with most care being financed through large corporations. The unemployed and even about 30% of employed persons have no health insurance beyond their own out-of-pocket purchases. Many among those with health insurance are underinsured with minimal benefits and very large deductibles. Unfortunately, many of the uninsured and underinsured are among those most at risk for head and neck cancer and could benefit most from a screening program. These high-risk but poorly insured persons are left with the unlikely situation of funding their cancer screening through out-of-pocket expenditures. Different health care delivery systems and financing plans have different potentials for developing successful cancer screening programs, and a brief look at some of the differences is instructive.

Misalignment of payment with screening goals is a feature of certain delivery systems, including fee-for-service plans. An example is when the benefits from cost reductions by reduced treatment through earlier diagnoses accrue to a third-party insurer, whereas the cost of the efforts of earlier diagnoses is borne largely by providers in the plan. Another organizational level misalignment of payment with screening goals occurs with reimbursement variation by provider type. Reimbursement rates are generally higher for physicians who are specialists than for primary care providers. Such organizational forces help drive decisions about whether a provider specializes, where they locate their practice, and how they practice. This, in part, helps to explain other outcomes that affect screening rates, including provider shortages in rural and inner city locations.[56]

In a large employer-funded health care system, providers play little to no role in decisions about coverage policies and reimbursement levels. Science-based policy is also rare in this system. Such decisions are largely made under market forces involving employers and third-party insurers with some input from government regulators.

As a result, individual provider behavior, knowledge, and training, though important, are potentially secondary to organizational forces in determining screening behavior. For example, physicians in the Department of Veterans Affairs were much more likely to perform cancer screening as a result of system-wide policies than because of their individual knowledge or attitudes concerning screening.[57] An additional result of the way that health care is financed in the United States, and a potential organizational barrier to screening, is that the highest cost of cancer screening in the industrialized world is found in the United States.[58]

One sector in which payment policy for cancer screening follows science-based guidelines consists of "equal access" providers such as the Veterans Administration, staff model health maintenance organizations, and safety net groups. Although this sector is relatively small, it can serve as an example of cancer screening outcomes that may occur when services are science-based and access barriers are low. For example, racial/ethnic disparities in cancer screening rates are measurably lower in this sector than in other provider settings.[59]

Health maintenance organizations have been found to be more likely to have cancer screening guidelines, systems for screening delivery, and screening monitoring.[60] Such organizations are associated with better preventive and screening outcomes than other delivery models.[61] Several characteristics of health maintenance organizations are associated with improved cancer screening outcomes including centralized administrations, economies of scale, goal-setting, audits, and formal feedback and provider discussion about practices and policies. All these characteristics point to greater ease in instituting changes for an improved cancer screening at the organizational level than interventions focused solely on patients or providers.[62]

Some examples of national interventions to improve screening for other cancer sites may serve as models for improving head and neck cancer screening. Legislation mandating mammography coverage by private insurers has been rolled out across all 50 states beginning in 1987 and correlates with substantial increases in its use.[63] Medicare Part B, which provides nearly universal coverage for Americans 65 years and older, has had a substantial impact on the use of cancer screening services. The National Breast and Cervical Cancer Early Detection Program is administered by the Centers for Disease Control and Prevention to provide screening for poor and uninsured women and is linked to the Medicaid program to provide follow-up care for those with positive results. This program provides an example of identifying persons with a high risk for the disease and a high risk for not receiving any cancer screening and combining it with a continuum of follow-up care—all directed from an organizational level. Another example is the increased screening rates and reduction in late-stage tumors of the colon subsequent to Medicare coverage for the relevant screening tests.[64] In all these examples of successes in screening of cancers from other anatomic sites, coverage determination is largely science-based, suggesting a strong need for conducting new research to support the use of head and neck cancer screening.

Summary and Future Issues

Efforts to develop new screening tests and diagnostic tools will play a role in the success of any cancer screening program. Screening methods that are less invasive, that result in earlier detection, lower costs, lower false-positive and false-negative rates, and that simplify the training involved in their delivery will all result in changes in the success of a screening program. New screening tests and methods may also result in a shift of provider types needed to screen, availability of the screening across population groups, acceptability and perceived value of the screening by patients, and ability to demonstrate clear reductions in morbidity and mortality when added to a screening program.

However, regardless of the screening tests and diagnostic tools available, at a minimum all of the following steps must occur for a successful cancer screening program: (1) organizational structure must support bringing the provider and patient together in a timely manner for the purpose of a cancer screening; (2) a provider must be qualified to do the cancer screening and offer it to the patient; (3) the patient must perceive the process to be acceptable and potentially beneficial; (4) with these three steps accomplished, appropriate follow-up care must then be available before the ultimate outcomes of reductions in morbidity and mortality from head and neck cancers are observed.

We have seen that interventions at the three levels of patient, provider, and organizational system are possible to improve cancer screening rates. Increasing the awareness and knowledge of head and neck cancer signs, symptoms, and risk factors are some of the ways to improve screening rates at the patient level. Simple reminder systems, appropriate payment, and appropriate training may result in improvements at the provider level. But changes at the organizational level are likely to produce the most substantial improvements in head and neck cancer screening rates. The ability to produce screening guidelines and monitor compliance, to align payment with importance of the screening, and to ensure appropriate training and patient education all are features more easily accomplished under certain types of health care delivery systems, including single-payer or equal-access health maintenance delivery systems. Note that preventive health messages to reduce or eliminate exposure to risk factors for head and neck cancer can be delivered during screening and can represent another avenue for reducing morbidity and mortality through population screening.

For organizational change to occur, research must be accomplished to ascertain whether there are clear benefits to head and neck cancer screening. Only then can these powerful organizational factors be brought fully into play. As depicted in Figure 3-7, having a relevant science base in place will then allow the development of guidelines and supportive legislation to ensure implementation and availability of the screening programs throughout the population. With screening guidelines and/or legislation in hand, organizational level factors can finally be mobilized to remove barriers to care and put appropriate resources into the establishment of a successful head and neck cancer screening program. This is the same basic formula followed with measurable success for the screening of other sites such as cancers of the colon, breast, and cervix. Legislative action can not only mandate head and neck cancer screening to specific groups but shape scope-of-practice acts and constructive-liability systems to allow unencumbered implementation of the programs.

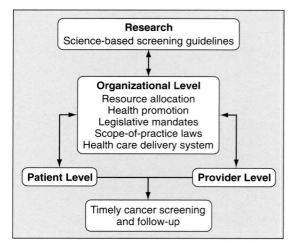

Figure 3-7. The role of research in achieving timely head and neck cancer screening.

References

1. Balas EA, Boren SA: Managing clinical knowledge for health care improvement. Yearbook of Medical Informatics. National Library of Medicine, 2000, pp 65–70.
2. Horowitz AM, Alfano MC: Performing a death-defying act. J Am Dent Assoc 132(Suppl):5S–6S, 2001.
3. Warnakulasuriya KA, Ekanayake AN, Sivayoham S, et al: Utilization of primary health care workers for early detection of oral cancer and precancer cases in Sri Lanka. Bull World Health Org 62(2):243–250, 1984.
4. Warnakulasuriya KA, Nanayakkara BG: Reproducibility of an oral cancer and precancer detection program using a primary health care model in Sri Lanka. Cancer Detect Prev 15(5):331–334, 1991.
5. Ikeda N, Downer MC, Ishii T, et al: Annual screening for oral cancer and precancer by invitation to 60-year-old residents of a city in Japan. Community Dent Health 12(3):133–137, 1995.
6. Jullien JA, Downer MC, Zakrzewska JM, et al: Evaluation of a screening test for the early detection of oral cancer and precancer. Community Dent Health 12(1):3–7, 1995.
7. Downer MC, Evans AW, Hughes Hallet CM, et al: Evaluation of screening for oral cancer and precancer in a company headquarters. Community Dent Oral Epidemiol 23(2):84–88, 1995.
8. Ramadas K, Sankaranarayanan R, Jacob BJ: Interim results from a cluster randomized controlled oral cancer screening trial in Kerala, India. Oral Oncol 39(6):580–588, 2003.
9. Warnakulasuriya S, Ekanayake A, Stjernsward J, et al: Compliance following referral in the early detection of oral cancer and precancer in Sri Lanka. Community Dent Oral Epidemiol 16(6):326–329, 1988.
10. Warnakulasuriya S, Pindborg JJ: Reliability of oral precancer screening by primary health care workers in Sri Lanka. Community Dent Health 7(1):73–79, 1990.
11. Mehta FS, Gupta PC, Bhonsle RB, et al: Detection of oral cancer using basic health workers in an area of high oral cancer incidence in India. Cancer Detect Prev 9(3-4):219–225, 1986.
12. Healthy People 2010. U.S. Department of Health and Human Services. Washington, DC: Government Printing Office, 2000.
13. American Cancer Society Cancer prevention and early detection. 4-04-2006. Available at: www.cancer.org/docroot/PED/content/PED_2_3X_Early_Detection.asp.
14. Hawkins RJ, Wang EE, Leake JL: Preventive health care, 1999 update: prevention of oral cancer mortality. The Canadian Task Force on Preventive Health Care. J Can Dent Assoc 65(11):61, 1999.
15. U.S. Preventive Services Task Force 1996: Screening Oral Cancer. Agency for healthcare research and quality. September 01, 1996. Available at: http://www.ahcpr.gov/clinic/uspstf/uspsoral.htm.
16. Sankaranarayanan R, Fernandez Garrote L, Lence Anta J, et al: Visual inspection in oral cancer screening in Cuba: a case-control study. Oral Oncol 38(2):131–136, 2002.
17. Kujan O, Glenny AM, Oliver RJ, et al: Screening programmes for the early detection and prevention of oral cancer. Cochrane Database Syst Rev Jul 19;3:CD004150, 2006.
18. Horowitz AM, Nourjah PA: Factors associated with having oral cancer examinations among US adults 40 years of age or older. J Public Health Dent 56(6):331–335, 1996.
19. Macek MD, Reid BC, Yellowitz JA: Oral cancer examinations among adults at high risk: findings from the 1998 National Health Interview Survey. J Public Health Dent 63(2):119–125, 2003.
20. Rothman K, Keller A: The effect of joint exposure to alcohol and tobacco on risk of cancer of the mouth and pharynx. J Chronic Dis 25(12):711–716, 1972.
21. Tomar SL, Logan HL, Porter CK, et al: Do Florida dentists examine their patients for oral cancer? [Abstract 44]. J Public Health Dent 63(Suppl 1):S42–S43, 2003.
22. Lavelle CL, Scully C: Criteria to rationalize population screening to control oral cancer. Oral Oncol 41(1):11–16, 2005.
23. Swan J, Breen N, Coates RJ, et al: Progress in cancer screening practices in the United States: results from the 2000 National Health Interview Survey. Cancer 15;97(6):1528–1540, 2003.
24. Kagawa-Singer M: Addressing issues for early detection and screening in ethnic populations—an update. Oncol Nurs Forum 27(9 Suppl):62–63, 2000.
25. Breen N, Wagener DK, Brown ML, et al: Progress in cancer screening over a decade: results of cancer screening from the 1987, 1992, and 1998 National Health Interview Surveys. J Natl Cancer Inst 93(22):1704–1713, 2001.
26. Tromp DM, Brouha XD, Hordijk GJ: Patient and tumour factors associated with advanced carcinomas of the head and neck. Oral Oncol 41(3):313–319, 2005.
27. Kumar S, Heller RF, Pandey U, et al: Delay in presentation of oral cancer: a multifactor analytical study. Natl Med J India 14(1):13–17, 2001.
28. Drilea SK, Reid BC, Li CH, et al: Dental visits among smoking and nonsmoking US adults in 2000. Am J Health Behav 29(5):462–471, 2005.
29. Kerawala CJ: Oral cancer, smoking and alcohol: the patient's perspective. Br J Oral Maxillofac Surg 37:374–376, 1999.
30. Lowry RJ, Craven MA: Smokers and drinkers awareness of oral cancer: a qualitative study using focus groups. Br Dent J 187:668–670, 1999.
31. Warnakulasuriya KA, Harris CK, Scarrott DM, et al: An alarming lack of public awareness towards oral cancer. Br Dent J 187:319–322, 1999.
32. Canto MT, Horowitz AM, Goodman HS, et al: Maryland veterans' knowledge of risk factors for and signs of oral cancers and their use of dental services. Gerodontology 15:79–86, 1998.
33. Horowitz AM, Moon HS, Goodman HS, et al: Maryland adults' knowledge of oral cancer and having oral cancer examinations. J Public Health Dent 58:281–287, 1998.
34. Stahl S, Meskin LH, Brown LJ: The American Dental Association's oral cancer campaign: the impact on consumers and dentists. J Am Dent Assoc 135(9):1261–1267, 2004.
35. Papas RK, Logan HL, Tomar SL: Effectiveness of a community-based oral cancer awareness campaign (United States). Cancer Causes Control 15(2):121–131, 2004.
36. Mandelblatt J, Kanetsky PA: Effectiveness of interventions to enhance physician screening for breast cancer. J Fam Pract 40(2):162–171, 1995.
37. Mandelblatt JS, Yabroff KR, Kerner JF: Equitable access to cancer services: a review of barriers to quality care. Cancer 86(11):2378–2390, 1999.
38. Lemon S, Zapka J, Puleo E, et al: Colorectal cancer screening participation: comparisons with mammography and prostate-specific antigen screening. Am J Public Health 91(8):1264–1272, 2001.
39. Reid BC, Warren JL, Rozier G: Comorbidity and early diagnosis of head and neck cancer in a Medicare population. Am J Prev Med 27(5):373–378, 2004.
40. Reid BC, Rozier RG: Continuity of care and early diagnosis of head and neck cancer. Oral Oncol 42(5):510–516, 2006.
41. Canto MT, Horowitz AM, Drury TF, et al: Maryland family physicians' knowledge, opinions and practices about oral cancer. Oral Oncol 38(5):416–424, 2002.
42. Goodman HS, Yellowitz JA, Horowitz AM: Oral cancer prevention. The role of family practitioners. Arch Fam Med 4(7):628–636, 1995.
43. Lurie N, Slater J, McGovern P, et al: Preventive care for women. Does the sex of the physician matter? N Engl J Med 329:478–482, 1993.
44. Lantz PM, Weisman CS, Itani Z: A disease-specific Medicaid expansion for women. The breast and cervical cancer prevention and treatment act of 2000. Womens Health Issues 13:79–92, 2003.
45. Bloom B, Gift HC, Jack SS: Dental services and oral health: United States. Vital Health Stat 1992;10(183), 1992.
46. Adams PF, Benson V: Current estimates from the National Health Interview Survey, 1989. DHHS Publ No. (PHS) 90-1504. Hyattsville, MD: National Centers for Health Statistics, 1990.
47. Yellowitz JA, Goodman HS: Assessing physicians' and dentists' oral cancer knowledge, opinions and practices. J Am Dent Assoc 126(1):53–60, 1995.
48. Holmes JD, Dierks EJ, Homer LD, et al: Is detection of oral and oropharyngeal squamous cancer by a dental health care provider associated with a lower stage at diagnosis? J Oral Maxillofac Surg 61(3):285–291, 2003.
49. Horowitz AM, Goodman HS, Yellowitz JA, et al: The need for health promotion in oral cancer prevention and early detection. J Public Health Dent 56:319–330, 1996.

50. Allison P, Franco E, Feine J: Predictors of professional diagnostic delays for upper aerodigestive tract carcinoma. Oral Oncol 34:127–132, 1998.

51. Burack RC, Gimotty PA: Promoting screening mammography in inner-city settings. The sustained effectiveness of computerized reminders in a randomized controlled trial. Med Care 35:921–931, 1997.

52. Harris RP, O'Malley MS, Fletcher SW: Prompting physicians for preventive procedures: a five year study of manual and computer reminders. Am J Prev Med 6:145–152, 1990.

53. Rimer BK: Interventions to enhance cancer screening: a brief review of what works and what is on the horizon. Cancer 83(Suppl 8):1770–1774, 1998.

54. Downer MC, Jullien JA, Speight PM: An interim determination of health gain from oral cancer and precancer screening: 2 Developing a model of population screening. Community Dental Health 14:72–75, 1997.

55. Downer MC, Jullien JA, Speight PM: An interim determination of health gain from oral cancer and precancer screening: 3 Pre-selecting high risk individuals. Community Dental Health 15:227–232, 1998.

56. Wolfe BL: Reform of health care for the nonelderly poor. In Danzinger S, Sandefur G, Weinberg D (eds): Confronting Poverty: Prescriptions for Change. Cambridge, MA: Harvard University Press, 1994, pp 253–288.

57. Ward MM, Vaughn TE, Uden-Holmen T, et al: Physician knowledge, attitudes and practices regarding a widely implemented guideline. J Eval Clin Pract 8:155–162, 2002.

58. Bell CM, Crystal M, Detsky AS, et al: Shopping around for hospital services: a comparison of the United States and Canada. JAMA 279:1015–1017, 1998.

59. Shavers VL, Brown ML: Racial and ethnic disparities in the receipt of cancer treatment. J Natl Cancer Inst 94:334–357, 2002.

60. Klabunde CN, Riley GF, Mandelson MT, et al: Health plan policies and programs for colorectal cancer screening: a national profile. Am J Manag Care 10:273–270, 2004.

61. Landon BE, Zaslavsky AM, Bernard SL: Comparison of performance of traditional Medicare versus Medicare managed care. JAMA 291:1744–1752, 2004.

62. Stone EG, Morton SC, Hulscher ME, et al: Interventions that increase use of adult immunization and cancer screening services; a meta-analysis. Ann Intern Med 136:641–651, 2002.

63. McKinney MM, Marconi KM: Legislative interventions to increase access to screening mammography. J. Community Health 17:333–349, 1992.

64. Gross CP, Andersen MS, Krumholz HM, et al: Relation between Medicare screening reimbursement and stage at diagnosis for older patients with colon cancer. JAMA 296(23):2815–2822, 2006.

4

Strategies for Oral Cancer Detection

Joel B. Epstein and James J. Sciubba

K E Y   P O I N T S

- Approximately two thirds of head and neck cancers are diagnosed at an advanced stage of disease.
- Early detection has an impact on prognosis.
- Detection requires head and neck and mucosal visual examinations and palpation.
- Adjuncts to facilitate early detection of head and neck cancer and premalignant lesions are needed.
- Adjuncts may facilitate biopsy site selection and margin delineation of mucosal disease.
- Vital tissue staining (in vivo) has shown usefulness in facilitating detection, biopsy site selection, and margin delineation.
- Imaging technologies and exfoliative cell collection with molecular technology are in development.

Introduction

Oral and oropharyngeal cancer statistics continue to demonstrate the value and positive impact of achieving an early diagnosis of the condition, with one person in four (approximately one person per hour) dying of the disease and survivors often suffering functional and cosmetic as well as psychosocial difficulties. In the United States, approximately 30,000 patients per year are diagnosed with oral cavity or oropharyngeal squamous cell carcinoma (OSCC). This represents 3% of all cancers.[1-3] The baseline annual risk is approximately 1 in 10,000 of the adult U.S. population.[4]

Although 84% of patients with oropharyngeal cancers survive at least 1 year after diagnosis, approximately 50% die within 5 years.[5,6] Ninety-five percent of OSCC cases occur in patients over 40 years of age, and well-known risk factors include tobacco and alcohol use.[6,7] Human papillomavirus (most commonly HPV 16) has been reported in 18.9% of oropharyngeal cancers and a lower percentage of oral cavity cancers and represents an additional risk factor.[8] The impact on the patient and his or her family in having the disease recognized and treated promptly while early in its stage or while preinvasive is enormous. Yet statistics continue to show that a significant proportion of oral cancer patients present initially with advanced-stage disease, thus complicating their management, function, quality of life, and lifespan.

Clinical Mucosal Alterations

Oral mucosal alterations serving as possible harbingers of oral premalignant disease or transformation include leukoplakia, erythroplakia (erythroplasia), and erythroleukoplakia (speckled leukoplakia). The reported risk of developing dysplastic alterations within this group of lesions varies widely, with one study noting a transformation rate ranging from 6.5% for homogeneous leukoplakias to 23.4% for erythroplakia[9] (Figs. 4-1 through 4-3). Particular attention must be directed to erythroplakias, in which a particularly high rate of dysplasia or frank carcinoma is present at the time of the initial diagnosis.[10,11]

Eighty-five percent of oral premalignant lesions (OPLs) and/or malignancies may present as a white lesion (leukoplakia).[11–13] When examined microscopically, 20% of cases of leukoplakia may show hyperkeratosis with dysplasia.[14] It is interesting that the least common sites for leukoplakia—the lateral tongue and the floor of the mouth—are the sites most likely to harbor dysplasia (25% and 50%, respectively).[14] Although more rare, approximately 90% of erythroplakic lesions represent severe dysplasia or carcinoma at the time of diagnosis.[10,15]

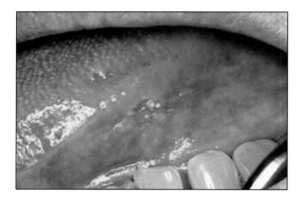

Figure 4-1. A diffuse and homogeneous form of leukoplakia is present over the ventral tongue with indistinct borders, soft texture, and a solitary ulceration at the superior margin. Upon further study it was shown to be a severe epithelial dysplasia.

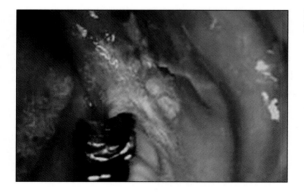

Figure 4-2. A thickened and nodular leukoplakia extends from the attached gingiva into the mucobuccal fold.

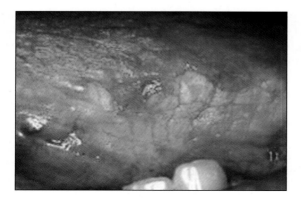

Figure 4-3. An erythroleukoplakia along the lateral tongue margin is characterized by a centrally erythroplastic region surrounded in part by a heavily keratotic component, which microscopically was noted to represent a superficially invasive squamous cell carcinoma.

An unusual and important form of leukoplakia, proliferative verrucous leukoplakia, was defined in 1985 by Hansen and colleagues.[16] In this unique form of mucosal disease, an unusually high rate of malignant transformation is seen in association with expanding, elevated/exophytic white tissue changes with corresponding fissure formation over multiple sites. These changes are often in a discontinuous or separated distribution (Fig. 4-4). In a long-term follow-up study, it was confirmed that this form of leukoplakia is a high-risk lesion for transformation to cancer, with women affected more frequently than men, despite a considerably lower incidence of cigarette or smokeless tobacco use.

Understanding the clinical and biologic nature of oral mucosal alterations with premalignant potential capable of transformation to invasive cancer is crucial to early diagnosis through screening and examinations. Early recognition of subtle or obvious clinical alterations during routine or periodic examinations is important, but statistics point toward either a lack of recognition of these lesions at early phases or a failure of many individuals to comply with screening recommendations. A variety of effective clinical tools have been designed to aid physicians and dentists in the evaluation of subtle oral mucosal alterations that may represent the initial phases of cancer or precursor lesions.[17]

The gold standard tool is tissue biopsy. Newer tools that are easy to use may assist in the selection of lesions for biopsy with impressive levels of sensitivity and specificity. These tools assist in the detection of alterations that are not appreciated by the naked eye on routine tissue examination or they better characterize those changes that *are* visible. Boxes 4-1 and 4-2 present desirable characteristics of adjunctive approaches for lesion identification, and Box 4-3 presents conditions in which adjuncts

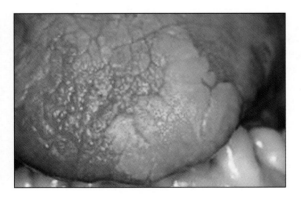

Figure 4-4. Widespread alteration over the dorsal and lateral margins of the tongue with a generally thickened, papillary to verrucous surface and uneven contour characterize this form of leukoplakia.

Box 4-1. Requirements of Adjunctive Tests for Patient Examination

---

Inexpensive, easy to use

Well tolerated, noninvasive

Rapid-acting, real-time clinical information

Used as adjunct to other imaging techniques and cellular techniques

No impact on histologic interpretation

Enhance visibility of mucosal lesions that may harbor dysplasia, CIS/SCC

Sensitive and specific for dysplasia/CIS/SCC; assist in differentiating dysplastic/malignant change from inflammatory lesions

---

CIS, carcinoma in situ; SCC, squamous cell carcinoma

Box 4-2. Usefulness of Adjuncts for Detection of Oral Mucosal Lesions

Increase visibility and detection of oral mucosal lesions

Accelerate decision for biopsy

Aid in biopsy site selection

Assist in detection of margin of abnormal tissue: may disclose larger area of retention than seen with standard clinical exam

Correlate with phenotypic change in oral lesions at risk of cancer and with carcinoma

Correlate with genetic/molecular markers in oral premalignant and malignant lesions

Predict risk of progression to cancer, including in histologically benign and mildly dysplastic tissue

Box 4-3. Lesions and Conditions in Which Adjuncts May Provide Additional Information

Difficult diagnostic presentations:

Clinically minimal/occult mucosal lesions

Multiple sites of leukoplakia; synchronous SCC

Irregular leukoplakia/erythroplakia

Lichenoid mucosal changes

Submucous fibrosis

Mucosal appearance following cancer treatment: persistent/recurrent SCC; premalignant lesions

Immunosuppressed patients: hematopoietic cell transplantation, solid organ transplantation, therapy of immune disease (e.g., rheumatoid arthritis, lupus erythematosus); HIV

may be of particular usefulness. Adjuncts to the oral examination that may enhance identification of lesions of concern are reviewed below.

The risk profile for developing oral cancer is known, but the rate of death has remained virtually unchanged over the past three decades.[5] There are not yet sufficient data to state that screening and early detection of OPL and cancer result in a clear decrease in mortality rate from this disease.[18,19] It is clear that regular visual screening programs can increase the detection of oral surface lesions that may be either malignant or premalignant.[20,21] Five-year survival rates would be expected to improve if OSCC is detected earlier,[5,6] when it requires less aggressive treatment with reduced morbidity and reduced cost of care. The potential valuable role of early detection and adjuncts to clinical examination have been documented in outcomes of other diseases.

History and Examination

A comprehensive history and head and neck and oral examinations are practical during routine dental office visits and require only a few minutes to perform since the oral exam does not include endoscopy.[17,22,23] Unfortunately, the head and neck and oral examinations may not always be performed as routinely or as frequently as recommended,[24,25] even though a standard visual examination for suspicious lesions is critical for identifying and diagnosing mucosal disease. The history should include attention to known risk factors, history of upper aerodigestive tract cancer, and potential symptoms. The examination includes a general head and neck exam, with palpation of cervical lymph nodes, oral inspection, and palpation of the oral cavity. To assess subtle tissue changes in texture or color (particularly erythroplakia), a bright white light source is required, and a halogen light source is recommended.

Chemiluminescence

Chemiluminescence was developed as an adjunct to the Pap smear of the uterine cervix after an acetic acid wash.[26-29] The use of chemiluminescent illumination in cervical examination increases the sensitivity of detection of dysplastic and malignant lesions, with a modest decrease in specificity.[28] In a study of 3300 female patients,[29] negative predictive values (NPV) for squamous cell cancer (SCC) of 94.7% were identified by Pap smear alone. These values rose to 99.1% with the addition of chemiluminescence. Because visual presentation of cervical and oral/pharyngeal lesions, including SCC, may be similar with beneficial contribution by chemiluminescence,[30] this technology was applied to the oral cavity examination. The use of acetic acid followed by chemiluminescent illumination for the identification of oral mucosal lesions has been reported to result in an improvement in visual lesion parameters in several studies involving several institutions.[31-33]

In a preliminary study of chemiluminescence of 26 lesions, enhanced visibility of the lesions was reported, but discrimination of white lesions due to keratotic, inflammatory, or dysplastic lesions was not achieved.[31]

Kerr and colleagues[32] examined 501 consecutive subjects over age 40 years with a positive tobacco history who underwent a standard visual examination with conventional incandescent lighting followed by examination with chemiluminescent lighting. With standard visual examination of 270 subjects, a total of 410 mucosal lesions were detected, of which 127 were deemed clinically "suspicious" for OPL or SCC based on definitions of the World Health Organization. Ninety-eight of these lesions were also visualized by chemiluminescent lighting, and an additional six lesions were seen that were not detected previously by visual examination. Chemiluminescence resulted in enhanced visibility of white but not red lesions ($P < .01$). The white lesions were brighter, sharper, and smaller with chemiluminescent lighting compared with incandescent illumination.

Chemiluminescent light examination was also assessed in a multicenter study of 134 subjects made up of those referred for evaluation of newly identified oral mucosal lesions or for follow-up of previously treated upper aerodigestive tract cancer.[33] A total of 138 lesions were identified with incandescent light (123 or 89%) and clinically diagnosed as leukoplakia. Ninety-eight percent (or 135) of the lesions identified on standard lighting were also seen by chemiluminescence using ViziLite (Zila, Inc, Phoenix, AZ) illumination. Of the three lesions not seen with chemiluminescence, two were red with clinical features that were not suspicious for malignancy and the third was a leukoplakia that was on the lower gingiva and was later diagnosed on biopsy as lichen planus. Two lesions were visible only with ViziLite, and both were later confirmed to be benign. There were no statistically significant differences in lesion detection ($P > .10$) with chemiluminescence. However, subjective clinical visibility of the identified lesions was judged to be enhanced with ViziLite in 54.1% of lesions. Increased sharpness of the lesion margin was seen in 48.1%, and increased report of lesion texture was seen in 35.6%. Lesion visibility based on brightness, sharpness, and texture was enhanced using ViziLite ($P < .001$), whereas a slight increase in the mean lesion size was not significant ($P = .06$).

Overall, chemiluminescent light following routine examination with incandescent light increases visibility of oral white and mixed red/white lesions, largely owing to an increase in the brightness of the lesions and a more distinct contrast at the border. Moreover, the surface texture of the lesions may also be enhanced.

Direct Fluorescence Imaging (Autofluorescence)

Autofluorescence is a characteristic of all tissue and has been assessed for changes that may occur in carcinogenesis. Single-center studies have reported use of a simple, hand-held device (VELscope, LED Dental, Inc, British Columbia, Canada) for direct visualization of autofluorescence of oral tissue. A pilot study of 44 patients reported that VELscope showed a 98% sensitivity and 100% specificity compared with histologic findings in discriminating normal mucosa from severe dysplasia/carcinoma in situ (CIS)/SCC.[34] Although the authors suggested the potential to use the device as an adjunct for oral cancer screening, biopsy guidance, and margin delineation,[34] this was not a true screening study, and the suggested use in screening was not reflected in the design in this pilot trial.

In a second report of three cases from the same institution, the authors reported identification of occult lesions that the clinicians had not noted during routine examination.[35] A study of fluorescence of 20 surgical specimens of OSCC was conducted at the same institution.[36] All tumors showed loss of fluorescence, and in all but one case fluorescence loss extended beyond the borders of the clinical lesion from 4 to 25 mm. Multiple biopsies were assessed from the 20 OSCC cases: 36 biopsies were from fluorescence-positive regions; of these, 89% showed histologic abnormality (7 OSCC/CIS, 10 severe dysplasia; 15 mild/moderate dysplasia) compared with 1 of 66 fluorescence-negative specimens. Molecular assessment of biopsies of the margins showed loss of heterozygosity (LOH) in sites previously associated with tumor recurrence (3p and/or 9p) in 12 of 19 fluorescence-lost versus 3 of 13 fluorescence-retained specimens ($P = .04$). These results suggest that fluorescence may assist in margin evaluation in patients with diagnosed OSCC.

An extensive literature review of autofluorescence for imaging in oral oncology with emphasis on human trials was published.[37] The mechanism of autofluorescence has been related primarily to connective tissue fluorophores in the tissue matrix or in cells, including collagen, elastin, keratin, and NADH (the reduced form of nicotinamide adenine dinucleotide) and may be primarily attributed to oxy- and deoxyhemoglobin. Scattering occurs from irregularities in the index of refraction caused by cell structures, including nuclei and organelles, epithelial thickness and keratin, blood concentration (hemoglobin), and collagen content. Thus, there is variation in fluorescence owing to changes in connective tissue and epithelium. Cell metabolism that may be increased in malignant disease may lead to altered NADH. The evaluation of autofluorescence in the oral cavity may be complicated by the complex oral flora, which may contain microorganisms that also fluoresce, as seen in one study in which fluorescent material could be wiped off the mucosal surface resulting in a change in imaging.[38] This study also showed that though sensitive, autofluorescence shows ambiguous results for SCC of the dorsum tongue and where plaque was present. Furthermore, the ability of autofluorescence to distinguish between inflammatory and premalignant and malignant tissue changes has not been clearly documented. These variables present challenges in the use of autofluorescence in the oral environment.

The key issue is the potential of this technology to distinguish OPL/SCC from benign and healthy oral tissues in the complex oral environment, and indeed additional studies are necessary. It is possible that bacterial retention and activity at sites of SCC enhance autofluorescence. However, although sensitivity in single-center studies looks promising, the potential for false-positives has yet to be determined in large populations and is likely to be high.

The risk of false-negative results must also be determined. If a lesion is malignant, autofluorescence may provide additional information about lesion margin. DeVeld and colleagues[37] note that overall the sensitivity of autofluorescence may be useful in addition to accurate clinical examination, but specificity was a concern because of the difficulty in distinguishing premalignant from benign lesions and because of variability in autofluorescence. The authors anticipate that larger studies and clinical use will lead to increased false-positive results and more variations in outcome. In their own study, DeVeld and colleagues[37] reported that they could not distinguish different types of lesions, which they related to variable degrees of keratinization, hyperplasia of the epithelium, and variation in blood content of the tissue, which is often increased in inflammatory lesions. In addition, they could not distinguish the role of oral microbes in fluorescence. They also note the potential influence of tissue pigmentation and the effects of tobacco and alcohol use in patients upon tissue autofluorescence.

Toluidine Blue

Toluidine blue (TBlue) stain has been shown to be selective for staining of premalignant and malignant mucosal lesions (Fig. 4-5). A meta-analysis of the literature to 1989 assessing the effectiveness of TBlue in identifying OSCC revealed sensitivity ranging from 93.5% to 97.8% and specificity ranging from 73.3% to 92.9%.[39] A study in Sri Lanka using TBlue in a single examination protocol of 102 subjects with undiagnosed oral lesions revealed 18 cases of OSCC, of which 7 were detected only after TBlue staining.[40]

Epstein and others[41] assessed the usefulness of TBlue as a diagnostic aid in 46 patients with prior upper aerodigestive tract cancer. All visual lesions or lesions identified with TBlue were biopsied. Seventy-eight percent of the lesions diagnosed as CIS or SCC were identified upon clinical examination. whereas 100% were identified after TBlue ($P = .02$) with no false-negatives. In this high-risk population, TBlue had a sensitivity of 100% and specificity of 51%. TBlue and clinical examination resulted in a similar number of false-positive results (33%), although application of TBlue was more accurate (68%) than clinical examination (59%). False-positive rates of TBlue retention associated with traumatic or inflammatory conditions were decreased by delaying until confirmation of staining at a second exam approximately 14 days later. This approach resulted in an accuracy of over 80% for detecting malignant and dysplastic lesions.[42–46]

A multicenter surveillance study of 668 patients previously treated for upper aerodigestive tract cancer was conducted by experienced clinical providers.[47] Clinical examination was conducted by one observer and followed by an examination after TBlue rinse application by a provider blinded to the finding of the first observer. Patients returned for follow-up if mucosal change was seen at the first visit or if TBlue was retained; all lesions identified on the second visit were biopsied. A total of 96 biopsies were completed in 81 patients, and 30 lesions received a histologic diagnosis of SCC/CIS. Twelve lesions were described as clinically suspicious (sensitivity 40.0%), whereas 29 of the lesions retained TBlue (sensitivity 96.7%; $P = .0002$).

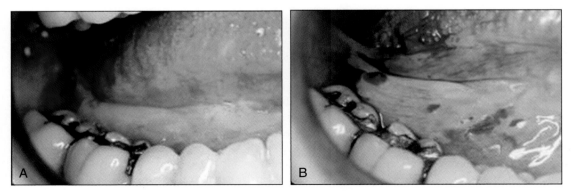

Figure 4-5. Positive uptake of toluidine blue dye highlights an area of leukoplakia (**A**) that is rimmed with blue dye uptake (**B**).

Most of the lesions considered clinically suspicious were not SCC (20/59, 33.9%), and only 57.9% (11/19) thought clinically to represent cancer were diagnosed as SCC on biopsy. Only 2 of 14 (14.3%) of erythroplakic lesions and 2 of 12 (16.7%) initially diagnosed as nodular/benign leukoplakia were histopathologically CIS/SCC. Greater sensitivity of TBlue compared with visual examination was associated with an increase in the number of false-positive results from 21 to 60. Biopsies of an additional 56 lesions were conducted based on TBlue staining, 31 of which represented significant pathology (14 dysplastic lesions; 17 SCC or CIS). This study showed that sensitivity of TBlue was much higher than with visual examination alone in identifying lesions subsequently diagnosed as SCC or CIS (97.3% versus 37.8%), whereas specificity was similar (visual exam 97.1%, TBlue 90.7%). The increased sensitivity of TBlue was attributed to 12 biopsy-positive lesions that were not identified on visual examination. These lesions were clinically smaller and therefore more likely to be difficult to identify. In a previous single-center study,[28] the predictive value of the clinical exam was similar to that of the multicenter study (43.8% versus 36.4%),[47] but the TBlue predictive value was considerably higher (50.9% versus 32.6%), indicating a relatively larger number of false-positives in the multicenter study.

TBlue may also be useful in assessing the extent of a lesion, lesion margins, and other sites of involvement not seen on clinical examination.[28,40,43-50] Assessment of the margins was studied in 50 consecutive patients with OSCC prior to resection.[48] TBlue identified positive resection margins in three cases and identified three cases of second primary SCC that were not identified on visual examination.[48]

Another paper assessed TBlue in 14 patients with SCC, stained preoperatively, and resected with a 1-cm margin of either extent of stain or clinical disease.[51] Only if intense TBlue stain was not seen was the result termed negative. This differs from other studies in which stain uptake was termed positive (intense), equivocal (minimal retention), or negative (no retention); therefore, the results of other studies cannot be directly compared. TBlue was positive at all sites of SCC, confirming previous studies of SCC. However, 10 sites of CIS or severe dysplasia were not reported as positive, but the number with minimal stain was not reported.[51] The authors of this study stated that dysplasia was not stained, which differs from findings in other studies (see previous text).

Biopsy site selection may be difficult in large variably erythroleukoplakic lesions and in patients following head and neck cancer therapy. Also, radiation therapy may lead to delayed healing if tissue biopsy or trauma occurs, which may make clinicians hesitant to biopsy. Therefore, patients with prior upper aerodigestive tract cancer who are at highest risk of new second cancers or recurrent disease are more difficult to assess clinically. TBlue may promote biopsy in postradiation patients, aid in site selection of biopsy, and improve the diagnostic yield.[28,39,42,43,45-47,52] False-negative results are critical in cancer management, and TBlue has consistently shown low false-negative rates.[26,45,46]

Molecular/genetic change in epithelial lesions is the basis of development of OPL and progression to cancer (Figs. 4-6 through 4-8). Analysis of loss of heterozygosity of selected chromosomal segments using polymerase chain reaction (PCR) can be used to document genetic alterations in oral mucosal lesions that predict risk of cancer progression in OPLs and to help identify patients with an increased risk of recurrence or spread of malignant disease after treatment.[53] Continuing studies have documented preferential TBlue binding in lesions with sites of molecular change associated with cancer or risk of progression to cancer.

TBlue staining has been shown to be related to genetic changes (allelic loss or loss of heterozygosity) that are associated with progression of OPLs to cancer even in histologically benign lesions and lesions with mild dysplasia.[53,55,56] TBlue has been

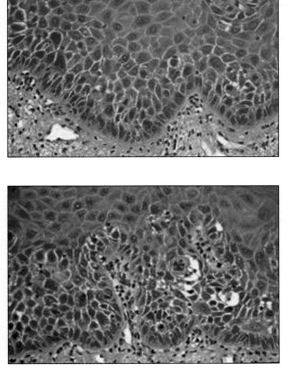

Figure 4-6. Mild epithelial dysplasia with basal and parabasal cellular atypia.

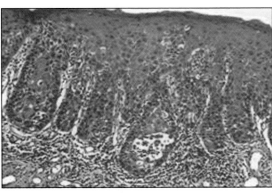

Figure 4-7. Moderate epithelial dysplasia characterized by nuclear hyperchromatism, inverted nuclear-cytoplasmic ratio, and an atypical mitotic figure. These changes extend to approximately 50% of the epithelial thickness.

Figure 4-8. Severe epithelial dysplasia is characterized by abnormal cytologic features extending through the epithelial thickness, but not extending beyond the basement membrane.

shown in a cross-sectional study to stain oral mucosal lesions that exhibit loss of heterozygosity for regions containing genes thought to be important in oral carcinogenesis.[54] A longitudinal, prospective study of 100 patients with OPLs followed up for a mean of 44 months confirmed and extended these findings.[56] Fifteen of the 100 OPLs progressed to OSCC, of which 4/19 arose from lesions with histologic hyperplasia, 4/64 from low-grade dysplasia, and 7/17 from high-grade dysplasias. Most of the cancers (60%) developed at the site of the index biopsy, marked by TBlue, and the remaining 40% arose within a 2-cm region. Only 5% of the TBlue-negative lesions progressed, whereas 33% of the TBlue-positive lesions developed OSCC ($P = .0002$). In addition, time to progression to cancer was significantly less for TBlue-positive lesions ($P < .01$), and the hazard ratio for developing OSCC was more than six times greater in TBlue-positive cases (6.67; 95% CI: 1.87–23.70; $P = .0008$). Positive TBlue staining was seen in 26% of nondysplastic lesions, in 23% of lesions with mild/moderate dysplasia, and in 94% with severe dysplasia ($P < .0001$). Furthermore, TBlue retention was shown to predict risk of progression for OPLs even with benign histology or minimal dysplasia, and it was associated with a high-risk molecular pattern (loss of heterozygosity at 3p and/or 9p plus any other arm—[40% versus 14%], $P = .023$). This prospective trial supported the studies that reported TBlue retention in "molecularly positive lesions," even in those diagnosed histologically as benign or mildly dysplastic lesions. These two studies suggest that lesions stained with TBlue demonstrate allelic loss in histologically benign lesions, suggesting that previously reported "false-positive toluidine blue staining" may represent true molecularly positive findings based on allelic loss.[55] These studies show the potential usefulness of Tblue to identify both OPLs and SCC.

Chemiluminescence and Toluidine Blue

A recent study examined the adjunctive value of a chemiluminescent light source (ViziLite, Inc.) and the application of pharmaceutical-grade TBlue (TBlue[630]) to assess lesions identified during the conventional oral soft tissue examination.[57] Lesions deemed clinically suspicious by visual examination under incandescent light were further assessed under chemiluminescence followed by TBlue stain. Each clinically identified lesion was biopsied and diagnosed based on routine histopathology. Ninety-seven clinically suspicious lesions were identified in 84 patients. The chemiluminescent exam identified all oral lesions previously identified on incandescent light examination and found improved brightness and/or sharpness of margins in 61.8% of identified lesions, features that may assist in detection. Biopsied lesions that also had the TBlue stain retention reduced the false-positive rate by 55.26% while maintaining a 100% negative predictive value. This trial showed that chemiluminescence may facilitate lesion identification by an increase in visibility, and TBlue stain retention was associated with a potential large reduction in biopsies showing benign histology (false-positive biopsy results) while maintaining a 100% negative predictive value for the presence of severe dysplasia or cancer. The addition of TBlue to the examination would have resulted in a 55.26% reduction in the number of false-positive biopsies, while maintaining a diagnosis of all lesions with severe dysplasia and OSCC. This study was conducted by clinical experts and the results may not be applied uniformly to the general population of practitioners.[57]

The Oral Brush Biopsy

In patients who have an obvious neoplasm or in whom a neoplasm is strongly suspected, a tissue biopsy performed with standard scalpel or punch biopsy technique is the method of choice. This gold standard retains its preeminence for accuracy in the proper hands.

In cases of less than obvious but observable mucosal change, however, the brush biopsy methodology has been shown to have a correspondingly high degree of specificity, sensitivity, and positive predictive value together with ease of use and a rapid learning curve.[58–60] Scheifele and colleagues[61] confirmed earlier studies in which the sensitivity and specificity of the brush biopsy procedure were confirmed. Some studies report a high false-positive rate, and false-negative findings have also been reported.[62,63] Any positive or atypical result requires follow-up and biopsy. Key to the diagnostic success of the oral brush biopsy is obtaining a full-thickness sampling of the oral epithelium from a representative site. This may be accomplished by using a specially designed stiff circular brush that, when applied to the observed mucosal lesion, is twisted several times until bleeding points (microbleeding) are noted. This microbleeding confirms that the clinician has penetrated the superficial lamina propria

and obtained a full sampling of the entire epithelial surface layer. The epithelial cells and other cell types that were obtained can then be easily transferred to a glass slide, fixed, and processed. Phenotypic change can be evaluated for the presence or absence of dysplastic cellular changes indicative of the degree of cytologic alteration.

This cellular analysis uses sophisticated image recognition software that is capable of recognizing alterations of nuclear volumes, staining characteristics, cytoplasmic volume, and nuclear chromatin. These individual changes are recorded by the imaging software, which are then confirmed or negated by a pathologist, who then creates the report of findings. This analysis might then demand a definitive scalpel biopsy or allow continued observation only or an elective removal or management of a now highly likely benign lesion.

Salivary Diagnostics

Recent studies have described the use of salivary fluid (whole saliva) for a potentially wide variety of diseases and conditions, including the diagnosis of oral mucosal dysplastic disease and carcinoma.

The prospect that salivary fluid may serve as the medium for the diagnosis of oral cancer and precancer holds great interest. The hypothesis is based on the presence of salivary biomarkers in the form of mRNA transcripts or signatures. By utilizing DNA microarray gene expression profiling technology, it is proposed that it will be possible to monitor or capture the onset and progression of oral cancer or precancer as well as to monitor patients after treatment.[64] In early studies, it has been demonstrated that four genes within the salivary transcriptome core were able to predict and discriminate whether saliva collected was from a healthy subject or from a patient with oral cancer.[65] These gene products included interleukin-8 (IL-8), ornithine decarboxylase, spermidine acetyltransferase, and IL-1{b}, with consistent results in the ability to discriminate.

In addition, other investigators report, by way of whole saliva analysis, a link between the presence of OSCC and elevated levels of reactive nitrogen species and substantially reduced salivary antioxidants. In addition, higher levels of salivary carbonylation levels and DNA oxidation markers were detected in saliva of oral cancer patients.[66,67]

Discussion

Early detection of OPLs and SCC is expected to have a significant impact on prognosis. Early detection relies on the ability to identify potential sites of abnormality, to differentiate OPLs from benign, reactive, and inflammatory conditions, to make the decision to perform a biopsy, to select a biopsy site, and to make an accurate pathologic diagnosis. Each of these steps is subject to variability.[68,69]

Examination of mucosal lesions aided by TBlue staining enhances prediction of epithelial dysplasias progressing to OSCC as well as progression of even nondysplastic and mildly dysplastic lesions based on associated high-risk loss of heterozygosity molecular profile. This suggests the potential clinical value of TBlue in evaluation of OPLs as well as in patients with CIS and SCC.[56] Indeed, TBlue has been shown to assist in identifying OPLs and margins of dysplastic/malignant tissue that may not be readily apparent clinically. In addition, TBlue staining is associated with loss of heterozygosity profile that is associated with SCC and risk of progression of OPLs to OSCC.

The finding of loss of regions of chromosomes containing presumptive tumor suppressor genes in a TBlue-stained group, but not in the negative group, suggests the molecular mechanism of TBlue staining. Therefore, TBlue staining may have predictive value for cancer transformation, associated with the loss of heterozygosity findings previously confirmed as being associated with OSCC and OPLs at risk of progression to cancer. Thus, TBlue may provide clinicians with an additional tool for judging cancer risk of OPLs and can guide the management of these lesions (e.g., monitoring or intervention with surgery and/or chemoprevention). It is possible that in studies in which loss of heterozygosity was not assessed, binding of TBlue reveals lesions with advanced loss of heterozygosity or loss of more than two arms with risk of progression to cancer. Some lesions with dysplasia do not retain stain, whereas other lesions that appear clinically and histologically benign, and yet represent true molecularly positive lesions with high risk of progression to cancer due to genetic profile. Patients with these lesions require careful follow-up and treatment. Furthermore, even when OPLs are identified, predicting the risk of progression to cancer has been unreliable, other than that based on degree of dysplasia, in which a greater degree of severity of dysplasia may correspond to increased risk of progression. TBlue retention is associated with molecular clones at an increased risk of progression even in histologic diagnoses of benign hyperplasia or mild dysplasia.

Chemiluminescence has been shown in studies to enhance the characteristics of oral lesions, which may increase detection due to increased visibility. The utility of chemiluminescence is enhanced when used in combination with TBlue. Further research on tissue autofluorescence is needed.

The oral brush biopsy technique offers the clinician an alternative to the more formal tissue biopsy in instances in which the identified mucosal alteration does not merit the clinical suspicion of a cancerous lesion. This technique may offer sensitivity and specificity and a minimally invasive approach with no local anesthesia, suturing, or cautery and no postoperative discomfort for initial evaluation of a lesion. It may also be useful in follow-up of OPLs.

A further use of the brush biopsy tool may be to provide cellular material for molecular analysis in that it lends whole and intact epithelial cells that may be transferred to a glass slide and easily fixed or in a fluid transport medium, where the sample is suspended for subsequent centrifugation, as the case may be.

Application of salivary diagnostics remains in the future but offers the promise of accuracy, ease of use, and a true screening tool. Clinical trials and further study, however, need to be carried out before this technology can be accepted and used clinically.

Future studies using molecular analysis and possibly DNA-cytometric analysis of exfoliated cells may help differentiate atypical and reactive or regenerative cells from those that are truly dysplastic or neoplastic in nature.[70,71]

Summary

Cancer development is a complex molecular process, eventually resulting in sufficient genetic or epigenetic change that leads to histologic phenotypic change and ultimately to clinical change. Clinical visualization of mucosal lesions is required to allow the next steps in diagnosis. Two visual adjunctive devices are approved by the FDA, using chemiluminescence and autofluorescence. Single-center and multicenter trials have used chemiluminescence with consistent evidence that visualization of white lesions is enhanced and may facilitate identification of oral mucosal lesions. Early studies of autofluorescence suggest that this imaging may be effective. However, many technical issues need to be overcome for oral use, and although sensitivity may be increased, most trials show low specificity.

Toluidine blue (TBlue) staining may provide clinicians with an additional tool for judging cancer risk of oral premalignant lesions (OPLs) and may guide the management of these lesions (e.g., monitoring or intervention with surgery and/or chemoprevention). TBlue is useful in the clinical management of patients and has been shown to assist in lesion identification, biopsy site selection, and margin identification of OPLs and oropharyngeal squamous cell carcinoma (OSCC). TBlue may be valuable in the clinical assessment of high-risk patients and in those in whom OPLs have been identified, and it may guide treatment and assess follow-up response to treatment. The clinical implications are that TBlue can facilitate visualization of lesions, accelerate the decision to biopsy, aid in biopsy site selection, provide additional information on margins of lesions, and reflect the loss of heterozygosity (LOH) profile with risk of progression of even histologically benign lesions or lesions with mild dysplasia. The combined use of chemiluminescence and TBlue has been shown to identify lesions with severe dysplasia, carcinoma in situ, and squamous cell carcinoma, with a reduction in the number of unnecessary biopsies.

References

1. Silverman S Jr: Oral Cancer, 5th ed. Hamilton, ON: BC Decker [sponsored by the American Cancer Society] 2003, p 9.
2. Weber RS, Duffey DC: Head and neck cancer. In Townsend CM (ed): Sabiston Textbook of Surgery, 16th ed. Philadelphia: Saunders, 2001, pp 533–553.
3. Jemal A, Murray T, Ward E, et al: Cancer statistics, 2005. CA Cancer J Clin 55:10–30, 2005.
4. Burzynski NJ, Firriolo FJ, Butters JM, Sorrell CL: Evaluation of oral cancer screening. J Cancer Educ 12:95–99, 1997.
5. Silverman S Jr: Demographics and occurrence of oral and pharyngeal cancers. The outcomes, the trends, the challenge. J Am Dent Assoc 132(Suppl):7S–11S, 2001.
6. American Cancer Society: Cancer Facts and Figures 2006. Atlanta: American Cancer Society, 2006. Available at: www. cancer.org/downloads/STT/CAFF2006PWSecured.pdf
7. Blot WJ, McLaughlin JK, Winn DM, et al: Smoking and drinking in relation to oral and pharyngeal cancer. Cancer Res 48(11):3282–3287, 1988.
8. Herrero R, Castellsague X, Pawlita M, et al, for the IARC Multicenter Oral Cancer Study Group. Human papillomavirus and oral cancer: the International Agency for Research on Cancer multicenter study. J Natl Cancer Inst 95(23):1772–1783, 2003.
9. Silverman S, Jr, Gorsky M, Lozada F: Oral leukoplakia and malignant transformation: a follow-up study of 257 patients. Cancer 53:563–568, 1984.
10. Shafer WF, Waldron CW: Erythroplakia of the oral cavity. Cancer 36:1021–1028, 1975.
11. Mashberg A, Samit AM: Early diagnosis of asymptomatic oral and oropharyngeal cancer. CA: Cancer J Clin 45:328–351, 1995.
12. Hawkins RJ, Wang EFL, Leake JL, the Canadian Task Force on Preventive Health Care. Preventive Health Care, 1999 Update: Prevention of Oral Cancer Mortality. J Can Dent Assoc 65:617–627, 1999.
13. Neville BW, Damm, DD, Allen CM, Bouquot JE: Oral and Maxillofacial Pathology, 2nd ed. Philadelphia: WB Saunders, 2002.
14. Waldron CW, Shafer WF: Leukoplakia revisited: a clinicopathologic study of 3256 oral leukoplakias. Cancer 36:1386–1392, 1975.
15. Neville BW, Day TA: Oral cancer and precancerous lesions. CA Cancer J Clin 52:195–205, 2002.
16. Hansen L, Olson JA, Silverman S, Jr: Proliferative verrucous leukoplakia. A follow-up study of 54 cases. Oral Surg Oral Med Oral Pathol: 285–298, 1985.
17. Sciubba JJ: Oral cancer and its detection. History taking and the diagnostic phase of management. J Am Dent Assoc 132:12S–15S, 2001.
18. Kujan O, Gilenny AM, Duxbury AJ, et al: Cochrane Database Systematic Review 2003; 4:CD004150.
19. Patton LL: The effectiveness of community-based oral screening and utility of adjunctive diagnostic aids in the early detection of oral cancer. Oral Oncol 39:708–723, 2003.
20. Kerr AR: Life saving oral cancer screening. NY State Dent J 66(7):26–30, 2000.
21. Nagao T, Warnakulasuriya S: Annual screening for oral cancer detection. Cancer Detect Prev 27:333–337, 2003.
22. Glazer HS: Spotting trouble: without an oral cancer screening, no dental exam is complete. AGD Impact 31(8):18–19, 2003.
23. Schmidt BL, Dierks EJ, Homer L, Potter B: Tobacco smoking history and presentation of oral squamous cell carcinoma. J Oral Maxillofac Surg 62(9):1055–1058, 2004.
24. Horowitz AM, Alfano MC: Perform a death-defying act: the 90-second oral cancer examination. J Am Dent Assoc 132(Suppl):5S–6S, 36S–40S, 2001.
25. Macek MD, Reid BC, Yellowitz JA: Oral cancer examinations among adults at high risk: findings from the 1998 National Health Interview Survey. J Public Health Dent 63:119–125, 2003.
26. Chang JI, Ou CH, Wu KM: The evaluation of cervical cancer screening by combining speculoscopy with Papanicolaou smear examination in Taiwan. Chung Hua i Hsueh Tsa Chih—Chin Med J 65(9):430–434, 2002.
27. Ciatto S: The Italian experience of a Pap test and speculoscopy based screening programme. J Med Screen 8(1):54, 2001.
28. LoGiudice L, Abbiati R, Boselli F, et al: Improvement of Pap smear sensitivity using a visual adjunctive procedure: a co-operative Italian study on speculoscopy (GISPE). Eur J Cancer Prev 7(4):295–304, 1998.
29. Yu BK, Kuo BI, Yen MS, et al: Improved early detection of cervical intraepithelial lesions by combination of conventional Pap smear and speculoscopy. Eur J Gynaecol Oncol 24(6):495–499, 2003.
30. Kurman RJ, Henson DE, Herbst AL, et al: Interim guidelines for management of abnormal cervical cytology. The 1992 National Cancer Institute Workshop. JAMA 271(23):1866–1869, 1994.
31. Farah CS, McCullough MJ: A pilot case control study on the efficacy of acetic acid wash and chemiluminescence illumination (ViziLite™) in the visualization of oral mucosal white lesions. Oral Oncol 43(8):820–824, 2006.
32. Kerr AR, Epstein JB, Sirois DA: Clinical evaluation of chemiluminescent lighting, an adjunct for oral mucosal examination. J Clin Dent 17:59–63, 2006.
33. Epstein JB, Gorsky M, Lonky S, et al: The efficacy of oral Lumenoscopy™ (ViziLite(®)) in visualizing oral mucosal lesions. Spec Care Dent 26:171–174, 2006.
34. Lane PM, Gilhuly T, Whitehead P, et al: Simple device for the direct visualization of oral-cavity tissue fluorescence. J Biomed Optics 11:(2), 2006.
35. Poh CF, Ng SP, Williams PM, et al: Direct fluorescence visualization of clinically occult high-risk oral premalignant disease using a simple hand-held device. Head Neck 29(1):71–76, 2007.
36. Poh CF, Zhang L, Anderson DW, et al: Fluorescence visualization detection of field alterations in tumor margins of oral cancer patients. Clin Cancer Res 12:6716–6722, 2006.
37. De Veld DCG, Witjes MJH, Sterenborg HJCM, Roodenburg JLN: The status of in vivo autofluorescence spectroscopy and imaging for oral oncology. Oral Oncol 41:117–131, 2005.
38. Onizawa K, Saginoya H, Furuya Y, et al: Usefulness of fluorescence photography for diagnosis of oral cancer. Int J Oral Maxillofac Surg 28:206–210, 1999.

39. Rosenberg D, Cretin S: Use of meta-analysis to evaluate tolonium chloride in oral cancer screening. Oral Surg Oral Med Oral Pathol 67(5):621–627, 1989.

40. Warnakulasuriya KA, Johnson NW: Sensitivity and specificity of OraScan (R) toluidine blue mouth rinse in the detection of oral cancer and precancer. J Oral Pathol Med 25(3):97–103, 1996.

41. Epstein JB, Oakley C, Millner A, et al: The utility of toluidine blue application as a diagnostic aid in patients previously treated for upper oropharyngeal carcinoma. Oral Surg Oral Med Oral Pathol Oral Radiol Endod 83(5):537–547, 1997.

42. Mashberg A: Reevaluation of toluidine blue application as a diagnostic adjunct in the detection of asymptomatic oral squamous carcinoma: a continuing prospective study of oral cancer III. Cancer 46(4):758–763, 1980.

43. Mashberg A: Tolonium (toluidine blue) rinse—a screening method for recognition of squamous carcinoma. Continuing study of oral cancer IV. JAMA 245(23):2408–2410, 1981.

44. Pizer ME, Dubois DD: An assessment of toluidine blue for the diagnosis of lip lesions. Va Med 106(11):860–862, 1979.

45. Moyer GN, Taybos GM, Pelleu GB, Jr: Toluidine blue rinse: potential for benign lesions in early detection of oral neoplasms. J Oral Med 41(2):111–113, 1986.

46. Mashberg A, Samit AM: Early detection, diagnosis, and management of oral and oropharyngeal cancer. CA Cancer J Clin 9(2):67–88, 1989.

47. Epstein JB, Feldman R, Dolor RJ, Porter SR: The utility of tolonium chloride rinse in the diagnosis of recurrent or second primary cancers in patients with prior upper aerodigestive tract cancer. Head Neck 25(11):911–921, 2003.

40. Warnakulasuriya KA, Johnson NW: Sensitivity and specificity of OraScan toluidine blue mouthrinse in the detection of oral cancer and precancer. J Oral Pathol Med 25(3):97–103, 1996.

48. Onofre MA, Sposto MR, Navarro CM: Reliability of toluidine blue application in the detection of oral epithelial dysplasia and in situ and invasive squamous cell carcinomas. Oral Surg Oral Med Oral Pathol Oral Radiol Endod 91(5):535–540, 2001.

49. Epstein JB, Scully C, Spinelli J: Toluidine blue and Lugol's iodine application in the assessment of oral malignant disease and lesions at risk of malignancy. J Oral Pathol Med 21(4):160–163, 1992.

50. Portugal LG, Wilson KM, Biddinger PW, Gluckman JL: The role of toluidine blue in assessing margin status after resection of squamous cell carcinomas of the upper aerodigestive tract. Arch Otolaryngol Head Neck Surg 122(5):517–519, 1996.

51. Kerawala CJ, Beale V, Reed M, Martin IC: The role of vital tissue staining in the marginal control of oral squamous cell carcinoma. Int J Oral Maxillofac Surg 29(1):32–35, 2000.

52. Mashberg A: Final evaluation of tolonium chloride rinse for screening of high-risk patients with asymptomatic squamous carcinoma. J Am Dent Assoc 106(3):319–323, 1983.

53. Sugimura T, Terada M, Yokota J, et al: Multiple genetic alterations in human carcinogenesis. Environ Health Perspect 98:5–12, 1992.

54. Epstein JB, Zhang L, Poh C, et al: Increased allelic loss in toluidine blue-positive oral premalignant lesions. Oral Surg Oral Med Oral Pathol Oral Radiol Endod 95(1):45–50, 2003.

55. Guo Z, Yamaguchi K, Sanchez-Cespedes M, et al: Allelic losses in OraTest-directed biopsies of patients with prior upper aerodigestive tract malignancy. Clin Cancer Res 7(7):1963–1968, 2001.

56. Zhang L, Williams M, Poh CF, et al: Toluidine blue staining identifies high-risk primary oral premalignant lesions with poor outcome. Cancer Res 65(17):8017–8021, 2005.

57. Epstein JB, Silverman S, Jr, Epstein JD, et al: Analysis of oral lesion biopsies identified and evaluated by visual examination, chemiluminescence and toluidine blue. Submitted January 2007.

58. Sciubba JJ and the U.S. Collaborative Oral CDx Study Group: Improving detection of precancerous and cancerous oral lesions: computer assisted analysis of the oral brush biopsy. J Am Dent Assoc 130:1445–1457, 1999.

59. Svirsky JA, Burns JC, Carpenter WM, et al. Comparison of computer-assisted brush biopsy results with follow up scalpel biopsy and histology. Gen Dent 50(6):500–503, 2002.

60. Petkas ZO, Keskin A, Gunham O, Karsioglu Y: Evaluation of nuclear morphometry and DNA ploidy status for detection of malignant and premalignant cytomorphometric measurements. J Oral Maxillofac Surg 64:828–835, 2006.

61. Scheifele C, Schmidt-Westhausen AM, Dietrich T, Reichart PA: The sensitivity and specificity of the Oral CDx technique: evaluation of 103 cases. Oral Oncol 40(8):824–828, 2004.

62. Poate TW, Buchanan JA, Hodgson TA, et al: An audit of the efficacy of the oral brush biopsy technique in a specialist oral medicine unit. Oral Oncol 40:829–834, 2004.

63. Potter TJ, Summerlin DJ, Campbell JH: Oral malignancies associated with negative trans epithelial brush biopsy. J Oral Maxillofac Surg 23:1943–1949, 2003.

64. Ziober AF, Patel KR, Alawi F, et al: Identification of a gene signature for rapid screening for oral squamous cell carcinoma. Clin Cancer Res 12(20 Pt 1):5960–5971, 2006.

65. Wong DT: Salivary diagnostics powered by nanotechnologies, proteomics and genomics. J Am Dent Assoc 137:313–321, 2006.

66. Bahar G, Feinmesser R, Shpitzer T, et al: Salivary analysis in oral cancer patients: DNA and protein oxidation, reactive nitrogen species and antioxidant profile. Cancer 109:54–59, 2007.

67. Nagler R, Baher G, Shpitzer T, Feinmesser R: Concomitant analysis of salivary tumor markers—a new diagnostic tool for oral cancer. Clin Cancer Res 12:3979–3984, 2006.

68. Fischer DJ, Epstein JB, Morton TH, Schwartz SM: Interobserver reliability in the histopathologic diagnosis of oral premalignant and malignant lesions. J Oral Pathol Med 33(2):65–70, 2004.

69. Fischer DJ, Epstein JB, Morton TH J., Schwartz SM: Reliability of histologic diagnosis of clinically normal intraoral tissue adjacent to clinically suspicious lesions in former upper aerodigestive tract cancer patients. Oral Oncol 41(5):489–496, 2005.

70. Mehrotra R, Gupta A, Singh M, Ibrahim R: Application of cytology and molecular biology in diagnosing premalignant or malignant oral lesions. Mol Cancer 23:5–11, 2006.

71. Acha A, Ruesga MT, Rodriguez MJ, et al: Applications of the oral scraped (exfoliative) cytology in oral cancer and precancer. Med Oral Patol Oral Cir Bucal 10:95–102, 2005.

5

Early Radiographic Detection of Head and Neck Cancer: Positron Emission Tomography

Heather A. Jacene

KEY POINTS

- 2-Fluoro-[18F]-deoxy-2-D-glucose positron emission tomography/computed tomography (FDG-PET/CT) is more useful than anatomic imaging for the evaluation of patients with head and neck cancer.
- FDG-PET/CT is currently indicated for the diagnosis, staging, and re-staging of head and neck cancer.
- For the detection of locoregional lymph node metastases from head and neck cancer, the sensitivity of FDG-PET/CT ranges from 67% to 91% with specificities from 80% to 100%.
- In up to 25% of people undergoing FDG-PET/CT, distant metastases or a second primary tumor may be detected.
- FDG-PET/CT should be performed at least 10 days after the completion of chemotherapy to avoid false-negative studies.
- FDG-PET/CT appears to be more accurate for the detection of recurrent head and neck cancer when obtained at least 8 weeks after the completion of radiation therapy. The optimum time to obtain a post-treatment FDG-PET/CT should be individualized to carefully consider possible imaging outcomes and the clinical scenario.
- Communication between the interpreting imaging physician and the referring physician is crucial for the most accurate interpretation of FDG-PET/CT scans.

Introduction

The early detection of cancer by imaging has relied on the detection of structural abnormalities by anatomic imaging for many years. Detection of cancer based on anatomy has several limitations. Structural abnormalities are often not detected until cancers have reached a size of 10 to 100 g, or until 10^{10} to 10^{11} cells are present[1] and anatomic imaging does not provide information about "what is in a mass." Detection of tumor depends on the difference in its radiographic appearance compared with the normal surrounding structures. In the postoperative patient, normal anatomy is often altered, thus decreasing the reliability of structural changes.

Metabolic tumor imaging with 2-fluoro-[18F]-deoxy-2-D-glucose positron emission tomography (FDG-PET) has ameliorated these difficulties and is rapidly becoming the standard imaging modality for a variety of tumor types. An obvious advantage of FDG-PET is its ability to detect tumor cells more independently from structural alterations.

There is now abundant literature on the use of FDG-PET for patients with head and neck cancer. Most of the early literature evaluated PET alone and included small, heterogeneous patient populations. Despite this, the technique proved to be more useful than anatomic imaging and is currently indicated for the diagnosis, staging, and re-staging of head and neck cancer. As with other malignancies, combined PET/CT has emerged as a powerful tool for the early diagnosis of cancer.

This chapter focuses on the role of FDG-PET and PET/CT imaging for the early detection of squamous cell carcinoma of the head and neck, including comparisons with anatomic imaging modalities. "Early detection" by imaging and how this affects patient management can be considered in several situations: (1) initial staging of locoregional lymph nodes, (2) staging for distant disease, (3) detection of synchronous primary tumors, and (4) early detection of residual or recurrent disease.

FDG-PET Imaging

Basic Principles

FDG-PET imaging is based on the principle that living cancer cells have increased rates of glucose utilization compared with normal cells, a phenomenon described by Warburg[2] in the 1950s. FDG is a glucose analog and, similarly, it is transported into cells through glucose transporters and phosphorylated by the enzyme hexokinase II. Once phosphorylated, FDG-6-phosphate is not metabolized further in the glycolytic pathway and is unable to diffuse across cell membranes. FDG-6-phosphate is essentially "trapped" within the cell. Cancer cells express higher levels of glucose transporters, primarily glucose transporter 1, and hexokinase II, and therefore accumulate more FDG (and glucose) compared with normal cells[3,4] (Fig. 5-1).

FDG is radiolabeled with the positron emitter ^{18}F, which allows visualization of the FDG once it is localized within a tumor (Fig. 5-2). After a positron (β^+ = posi-

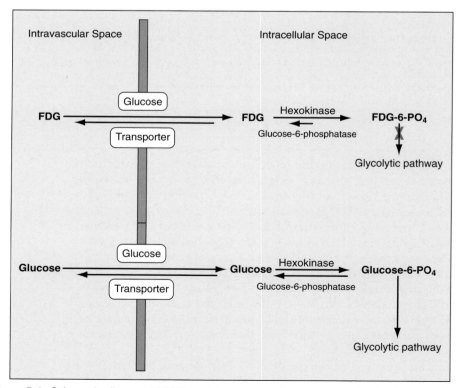

Figure 5-1. Schematic diagram of FDG and glucose entry into a cell. Similar to glucose, FDG is transported intracellularly via glucose transporters and phosphorylated by the enzyme hexokinase. FDG-6-phosphate is unable to cross cell membranes and is not metabolized further in the glycolytic pathway. In tumor cells, the level of the enzyme that de-phosphorylates FDG-6-phosphate is negligible and the molecule is essentially trapped within the cell.

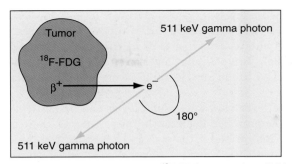

Figure 5-2. Schematic diagram of the detection of ^{18}F-FDG. A positron (β^+) is emitted from the site of ^{18}F-FDG accumulation within a tumor and travels a short distance. The positron annihilates with an electron (e$^-$) and the energy is converted into two 511 keV gamma photons approximately 180 degrees apart from each other. If the PET (positron emission tomography) camera detects the two opposing photons within a certain time frame, an event is recorded and is assumed to have occurred along the line connecting the positions where the photons were detected. Detection of multiple events forms the basis of image generation.

tively charged particle) is emitted, it travels a short distance (millimeters) before colliding with an electron (e$^-$ = negatively charged particle). The mass of the positron and electron is converted into energy in the form of two 511 keV gamma photons, approximately 180 degrees apart from each other. If the PET camera detects the two opposing photons within a certain time frame, an event is recorded and is assumed to have occurred along the line connecting where the photons were detected. Detection of multiple events forms the basis of image generation.

FDG-PET imaging is limited by lack of anatomic detail. The recent introduction of hybrid PET/CT scanners overcomes this limitation. Many clinical oncology studies have demonstrated advantages of hybrid PET/CT versus PET alone and software-fused PET and CT images acquired during separate imaging sessions. The hybrid scanners consist of a CT scanner directly in front of a PET scanner. Images are acquired sequentially without changing patient position. The CT scan is used for attenuation correction and anatomic correlation. At present, most new sales are PET/CT scanners, and at the time this manuscript was prepared, only one of the three major PET manufacturers was still offering stand-alone PET scanners.

FDG-PET and PET/CT Technique

Precise FDG-PET techniques and image acquisition protocols may vary slightly among institutions; however, certain aspects are generally followed to ensure the highest-quality studies and comparability between serial scans and scans obtained at different institutions. Consensus recommendations for FDG-PET image acquisition were recently published to better standardize the FDG-PET imaging technique for clinical trials,[5] but the recommendations can largely be applied in the clinical setting as well. Several aspects of the imaging technique are highlighted here because they are important both for imaging and for referring physicians to understand, especially in the setting of early detection of cancer.

Patient preparation is critical to ensure that images are of high quality. Preimaging instructions are usually provided by the imaging center, including a directive that patients should abstain from strenuous work or exercise for 24 hours before the study to decrease skeletal muscle uptake of FDG.

Patients should fast for at least 4 hours before arriving for their appointment, and serum glucose levels should be checked before FDG is administered. Glucose competes with FDG for uptake into cells, and tumor metabolism may be underestimated in the presence of high serum glucose levels.[6] The exact cutoff level below which serum glucose level must lie varies from institution to institution, but the recommended level for nondiabetic patients is less than 120 mg/dL and for diabetics between 150 and 200 mg/dL.[5] High serum insulin levels can also negatively alter FDG biodistribution by shunting FDG to the muscle, thus leaving less FDG available for tumor uptake.[7]

The need for controlled glucose levels and low insulin levels can be particularly challenging in some patients with uncontrolled diabetes. In these patients, there may be a need for careful review of the indication for the scan and adjustment of insulin/diabetic regimens in consultation with the referring physician. At our institution, patients refrain from taking regular insulin for at least 4 hours before the FDG injection and for 10 hours before longer-acting insulins. The consensus recommendations do not advise administration of insulin to adjust glucose levels at the time of the procedure; however, one study has evaluated the use of ultra short–acting insulin for this purpose and concluded that the images were not adversely affected with waiting times of at least 1 hour for FDG injection after insulin administration.[8] This option may be used in special situations, such as when a patient has traveled a long distance to obtain the scan.

After the intravenous injection of FDG, there is an uptake phase time during which patients are asked to sit quietly in a dimly lit room. Talking and reading should be discouraged because muscle uptake in the head and neck can result. The temperature of the room should not be too cold because this may stimulate brown fat uptake of FDG.[9] Uptake in muscle and brown fat can confound image interpretation. Standard imaging fields for head and neck cancer should include the entire head and neck region, most often extending from the vertex of the skull caudally.

When PET/CT is performed, the CT scan is used for both attenuation correction and lesion localization. Administration of intravenous contrast depends on the individual center. The addition of intravenous contrast improves the ability to differentiate blood vessels and lymph nodes and to examine the enhancement patterns of abnormal densities. When an intravenous contrast CT scan is used for attenuation correction, quantification of FDG uptake can be overestimated. This overestimation is most significant when the intravenous contrast CT scan is obtained in the arterial phase, but it is small when delayed-phase intravenous contrast CT scans are used.[10] If precise quantitation is necessary, CT attenuation correction should be performed with non-contrast scans. Clinically, the differences in quantitation are small, but scans should be performed the same way in the test-retest setting.

Normal FDG Biodistribution and Physiologic Variants in the Head and Neck

Figure 5-3 demonstrates the normal biodistribution of FDG. In the pre- and postoperative head and neck, a wide range of normal variation of FDG uptake exists (Fig. 5-4). The advent of combined PET/CT imaging has led to the description of these normal variations and physiologic patterns of FDG uptake.[11] Several notable benign physiologic patterns of FDG uptake are particular to the head and neck region, brown adipose tissue (brown fat), skeletal muscle, and vocal cord uptake.

FDG uptake in brown fat in adult humans was first described in 2003 by Cohade and colleagues.[9] In hibernating mammals and newborns, brown fat functions as a thermogenic organ for maintenance of body temperature.[12] The hallmark of brown fat FDG uptake is the finding of foci of intense FDG activity that fuses to fat density on the CT scan without an associated CT abnormality[9] (Fig. 5-5). Without comparison with CT, the activity can be misinterpreted as lymph node metastases, although presently the pattern of uptake should be well recognized. Brown fat uptake has been

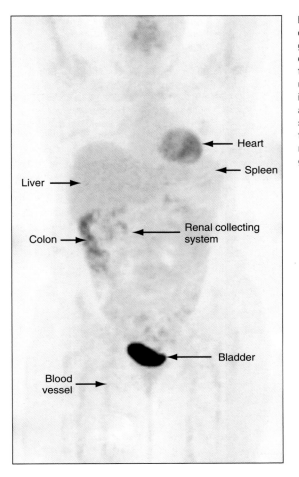

Figure 5-3. Normal biodistribution of FDG. High levels of FDG uptake are usually seen in the cerebral cortex, basal ganglia, and thalami (not shown). Unlike glucose, FDG is excreted in the urine accounting for the high uptake seen in the renal collecting systems and urinary bladder. FDG uptake in the heart is variable, and skeletal muscle uptake is usually low in the resting state. Working muscle accumulates FDG in correlation with work level. The liver, spleen, and blood pool have low-level FDG uptake, whereas the bone marrow, lung, and white adipose tissue have negligible uptake. FDG uptake in the rest of the gastrointestinal tract is variable.

reported to be associated with colder outdoor temperatures and tends to be visualized more often in thinner patients.[9]

Skeletal muscle uptake of FDG varies according to the activity level of the muscle. Muscle activity is usually linear and symmetric, but it can be focal and asymmetric (see Fig. 5-4F, *crosshairs*). Neck dissection and reconstruction are often causes of asymmetric and focal uptake that can be confused with malignancy. In these cases, the visualized muscle uptake is usually compensatory because of an increase in workload. It is imperative that the reader have a good understanding of the type of neck dissection or reconstruction performed, and excellent communication between the reader and the surgeon is often necessary for accurate image interpretation. FDG uptake in various muscles in the head and neck has been described, including the longus coli, pterygoid, masseter, sternocleidomastoid, scalene, cricoarytenoid, and temporalis muscles.[13-17] Unilateral spinal accessory nerve injury after head and neck surgery can lead to asymmetrically increased FDG activity in the trapezius muscle on the ipsilateral side. This resolves as the nerve recovers.[18]

Finally, the vocal cords normally have low levels of FDG activity (see Fig. 5-4E). However, a good example of asymmetric but physiologic uptake occurs when one of the vocal cords becomes paralyzed. The normal cord has increased FDG activity whereas the paralyzed cord does not (Fig. 5-6). The uptake in the normal cord is physiologic and compensatory and should not be confused with malignancy. The abnormal vocal cord may appear medially displaced on the corresponding CT scan, or the patient may have clinical evidence of vocal cord paralysis (i.e., hoarseness).

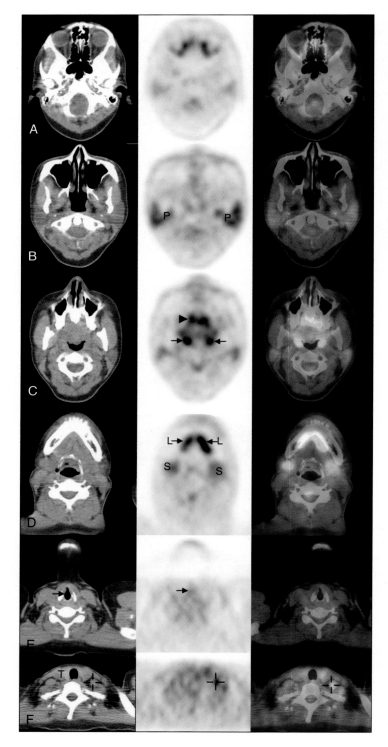

Figure 5-4. Description of normal FDG uptake in the head and neck region. **A,** The extraocular muscles have intense FDG uptake usually in a linear pattern. **B–D,** The palatine tonsils (*arrows*) and soft palate (*arrowhead*) are visualized in most patients and have intense FDG activity. The parotid glands (P), submandibular glands (S), and sublingual glands (L) are seen in about 50% to 75% of patients and have moderate uptake (greater than the blood pool). The tongue has minimal FDG uptake (not shown). The level of FDG uptake in the tonsils and sublingual glands decreases with increasing age. **E–F,** Normal vocal cords (*arrows*) and thyroid gland (T) have minimal- to low-level uptake. (Left panels, CT; center panels, PET; right panels, fused images.)

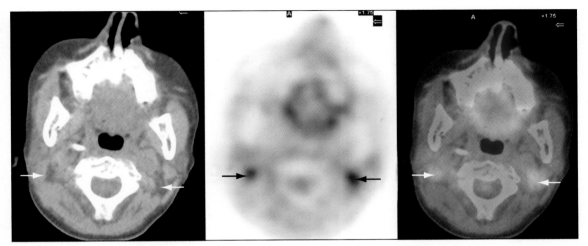

Figure 5-5. Physiologic FDG uptake in brown adipose tissue (brown fat).   There are foci of intense FDG activity in the posterior neck bilaterally (*arrows*) that fuse to fat on the CT scan. Hypermetabolism in brown fat is most commonly seen in the head, neck, and supraclavicular areas, but can also be seen in the paraspinal and intra-abdominal regions. (Left panel, CT; center panel, PET; right panel, fused image.)

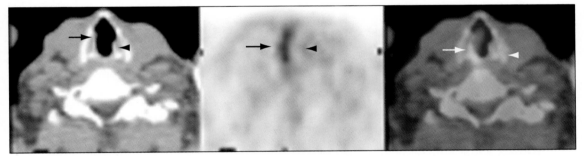

Figure 5-6. Asymmetric FDG activity in the vocal cords.   There is FDG activity fusing to the right vocal cord which is physiologic (*arrows*). The left vocal cord is paralyzed, showing medial lateralization (*arrowheads*), with decreased FDG activity. In this case, the left, not the right, vocal cord is abnormal. (Left panel, CT; center panel, PET; right panel. fused image.)

Initial Staging of Head and Neck Cancer

Lymph Node Staging

Accurate staging of cervical lymph nodes at diagnosis is of the utmost importance for patients with head and neck cancer. Lymph node status is a well-known independent prognostic indicator of survival, and initial management decisions are based on the presence of metastatic cervical lymph nodes in addition to primary tumor extent. Clinical head and neck examination has been shown to be inaccurate for assessing lymph node status in up to 45% of patients, and computed tomography (CT), magnetic resonance imaging (MRI), and ultrasonography also have limitations.

Similar to primary head and neck tumors, lymph node metastases from head and neck cancers accumulate FDG[19-24] (Fig. 5-7). The level of FDG activity within the lymph nodes can be variable, and standardized uptake values—a quantitative measure of FDG uptake—have been reported from the 2 to 7 range. FDG activity level can vary between the primary tumor and the nodal metastases and between nodal metastases in a single patient.[25]

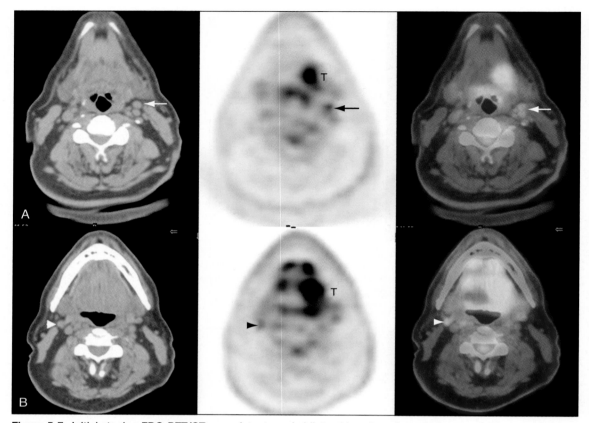

Figure 5-7. Initial staging FDG-PET/CT scan detects early bilateral lymph node metastases. A 63-year-old man with newly diagnosed squamous cell carcinoma of the tongue presented for initial staging FDG-PET/CT scan. MRI of the neck revealed left-sided cervical lymph nodes, which were suspicious for metastatic disease. **A,** There was intense FDG activity fusing to the left tongue primary cancer (T) and a borderline-sized left cervical lymph node (*arrows*). **B,** Abnormal FDG activity was also visualized in a normal-sized right level II lymph node (*arrowheads*), which was suspicious for metastatic disease. As a result, the patient underwent bilateral, rather than unilateral, neck dissections. Malignancy was found in bilateral neck lymph nodes at surgery. (Left panels, CT; center panels, PET; right panels, fused images.)

Table 5-1 presents a summary of the performance of FDG-PET and PET/CT for the nodal staging of head and neck cancer.[19–24,26–32] Most of the studies evaluated patients with untreated squamous cell carcinoma with a variety of primary tumor sites. For the detection of lymph node metastases, the sensitivity of FDG-PET ranged from 67% to 91%, and specificities ranged from 80% to 100%. Most studies compared FDG-PET with at least one standard anatomic imaging modality. Considered together, the sensitivity of MRI, CT, and ultrasound ranged from 36% to 82%, 58% to 90%, and 72% to 84%, respectively. The specificity of the anatomic imaging modalities ranged from 25% to 98%. Although there is a wide range of overlap in the sensitivities and specificities of the various imaging modalities, individual studies mostly demonstrated that FDG-PET was at least equivalent or superior to standard anatomic imaging in the detection of lymph node metastases in patients with head and neck cancer (Fig. 5-8).

There are fewer articles specifically discussing the use of combined FDG-PET/CT for lymph node staging in patients with an unoperated neck. Schwartz and colleagues[32] reported a sensitivity of 96% for lymph node staging with combined PET/CT versus 78% for contrast-enhanced CT. The specificities of the two modalities were equal (98.5%), but PET/CT was more likely to agree with pathology results in

Table 5-1. Performance of FDG-PET and PET/CT for the Nodal Staging of Head and Neck Cancer

Author (Year)	N	Primary Tumor and Indication*	Sensitivity (%)				Specificity (%)			
			PET	MRI	CT	US	PET	MRI	CT	US
PET alone										
Bailet[19] (1992)	16		71	58			98	98		
Laubenbacher[27] (1995)	22		90	78			95	71		
McGuirt[21] (1995)	38	25 previously untreated	81†	81†						
McGuirt[22] (1995)	49	Mucosal	83		90		82		79	
Braams[29] (1995)	12	Oral cavity	91	36			88	94		
Wong[24] (1997)	54	31 previously untreated	67	67			100	25		
Adams[28] (1998)	60		90	82	80	72	94	85	79	70
Stuckenson[36] (2000)	106	Oral cavity	70	64	66	84	82	69	74	68
DiMartino[20] (2000)	50	35 previously untreated	84		84	84	90		96	88
Hannah[26] (2002)	40		82		81		100		81	
PET/CT										
Gordin[30] (2007)	91	21 previously untreated	100				100			
Jeong[31] (2007)	47		80.3	91.8	90.2		92.8	98.9	93.9	
Schwartz[32] (2005)	20			96	98.5			98.5	98.5	

*Multiple primary head and neck squamous cell carcinoma sites and previously untreated disease unless specifically stated.
†Accuracy.
ECT, contrast-enhanced CT scan; MRI, magnetic resonance imaging; PET, positron emission tomography; US, ultrasonography.

this study than the contrast-enhanced CT. Jeong and associates[31] also found that PET/CT was more accurate than clinical exam, contrast-enhanced CT, and PET alone for initial lymph node staging.

More accurate staging with FDG-PET and PET/CT can impact patient care. Treatment modalities have been reported to be altered in 18% to 50% of patients.[18,29,30,33–35] The ultimate effect on outcome, however, remains in question.

FDG-PET and PET/CT do have several limitations in the evaluation of lymph node metastases. False-negative studies are primarily due to small foci of disease within lymph nodes. In one study, all lymph nodes larger than 12 mm were detected, but only 50% of those that were less than 6 mm were visualized on FDG-PET.[36] Inflammatory and reactive lymph nodes are the major source of false-positives. The level of FDG uptake in metastatic and reactive lymph nodes has been shown to have substantial overlap.[29] In addition, FDG-PET alone does not have high enough resolution to detect early bone and cartilage invasion by tumor.[37]

It is uncertain whether FDG-PET/CT will remain in the forefront as newer molecular and anatomic imaging techniques, including new radiotracers and contrast agents, are developed. Dammann and associates[38] recently reported a higher sensitivity for the detection of lymph node metastases with MRI versus FDG-PET, with equal specificities. MRI also provided more optimal anatomic localization.

Synchronous and Incidental Primary Tumors and Distant Metastases

FDG-PET for the early detection of distant metastases and second primary tumors is particularly useful in patients with head and neck cancers. Patients with head and neck cancer have an increased risk—4% per year—for synchronous or metachronous primary tumors.[39,40] The most common sites of synchronous primary tumors are

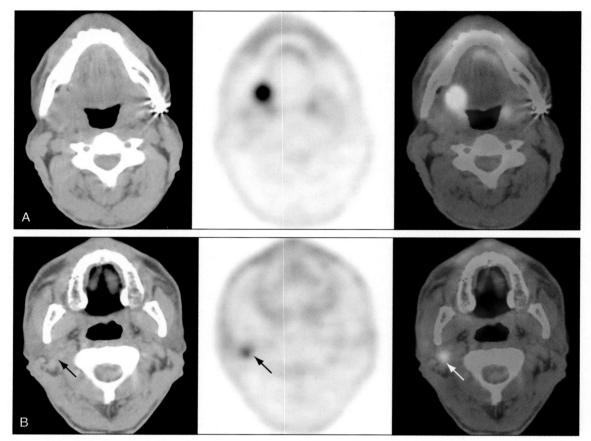

Figure 5-8. Early detection of lymph node metastases.   A 55-year-old man with a new diagnosis of invasive, moderately differentiated squamous cell carcinoma of the right tonsil presented for a staging FDG-PET/CT scan. **A,** The primary tumor in the right tonsillar/base of the tongue region had intense FDG activity. **B,** A normal-sized (9 mm) right level II cervical lymph node also had increased FDG uptake (*arrows*), suspicious for a lymph node (arrowheads) metastasis. At surgery, this node was found to contain metastatic disease. (Left panels, CT; center panels, PET; right panels, fused images.)

tobacco- and alcohol-exposed regions, such as lung, esophagus, and other parts of the upper aerodigestive tract. In addition, both advancing stage and diagnosis of a synchronous tumor are negative prognostic factors. Five-year survival rates decline from 48% to between 8% and 23% after diagnosis of a synchronous tumor.

The standard modalities available today for second primary cancer screening are primarily invasive and involve direct inspection of the most common areas at risk for a second primary tumor. Chest radiography is performed as part of the staging procedures. However, in the current era of imaging, CT scanning is the most sensitive technique for evaluating the lung fields.

Drawing definite conclusions from the literature regarding the usefulness of FDG-PET for the detection of metastases outside the head and neck and synchronous primaries is challenging. Moreover, it demonstrates our growing experience with PET over the past one and a half decades. In the small number of studies specifically addressing this topic,[36,41–47] the patient populations were heterogeneous in regard to primary tumor location and stage, and only a small percentage of patients were identified with distant metastases or second primary tumors. The studies often considered distant metastases, synchronous tumors, and incidental primary tumors as one group of FDG-avid lesions outside the head and neck. Despite these limitations, most authors advocate the whole-body PET or PET/CT technique for initial staging of

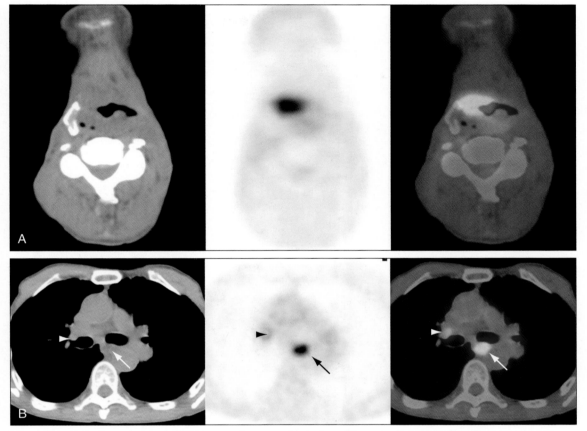

Figure 5-9. Detection of recurrent disease and a second primary malignancy by FDG-PET/CT. A 65-year-old man with a history of squamous cell carcinoma of the base of the tongue post-resection and radiation presented with a new tongue mass. **A,** FDG-PET/CT scan revealed an intense focus of FDG activity in the right tongue base with associated soft tissue asymmetry. Pathology revealed recurrent squamous cell carcinoma. **B,** Whole-body PET/CT images revealed a previously undetected second primary squamous cell carcinoma in the esophagus (*arrows*). An inflammatory hilar lymph node was also visualized (*arrowheads*). (Left panels, CT; center panels, PET; right panels, fused images.)

head and neck cancer rather than limiting the field of view (Fig. 5-9), which is consistent with current clinical practice.

Table 5-2 summarizes the key findings of the studies evaluating FDG-PET for the detection of distant disease at initial diagnosis. The study of Keyes and colleagues[41] produced negative results, and the authors concluded that the high false-positive rate did not warrant imaging the thorax in patients with head and neck cancer. In this article, the six false-positive exam results were due to artifacts or inflammation. Furthermore, to support their conclusions, the authors argued that in two of the three true-positive cases, the metastases were also detected by standard imaging modalities. The high false-positive rate in this early study might have been related to a lower threshold for calling a focus of activity suspicious for malignancy on PET alone.

Subsequent studies have reported a 7% to 25% rate of detection of either distant metastases from head and neck cancer or a second primary malignancy.[36,41–47] The most common locations of metastases reported are the lungs and the mediastinal lymph nodes. Second primary tumors have consistently been reported in the lung (Fig. 5-10). Stokkel and associates[46] found a second upper aerodigestive tract tumor in eight of nine patients with a simultaneous detected primary tumor by PET. This represented 15% of the total patient population (N = 54). Other locations reported

Table 5-2. Key Findings of the Studies Evaluating FDG-PET for the Detection of Distant Disease at Initial Diagnosis

Author (Year)	N	Pre-PET Stage III/IV	No. with Distant Metastases (DM) or Synchronous/ Second Primary (SP)	Comments
Keyes[41] (2000)*	56	8	3 DM	6 false-positive—artifact or inflammation 1 false-negative
Stokkel[46] (2000)*	54	Not given	9 SP (3 lung, 2 tongue, 1 tonsil, 1 pharynx, 1 thyroid, 1 pyriform sinus)	
Stuckenson[36] (2000)	106	Not given	10 DM or SP	
Teknos[47] (2001)	12	12	3 DM	2 patients whose metastases were undetected on other imaging
Kitagawa[42] (2002)†	26	Not given	1 DM; 2 colon cancer metastases	10 patients with inflammatory nodes
Sigg[45] (2003)	56	Not given		6.9%—important information for staging trunk 5.2%—changed plan 1—ulcerative colitis
Goerres[62] (2003)‡	34	27	3 DM (lung, mediastinal); 4 SP (2 broncogenic carcinoma, 1 prostate, 1 colon)	1 false-positive—degenerative changes Management was changed in 15% of patients due to PET or PET/CT
Koshy[43] (2005)	36	33	3 DM	All 3—curative to palliative intent
Nishiyama[44] (2005)	53	Not given	2 DM (lung, liver); 5 SP (2 gastric, 1 rectal, 1 pancreas, 1 thyroid)	3 false-positives (2 pneumonias; 1 chronic thyroiditis) 1 false-negative for prostate cancer 2 second primaries only detected by PET

All studies done for staging prior to initial therapy, except Sigg, which evaluated 76 scans in 56 patients—54 scans to detect recurrence.
Included cases of non–squamous cell carcinoma in the head and neck.
†*Oral cavity or oropharyngeal tumors only.*
‡*Oral cavity tumors only.*

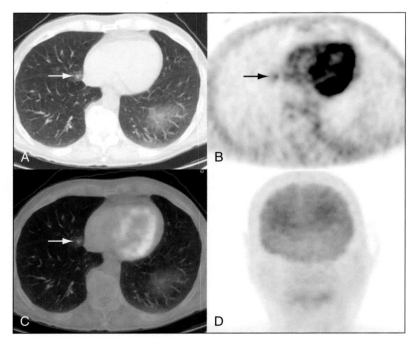

Figure 5-10. Detection of a synchronous primary malignancy by FDG-PET/CT. A 73-year-old man with a history of a T2N0 squamous cell carcinoma of the supraglottic larynx post-supraglottic laryngectomy presented for an FDG-PET/CT scan with new-onset weight loss. A new 1-cm noncalcified lung nodule with moderate FDG activity was identified (*arrows*, **A–C**). The differential diagnosis included an inflammatory nodule or malignancy. Given that it was a new finding from previous examinations, the nodule was resected and histology revealed a small, primary lung squamous cell carcinoma. No evidence of recurrent disease was identified in the head and neck region (**D**).

for incidental tumors include stomach, rectum, pancreas, and thyroid gland and metastases from colorectal and prostate cancer.

In a pilot study, Teknos and colleagues[47] found that PET was able to detect occult lung and mediastinal metastases that went undetected by CT scanning in a small number of patients (n = 2 of 3). Stuckenson and colleagues[36] reported that 10% of their patients had distant metastases or second primary tumors that were detected only by PET. Other studies in Table 5-2 required M0 status for entry into the study.

Note that truly early detection of synchronous lung or esophageal primaries with FDG-PET may be reduced owing to the inherent limitations of the technique. Small lung nodules and thin mucosal esophageal lesions may be below the resolution for detection by PET. In addition, the head and neck and gastroesophageal junction can have substantial physiologic FDG activity with considerable patient–to-patient variability, making it difficult to detect lesions with a high degree of specificity.

Detection of Recurrent Disease

Performance of FDG-PET for Detection of Recurrent Disease

Late detection of recurrence portends a poor clinical outcome after salvage surgery. Table 5-3 summarizes the literature on the use of FDG-PET for the early detection of recurrent head and neck cancer. Overall, sensitivities are good (92% to 100%), particularly when patients present with clinical symptoms and/or clinical or radiographic signs of recurrence.[37,48–51]

Higher sensitivities and accuracies for the detection of recurrent head and neck cancer have been reported with FDG-PET compared with CT/MRI and physical

Table 5-3. FDG-PET for the Detection of Recurrent Head and Neck Cancer

Author (Year)	N	Primary Site*	Suspicion of Recurrence	Therapy	Time Between End of Therapy and PET		Sensitivity (%)	Specificity (%)
					Mean	Range		
Lapela[48] (1995)	15		Clinical	RT Surgery (n = 11)	10 mo (median)	2–56 mo	93	43
Lowe[37] (1999)†	5/12	Laryngeal	No	RT	21 mo	5 mo–5 yr	100	Not done
Lonneux[49] (2000)	44		Clinical	Surgery; RT; chemotherapy; combination	60 wk	6–728 wk	96	61
Terhaard[50] (2001)	75	Larynx Hypopharyngeal	Clinical	RT	16.5 mo	4–67 mo	92	63
Wong[51] (2002)	143		Clinical or radiographic (70%)	Variety	6.9 mo		96	72
Yao[53] (2000)	53		Clinical or radiographic	Chemo-RT	15 wk (median)	5–29 wk	100	94
Porceddu[52] (2005)	39		Clinical or radiographic	Chemo-RT	12 wk (median)	8–32 wk	83	94
Rogers[57] (2004)	12		No	RT	1 mo	Not given	45	100
Gourin[54] (2006)	17	Oropharynx Larynx	No	Chemo-RT	Not given	8–10 wk	40	25
Andrade[55] (2006)	28		No	Chemo-RT	8 wk	4–15.7 wk	76.9	93.3
Nayak[56] (2007)	43		Not given	Chemo-RT	Not given	2–6 mo	88	91

*Multiple primary head and neck squamous cell carcinoma sites unless specifically stated.
†Five of 12 patients evaluated for recurrent disease
Chemo-RT, chemoradiation therapy; RT, radiation therapy.

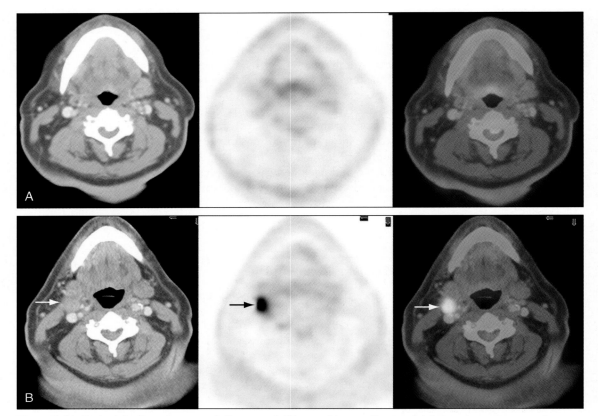

Figure 5-11. Early detection of recurrent disease.   A 65-year-old man with superficially invasive squamous cell carcinoma of the right lateral tongue underwent resection 4 years before presentation. **A,** The first re-staging FDG-PET/CT was negative for disease recurrence. **B,** Re-staging PET/CT with intravenous contrast scan 9 months later revealed a right level II cervical lymph node with intense FDG activity (*arrows*). The patient underwent level I–IV right neck dissection, and pathology revealed a single right level II node with metastatic squamous cell carcinoma. (Left panels, CT; center panels, PET; right panels, fused images.)

examination (Figs. 5-11 and 5-12).[49,51] Lonneux and associates[49] found higher sensitivities and accuracies for FDG-PET versus CT/MRI: 96% versus 73%, and 81% versus 64%, respectively. The five patients with recurrent laryngeal cancer in the study by Lowe and colleagues[37] did not have early disease recurrence detected by CT. Furthermore, Wong and associates[51] reported that 20% of the recurrences detected in their patients were unsuspected by physical exam, clinical symptoms, or conventional radiology.

The specificity of FDG-PET for detection of recurrent head and neck cancer is not high (43% to 72%), performing similarly to CT/MRI.[49] False-positive studies are mostly due to inflammation (Fig. 5-13), infection, and radiation injury/necrosis.[24,48,50,52,53] Severe dysplasia, histiocytic response, and foreign body giant cell reaction have also been reported as causes for false-positive PET studies[50,54] (Fig. 5-14). Specificity seems to be site-specific and is dependent on the timing of the FDG-PET after the completion of therapy that includes radiation. Specificity is higher (95% to 96%) for the detection of regional and distant metastases compared with local recurrence (79%)[51] and when performed more than 12 weeks after completion of therapy.[49]

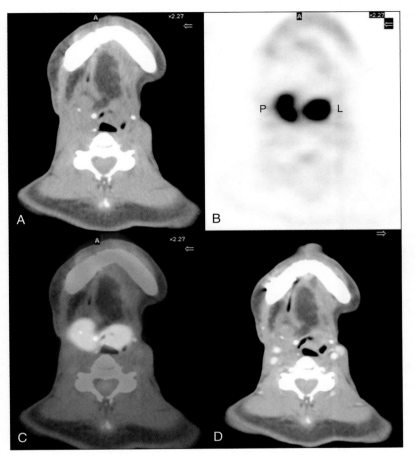

Figure 5-12. Recurrent head and neck cancer. A 54-year-old man with a history of recurrent right base of tongue squamous cell carcinoma after chemoradiation, bilateral neck dissection, and repeat salvage surgeries presented for a re-staging FDG-PET/CT scan. FDG-PET/CT scan with and without IV contrast demonstrated extensive metabolic activity in the right pharyngeal mass (P) and at the base of the left-sided reconstruction (L). The area of recurrent tumor on the right was not as extensive as the postoperative changes on the concurrent CT scan. (**A**, noncontrast CT; **B**, FDG-PET; **C**, fused image; **D**, IV contrast CT.)

The overall sensitivity and specificity of combined FDG-PET/CT for the detection of residual disease after definite chemoradiation have been reported to be 76.9% and 93.3%, respectively.[55] FDG-PET/CT was more accurate than contrast-enhanced CT (86% versus 68%). Contrast-enhanced CT had a higher false-positive rate than PET for detecting residual disease at the primary tumor site.

There is opposing literature regarding the use of quantitative analyses with standard uptake value for differentiation of recurrent disease versus benign processes. It is not surprising that substantial overlap of the standard uptake value has been demonstrated between benign and malignant lesions.[48] However, the standard uptake value may be helpful in patients scanned later than 12 weeks after the completion of therapy.[49] Of course, the standard uptake value should not be used in isolation to make this determination.

In the setting of suspected recurrent head and neck cancer, the results of FDG-PET scanning can affect and guide patient management. Lonneux and colleagues[49] proposed a conservative approach, with delay of biopsy, for patients with suspected recurrence and a negative PET scan (Fig. 5-15). A positive scan would be followed either by a repeat scan or biopsy, depending on the timing of the imaging study, before or after 12 weeks from the completion of therapy. By this approach, 21 of

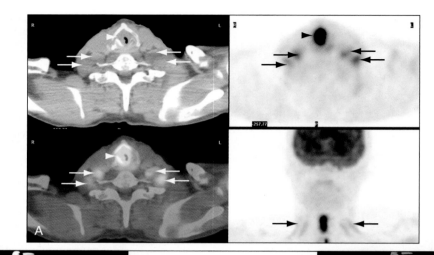

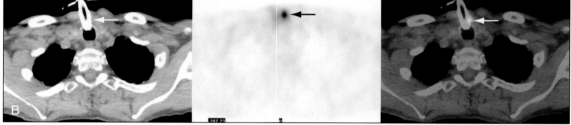

Figure 5-13. FDG uptake in muscles and postsurgical inflammation.   A 60-year-old man with laryngeal squamous cell carcinoma presented for a staging PET/CT scan. **A,** Intense FDG activity is visualized in the primary right laryngeal carcinoma (*arrowhead*). Symmetric activity is also visualized in the bilateral scalene muscles (*arrows*). The linear nature of the scalene muscle FDG uptake is well appreciated on the maximum intensity projection image (top left, CT; top right, FDG-PET; bottom left, fused images; bottom right, maximal intensity projection image.). **B,** Intense FDG activity is also visualized fusing to the left of the tracheostomy tube (*arrows*). This is not an additional focus of disease, but rather inflammation at the surgical site. (Left panel, CT; center panel, PET; right panel, fused image.)

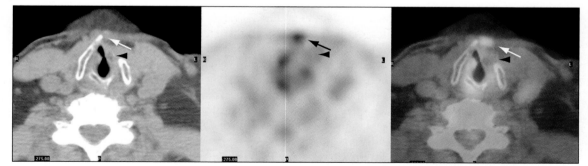

Figure 5-14. False-positive FDG PET/CT scan for recurrent malignancy.   A 70-year-old man with a history of squamous cell carcinoma of the left true vocal cord after left hemilaryngectomy and neck dissection presented for a re-staging FDG-PET/CT scan. FDG-PET/CT images revealed a 6.5-mm soft tissue nodule adjacent to the anterior edge of right thyroid cartilage (*arrows*). Postoperative changes are also seen (*arrowheads*). The nodule was resected, and pathology revealed fibrovascular tissue with extensive foreign body giant cell reaction and no tumor. (Left panel, CT; center panel, PET; right panel, fused image.)

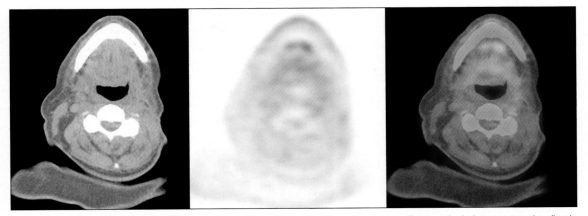

Figure 5-15. Negative FDG-PET/CT scan for recurrent head and neck cancer.   Postsurgical changes are visualized in the left neck; however, no abnormal focal areas of increased FDG activity are visualized in this patient with a history of oropharyngeal squamous cell carcinoma to suggest recurrent malignancy. (Left panel, CT; center panel, PET; right panel, fused image.)

38 patients in their series would have avoided an invasive procedure on the basis of a negative PET scan.[49]

The preceding study results were supported by Terhaard and colleagues,[50] who performed serial PET scans on their patients and correlated the results with the outcomes. All patients with a negative scan after treatment had negative laryngoscopies for at least 1 year after the FDG-PET scan. Two of the three patients with eventual recurrences were PET-positive at the time of recurrence. Eighteen patients with negative initial biopsies but an apparently positive PET scan had a repeat scan. Nine of the second scans were positive, suggesting local disease recurrence, and six patients were shown to have disease on subsequent biopsy. The other nine patients had decreasing FDG activity, and all remained disease free for 1 year after the follow-up PET scan. Considering the additional information from the follow-up PET scans, the sensitivity of PET for detection of recurrence rose from 92% to 97%, and a negative PET scan could exclude recurrent disease in 97% of patients. Specificity improved from 63% to 82%. It should be noted, however, that in this study, all PET scans were performed at a median of 16.5 months after the completion of radiation therapy, a time at which FDG-PET appears to perform better in general.

FDG-PET for Excluding Planned Neck Dissection After Definitive Radiation

The role of a planned neck dissection after definitive radiation therapy remains controversial because of the high rate of pathologic complete response in series of patients undergoing this surgery and because of a desire to avoid the added morbidity of unnecessary treatment. Given the apparent high negative predictive value of FDG-PET for the detection of recurrent/residual disease, the role of PET for excluding a planned neck dissection is a logical application to investigate, but the results are still debatable.

Yao and associates[53] reported on 53 patients (70 evaluable hemi-necks) with initial neck stage of N2a or greater head and neck cancer, who had a complete response of the primary tumor after definitive radiation therapy plus ($n = 46$) or minus ($n = 7$) chemotherapy. In this series, FDG-PET/CT scans were performed a median of 15 weeks after the completion of therapy and 21 necks were PET-negative and CT/MRI-positive. Four of these patients—three with residual lymphadenopathy greater than 3 cm—were negative for disease by neck dissection pathology. After a median follow-up of 27 months, all 17 of the other PET-negative patients followed up clinically (14 with residual nodes less than 2 cm) were negative for disease. The negative predictive value of FDG-PET for the detection of recurrent disease was 100%. The authors concluded that planned neck dissection could be eliminated in patients with negative post-treatment PET scan if nodes are smaller than 2 to 3 cm. Patients with nodes larger than 3 cm were few, and although those with negative PET scans did not recur for at least 2 years in this study, further data and correlation with outcomes are needed.[53] The researchers also speculated that the use of intensity-modulated radiation therapy may have contributed in part to the patients' high control rates and questioned whether the time period of waiting 12 weeks from completion of therapy to PET was outside the window for optimal planned neck dissection.

Porceddu and colleagues[52] found that after chemoradiation therapy for stage III/IV head and neck squamous cell carcinoma, FDG-PET had a 97% negative predictive value for the detection of residual nodal disease. Similar to Yao and associates,[53] the 39 patients in this series had a complete response of the primary tumor to chemoradiation but presented with 0.8- to 3.5-cm residual nodes on physical examination or CT scan. The median time from end of treatment to PET scanning was 12 weeks, and 79% had the PET scans performed between 8 and 12 weeks after chemoradiation. Five patients eventually failed at distant sites, one patient 6 months after the PET scan and four patients more than 1 year after therapy. The authors concluded that there is a low risk of recurrence if there is a complete response in the neck after radiation therapy and that residual tumor cells re-populate the nodes and can be detected by 8–12 weeks after therapy.[52]

More recently, the preceding results were confirmed by Nayak and colleagues[56] with the newer combined PET/CT technique. Forty-three patients with N2 disease or greater underwent FDG-PET/CT at baseline and then within 2 to 5 months after completing chemoradiation. The sensitivity, specificity and positive and negative predictive values for residual/recurrent disease were 88%, 91%, 70%, and 97%, respectively. In this series, four patients underwent a neck dissection for clinical reasons despite the negative PET scan, and the histology in the neck was negative for all. In addition, 86% of the patients were spared a neck dissection owing to the information provided by FDG-PET/CT.[56]

Not everyone is in agreement regarding the omission of a planned neck dissection because of several reports of higher false-negative rates for the detection of residual cancer with FDG-PET after the completion of radiation therapy. Rogers and associates[54] found that six of seven patients with a negative FDG-PET scan at 1 month after radiation therapy for stage III/IV head and neck squamous cell carcinoma harbored residual disease at planned neck dissection. In four cases, residual carcinoma was seen in the setting of necrosis, and viability of tumor could not be commented upon.[57]

More recently, Gourin and associates[54] evaluated 17 patients with stage N2 or N3 oropharyngeal or laryngeal carcinoma treated with primary chemoradiation therapy. PET/CT scans were performed within 8 to 10 weeks after the completion of therapy, and no patient had clinically apparent disease at the time of the PET scan or neck dissection. Three (of six) studies were falsely negative.

Although the above data leave some question as to whether a planned neck dissection can be omitted for patients with a negative PET scan after chemoradiation therapy, more data seem to be emerging that support the appropriateness of a conservative approach in patients with a negative scan performed at least 8 weeks after completion of therapy. Note that the designs of the positive and negative studies discussed previously do differ, and this may have affected the results. In the studies that do not advocate omitting surgery, post-therapy evaluations were performed at earlier time points. Both higher rates of false-positive studies—mostly due to inflammation—and false-negative studies can be seen during this time frame. The time course of effects of radiation therapy on glucose transporters and hexokinase, which are required for FDG uptake, are unknown. False-negative studies may be more likely to occur when the residual tumor foci are microscopic.[55] Furthermore, the patient populations were slightly different regarding the presence or absence of residual lymphadenopathy after radiation therapy.

PET/CT versus PET Alone and IV Contrast CT

In the post-therapy setting, interpretation of anatomic imaging is difficult as a result of altered anatomy. FDG-PET can be limited as well by post-therapy inflammation. Chen and associates[58] compared contrast-enhanced CT with FDG-PET/CT for the detection of residual disease in 30 patients with advanced squamous cell carcinoma of the head and neck treated with chemoradiation. Twenty-six patients had PET scans 8 weeks or less from the end of therapy, and 16 were obtained at 6 weeks or less. Contrast-enhanced CT showed the best accuracy for detecting residual disease at primary site with a lower false-positive rate, but PET/CT was better for detecting disease in neck nodes. False-negative studies were more likely to occur when the time between treatment and scanning was shorter.[58]

Other studies have also demonstrated the benefit of PET/CT over PET alone in head and neck cancer. Combined PET/CT decreases equivocal findings, has better accuracy for detecting cancer, and ultimately results in improved patient care.[33,59]

Timing of FDG-PET or PET/CT After Therapy

Although timing of the FDG-PET or PET/CT scan after therapy has been briefly discussed in several of the above sections, this topic is important and deserves special comment. Ideally, a waiting period of 1 month should be observed between the completion of chemotherapy and obtaining a PET scan. "Stunning" of residual viable tumor cells (viable cells having less uptake than expected) has been demonstrated as occurring in vitro, which may be due to alterations in the expression of the proteins involved in glucose metabolism.[60] Therefore, a delay in scanning is recommended to decrease the likelihood of false-negative scans. For practical purposes, if the 1-month wait period cannot be observed, then there should be a minimum duration of 10 days between the end of therapy and the post-chemotherapy FDG-PET scan.[60]

Most patients with head and neck cancer receive either radiation alone or radiation in combination with chemotherapy. Several groups have attempted to define the optimal time to obtain a PET scan after radiation therapy; however, the results are more variable compared with chemotherapy alone, and no definite consensus or recommendations have been published. It seems clear that false-positive and false-negative studies are more likely to occur if scans are obtained less than 8 weeks after the completion of therapy.

Explanations for false-negative scans after radiation therapy include microscopic disease that falls below the resolution of the PET scanner for detection and uncertainty as to whether residual tumor cells in a specimen are in fact viable. Whether radiation induces the same stunning effect seen with chemotherapy has not been elucidated.

FDG-PET scans 1 month after therapy have been reported to be falsely positive as a result of post-radiation inflammation. Higher levels of FDG uptake in a residual lymph node after radiation therapy are more likely to be associated with malignancy. Positive predictive values and specificity can be improved based on the threshold used for a positive PET scan. In fact, Kim and colleagues[61] found a high sensitivity and specificity for the detection of residual disease in primary tumors and nodes using a standardized uptake value of 3 as a malignancy threshold and support the use of early PET scanning 1 month after definitive radiation.

Proponents of early scanning argue that longer waiting times can result in a delay in diagnosis, which may affect therapy options, increased anxiety among patients who want to know the outcome of the therapy, and possible loss of patients to follow up. Therefore, the clinical context and consequences of inaccurate FDG-PET findings need to be carefully considered.

Conclusions

Metabolic tumor imaging with FDG-PET has emerged as a valuable tool for the evaluation of patients with head and neck cancer, particularly when obtained as a combined PET/CT scan. FDG-PET/CT detects early locoregional lymph node metastases that may appear normal on anatomic imaging, and it is useful for detecting early recurrences in the post-treatment setting when normal anatomy is often altered. In addition, FDG-PET/CT detects distant metastases and synchronous or second primary malignancies in a significant number of patients.

Attention to details for patient preparation prior to FDG-PET/CT scanning and image acquisition is critical for optimal images to be obtained. FDG-PET scanning after chemotherapy should be delayed at least 10 days to avoid false-negative studies. After chemoradiation, FDG-PET is more accurate with a longer delay (probably more than 8 weeks) from the end of therapy.

Regardless of the indication for FDG-PET/CT scanning, excellent communication between the referring physician and the imaging physician is essential. This should occur prior to imaging to ensure that the imaging physician is aware of the clinical history, particularly surgical history or altered anatomy, and also after imaging for review of the findings.

References

1. Kasamon YL, Jones RJ, Wahl RL: Integrating PET and PET/CT into the risk-adapted therapy of lymphoma. J Nucl Med 48(Suppl 1):19S–27S, 2007.
2. Warburg O: On the origin of cancer cells. Science 123:309–314, 1956.
3. Brown RS, Wahl RL: Overexpression of Glut-1 glucose transporter in human breast cancer. An immunohistochemical study. Cancer 72:2979–2985, 1993.
4. Brown RS, Leung JY, Kison PV, et al: Glucose transporters and FDG uptake in untreated primary human non-small cell lung cancer. J Nucl Med 40:556–565, 1999.
5. Shankar LK, Hoffman JM, Bacharach S, et al: Consensus recommendations for the use of 18F-FDG PET as an indicator of therapeutic response in patients in National Cancer Institute Trials. J Nucl Med 47:1059–1066, 2006.
6. Wahl RL, Henry CA, Ethier SP: Serum glucose: effects on tumor and normal tissue accumulation of 2-[F-18]-fluoro-2-deoxy-D-glucose in rodents with mammary carcinoma. Radiology 183:643–647, 1992.
7. Minn H, Leskinen-Kallio S, Lindholm P, et al: [18F]fluorodeoxyglucose uptake in tumors: kinetic vs. steady-state methods with reference to plasma insulin. J Comput Assist Tomogr 17:115–123, 1993.
8. Turcotte E, Leblanc M, Carpentier A, et al: Optimization of whole-body positron emission tomography imaging by using delayed 2-deoxy-2-[F-18]fluoro-D-glucose injection following IV insulin in diabetic patients. Mol Imaging Biol 8:348–354, 2006.
9. Cohade C, Mourtzikos KA, Wahl RL: "USA-Fat": prevalence is related to ambient outdoor temperature-evaluation with 18F-FDG PET/CT. J Nucl Med 44:1267–1270, 2003.
10. Nakamoto Y, Chin BB, Kraitchman DL, et al: Effects of nonionic intravenous contrast agents at PET/CT imaging: phantom and canine studies. Radiology 227:817–824, 2003.
11. Nakamoto Y, Tatsumi M, Hammoud D, et al: Normal FDG distribution patterns in the head and neck: PET/CT evaluation. Radiology 234:879–885, 2005.
12. Cannon B, Nedergaard J: Brown adipose tissue: function and physiological significance. Physiol Rev 84:277–359, 2004.
13. Ihn YK, Park YH, Chung SK: FDG uptake in benign asymmetric hypertrophy of the masticator muscles. Clin Nucl Med 31:221–222, 2006.
14. Jacene HA, Goudarzi B, Wahl RL: Scalene muscle uptake: a potential pitfall in head and neck PET/CT. Eur J Nucl Med Mol Imaging 35:89–94, 2008.
15. Jackson RS, Schlarman TC, Hubble WL, et al: Prevalence and patterns of physiologic muscle uptake detected with whole-body 18F-FDG PET. J Nucl Med Technol 34:29–33, 2006.
16. Kawabe J, Higashiyama S, Okamura T, et al: FDG uptake by tongue and muscles of mastication reflecting increased metabolic activity of muscles after chewing gum. Clin Nucl Med 28:220–221, 2003.
17. Lin EC: Focal asymmetric longus colli uptake on FDG PET/CT. Clin Nucl Med 32:67–69, 2007.
18. Osman M, Mosley C, El-Sadda W, et al: Prevalence and patterns of nerve injury in patients with head and neck cancer as detected with F18 FDG PET/CT [abstract]. In: 92nd Scientific Assembly and Annual Meeting of the Radiological Society of North America; Chicago, IL, 2005. Abstract #SST19-09.
19. Bailet JW, Abemayor E, Jabour BA, et al: Positron emission tomography: a new, precise imaging modality for detection of primary head and neck tumors and assessment of cervical adenopathy. Laryngoscope 102:281–288, 1992.
20. DiMartino E, Nowak B, Hassan HA, et al: Diagnosis and staging of head and neck cancer: a comparison of modern imaging modalities (positron emission tomography, computed tomography, color-coded duplex sonography) with panendoscopic and

histopathologic findings. Arch Otolaryngol Head Neck Surg 126:1457–1461, 2000.

21. McGuirt WF, Greven KM, Keyes JW, Jr, et al: Positron emission tomography in the evaluation of laryngeal carcinoma. Ann Otol Rhinol Laryngol 104:274–278, 1995.

22. McGuirt WF, Williams DW, 3rd, Keyes JW, Jr, et al: A comparative diagnostic study of head and neck nodal metastases using postiron emission tomography. Laryngoscope 105:373–375, 1995.

23. Minn H, Joensuu H, Ahonen A, et al: Fluorodeoxyglucose imaging: a method to assess the proliferative activity of human cancer in vivo. Comparison with DNA flow cytometry in head and neck tumors. Cancer 61:1776–1781, 1988.

24. Wong WL, Chevretton EB, McGurk M, et al: A prospective study of PET-FDG imaging for the assessment of head and neck squamous cell carcinoma. Clin Otolaryngol Allied Sci 22:209–214, 1997.

25. Haberkorn U, Strauss LG, Dimitrakopoulou A, et al: Fluorodeoxyglucose imaging of advanced head and neck cancer after chemotherapy. J Nucl Med 34:12–17, 1993.

26. Hannah A, Scott AM, Tochon-Danguy H, et al: Evaluation of 18 F-fluorodeoxyglucose positron emission tomography and computed tomography with histopathologic correlation in the initial staging of head and neck cancer. Ann Surg 236:208–217, 2002.

27. Laubenbacher C, Saumweber D, Wagner-Manslau C, et al: Comparison of fluorine-18-fluorodeoxyglucose PET, MRI and endoscopy for staging head and neck squamous-cell carcinomas. J Nucl Med 36:1747–1757, 1995.

28. Adams S, Baum RP, Stuckensen T, et al: Prospective comparison of 18F-FDG PET with conventional imaging modalities (CT, MRI, US) in lymph node staging of head and neck cancer. Eur J Nucl Med 25:1255–1260, 1998.

29. Braams JW, Pruim J, Freling NJ, et al: Detection of lymph node metastases of squamous-cell cancer of the head and neck with FDG-PET and MRI. J Nucl Med 36:211–216, 1995.

30. Gordin A, Golz A, Keidar Z, et al: The role of FDG-PET/CT imaging in head and neck malignant conditions: impact on diagnostic accuracy and patient care. Otolaryngol Head Neck Surg 137:130–137, 2007.

31. Jeong HS, Baek CH, Son YI, et al: Use of integrated 18F-FDG PET/CT to improve the accuracy of initial cervical nodal evaluation in patients with head and neck squamous cell carcinoma. Head Neck 29:203–210, 2007.

32. Schwartz DL, Ford E, Rajendran J, et al: FDG-PET/CT imaging for preradiotherapy staging of head-and-neck squamous cell carcinoma. Int J Radiat Oncol Biol Phys 61:129–136, 2005.

33. Schoder H, Yeung HW, Gonen M, et al: Head and neck cancer: clinical usefulness and accuracy of PET/CT image fusion. Radiology 231:65–72, 2004.

34. Fleming AJ, Jr, Smith SP, Jr, Paul CM, et al: Impact of [18F]-2-fluorodeoxyglucose-positron emission tomography/computed tomography on previously untreated head and neck cancer patients. Laryngoscope 117:1173–1179, 2007.

35. Ha P, Hdeib A, Goldenberg D, et al: The role of positron emission tomography and computed tomography fusion in the management of early-stage and advanced-stage primary head and neck squamous cell carcinoma. Arch Otolaryngol Head Neck Surg 132:12–16, 2006.

36. Stuckensen T, Kovacs AF, Adams S, et al: Staging of the neck in patients with oral cavity squamous cell carcinomas: a prospective comparison of PET, ultrasound, CT and MRI. J Craniomaxillofac Surg 28:319–324, 2000.

37. Lowe VJ, Kim H, Boyd JH, et al: Primary and recurrent early stage laryngeal cancer: preliminary results of 2-[fluorine 18]fluoro-2-deoxy-D-glucose PET imaging. Radiology 212:799–802, 1999.

38. Dammann F, Horger M, Mueller-Berg M, et al: Rational diagnosis of squamous cell carcinoma of the head and neck region: comparative evaluation of CT, MRI, and 18FDG PET. AJR Am J Roentgenol 184:1326–1331, 2005.

39. Tepperman BS, Fitzpatrick PJ: Second respiratory and upper digestive tract cancers after oral cancer. Lancet 2:547–549, 1981.

40. Warnakulasuriya KA, Robinson D, Evans H: Multiple primary tumours following head and neck cancer in southern England during 1961–98. J Oral Pathol Med 32:443–449, 2003.

41. Keyes JW, Jr, Chen MY, Watson NE, Jr, et al: FDG PET evaluation of head and neck cancer: value of imaging the thorax. Head Neck 22:105–110, 2000.

42. Kitagawa Y, Nishizawa S, Sano K, et al: Whole-body (18)F-fluorodeoxyglucose positron emission tomography in patients with head and neck cancer. Oral Surg Oral Med Oral Pathol Oral Radiol Endod 93:202–207, 2002.

43. Koshy M, Paulino AC, Howell R, et al: F-18 FDG PET-CT fusion in radiotherapy treatment planning for head and neck cancer. Head Neck 27:494–502, 2005.

44. Nishiyama Y, Yamamoto Y, Yokoe K, et al: FDG PET as a procedure for detecting simultaneous tumours in head and neck cancer patients. Nucl Med Commun 26:239–244, 2005.

45. Sigg MB, Steinert H, Gratz K, et al: Staging of head and neck tumors: [18F]fluorodeoxyglucose positron emission tomography compared with physical examination and conventional imaging modalities. J Oral Maxillofac Surg 61:1022–1029, 2003.

46. Stokkel MP, ten Broek FW, Hordijk GJ, et al: Preoperative evaluation of patients with primary head and neck cancer using dual-head 18fluorodeoxyglucose positron emission tomography. Ann Surg 231:229–234, 2000.

47. Teknos TN, Rosenthal EL, Lee D, et al: Positron emission tomography in the evaluation of stage III and IV head and neck cancer. Head Neck 23:1056–1060, 2001.

48. Lapela M, Grenman R, Kurki T, et al: Head and neck cancer: detection of recurrence with PET and 2-[F-18]fluoro-2-deoxy-D-glucose. Radiology 197:205–211, 1995.

49. Lonneux M, Lawson G, Ide C, et al: Positron emission tomography with fluorodeoxyglucose for suspected head and neck tumor recurrence in the symptomatic patient. Laryngoscope 110:1493–1497, 2000.

50. Terhaard CH, Bongers V, van Rijk PP, et al: F-18-fluoro-deoxy-glucose positron-emission tomography scanning in detection of local recurrence after radiotherapy for laryngeal/pharyngeal cancer. Head Neck 23:933–941, 2001.

51. Wong RJ, Lin DT, Schoder H, et al: Diagnostic and prognostic value of [(18)F]fluorodeoxyglucose positron emission tomography for recurrent head and neck squamous cell carcinoma. J Clin Oncol 20:4199–4208, 2002.

52. Porceddu SV, Jarmolowski E, Hicks RJ, et al: Utility of positron emission tomography for the detection of disease in residual neck nodes after (chemo)radiotherapy in head and neck cancer. Head Neck 27:175–181, 2005.

53. Yao M, Smith RB, Graham MM, et al: The role of FDG PET in management of neck metastasis from head-and-neck cancer after definitive radiation treatment. Int J Radiat Oncol Biol Phys 63:991–999, 2005.

54. Gourin CG, Williams HT, Seabolt WN, et al: Utility of positron emission tomography-computed tomography in identification of residual nodal disease after chemoradiation for advanced head and neck cancer. Laryngoscope 116:705–710, 2006.

55. Andrade RS, Heron DE, Degirmenci B, et al: Posttreatment assessment of response using FDG-PET/CT for patients treated with definitive radiation therapy for head and neck cancers. Int J Radiat Oncol Biol Phys 65:1315–1322, 2006.

56. Nayak JV, Walvekar RR, Andrade RS, et al: Deferring planned neck dissection following chemoradiation for stage IV head and neck cancer: The utility of PET-CT. Laryngoscope 117:2129–2134, 2007.

57. Rogers JW, Greven KM, McGuirt WF, et al: Can post-RT neck dissection be omitted for patients with head-and-neck cancer who have a negative PET scan after definitive radiation therapy? Int J Radiat Oncol Biol Phys 58:694–697, 2004.

58. Chen YK, Su CT, Ding HJ, et al: Clinical usefulness of fused PET/CT compared with PET alone or CT alone in nasopharyngeal carcinoma patients. Anticancer Res 26:1471–1477, 2006.

59. Zimny M, Wildberger JE, Cremerius U, et al: Combined image interpretation of computed tomography and hybrid PET in head and neck cancer. Nuklearmedizin 41:14–21, 2002.

60. Engles JM, Quarless SA, Mambo E, et al: Stunning and its effect on 3H-FDG uptake and key gene expression in breast cancer cells undergoing chemotherapy. J Nucl Med 47:603–608, 2006.

61. Kim SY, Lee SW, Nam SY, et al: The feasibility of 18F-FDG PET scans 1 month after completing radiotherapy of squamous cell carcinoma of the head and neck. J Nucl Med 48:373–378, 2007.

62. Goerres GW, Schmid DT, Grätz KW, et al: Impact of whole body positron emission tomography on initial staging and therapy in patients with squamous cell carcinoma of the oral cavity. Oral Oncol 39:547–551, 2003.

6

Chemoprevention of Head and Neck Cancer

Kavita Malhotra Pattani

KEY POINTS

- Despite advances in early detection and diagnosis of head and neck cancers, the overall survival rates have shown only marginal improvement. Field cancerization and the multistep carcinogenesis process are thought to play a key role.
- Chemoprevention is defined as the use of drugs or other natural, synthetic, or biologic agents to inhibit, delay, or reverse the stepwise carcinogenic progression to invasive cancer.
- Retinoids are a well-studied class of chemopreventive agents. They have offered promising data on their effects in reducing oral leukoplakias, in lowering second primary cancers, and in delaying recurrences. Further trials are underway to validate these findings.
- Numerous agents are in trial to identify those that prove to be effective and demonstrate low levels of toxicities and evoke good patient compliance.
- Recent investigations have emphasized the need for molecular and genomic (surrogate) biomarkers that can serve as intermediate end points.
- Well-defined risk stratification strategies will further improve and help tailor chemopreventive therapies.

Introduction

Head and neck cancers account for approximately 3% to 5% of all cancer in the United States. According to the American Cancer Society's publication *Cancer Facts & Figures 2009*, an estimated 48,010 people will develop head and neck cancer in 2009, with an estimated mortality of 11,260, making head and neck cancer an important public health problem.

Tobacco and alcohol are widely recognized as the leading risk factors for head and neck cancers. Historically, over 80% of head and neck cancers have been linked to tobacco use. Both tobacco and alcohol potentiate the carcinogenic effects of either alone and place people at a much greater risk for developing these cancers.

Unfortunately, despite the advances in early detection and diagnosis of head and neck cancers and the progress in multimodality treatment efforts including radiation, chemotherapy, and surgery, the overall survival rates for those with head and neck cancers have improved only marginally in the last three decades.[1] More important is that despite curative treatment options for treating head and neck cancers, patients are subsequently faced with significant morbidities and even debilitating changes. In 1953, Slaughter and associates[2] proposed the concept of *field cancerization* to describe the premalignant histologic changes observed adjacent to oral carcinomas. Many early head and neck cancers were observed to arise in patients with these areas of field cancerization. Consequently, lesions arising in fields of premalignant disease pose a dilemma for surgeons regarding the feasibility of complete and effective excision.

The extensive multifocal development of premalignant and malignant lesions is believed to result in an increased incidence of second primary cancers and locoregional recurrences. A large number of patients who are successfully treated for early lesions develop second primaries due to condemned mucosa. Second primaries are estimated to occur at an annual rate of 3% to 10% (derived from populations mainly consisting of cigarette smokers), resulting in significant threats to the long-term survival of patients.[3] Patients with stage I and II head and neck cancer are more likely to die from a second primary tumor than from their original cancers.[4] Patients with recurrence of disease or distant metastatic disease also experience a poor survival rate.

More recently, the multistep carcinogenesis process contributing to head and neck cancer is gaining tremendous interest. This includes genetic and epigenetic alterations and environmental and viral infectious causes. It has been suggested that cancer occurs through a series of genetic events that are necessary for solid epithelial tumors to arise.

Chemoprevention Strategies

The concept of preventive strategies to interrupt these processes has generated a great deal of interest. Chemoprevention, a term first used by Sporn and colleagues,[5] is defined as the use of drugs or other natural, synthetic, or biologic agents to inhibit, delay, or reverse the stepwise carcinogenic progression to invasive cancer. Chemoprevention studies use these fundamental premises to identify alterations or biomarkers to serve as intermediate endpoints in the trials. Chemoprevention has been studied with much success in breast cancer and familial adenomatous polyposis, thus affording considerable attention in head and neck cancer treatments.[6,7]

Chemopreventive strategies can target high-risk individuals, individuals with precancerous lesions, and/or the prevention of second primaries or recurrences. Over 2000 agents have been studied for chemopreventive effects. Specific molecular and cellular targeted therapies have aided in the clinical development of new agents. Extensively studied chemopreventive agents in head and neck cancer include retinoids, beta carotene, vitamin E, selenium, nonsteroidal anti-inflammatory drugs, epidermal growth factor receptor (EGFR)-tyrosine kinase and farnesyl transferase inhibitors (Box 6-1). This chapter reviews both well-studied and newer promising chemopreventive agents.

Box 6-1. Potential Chemopreventive Agents

Retinoids	Polyphenols
Vitamin A	Blackberries
Fenretinide	Pomegranate juice
Isotretinoin	
Etretinate	Gugglesterone
Beta carotene	Pioglitazone
Alpha-tocopherol	Molecularly targeted agents
Selenium	EGFR—TKIs
NSAIDS	EGFR—farnesyl
COX-2 inhibitors	EGFR—EKB-569
ASA	Transferase inhibitors
Curcumin	p53 gene
Bowman-Birkman inhibitors	ONYX-015
Green tea extract	Ad5CMV

ASA, aspirin; COX-2, cyclooxygenase 2; EGFR, epidermal growth factor receptor; NSAIDs, nonsteroidal anti-inflammatory drugs; TKIs, tyrosine kinase inhibitors.

Retinoids

The retinoids include vitamin A and its biologically active derivatives retinal and retinoic acid (RA) along with a repertoire of more than 3000 of its synthetic derivatives. The retinoid class has been studied for several years as potential chemopreventive agents.

Retinoids exert a majority of their effects by binding to specific receptors and modulating gene expression. This can result in potent consequences on premalignant and malignant cell growth, differentiation, and apoptosis. The development of new active retinoids and, more notably, the identification of two distinct families of nuclear retinoid receptors have led to an increased understanding of the molecular mechanism of retinoid action and effect on gene expression.

Once vitamin A (retinol) has been taken up by a cell, it can be oxidized to retinal and then retinal can be oxidized to retinoic acid. The conversion of retinal to retinoic acid is an irreversible step. Retinoic acid can bind to two different nuclear receptors (the retinoic acid receptors (RARs) or the retinoid X receptors [RXRs]) to play an important role in gene transcription by interacting with DNA response elements in the promoter regions of specific genes (Fig. 6-1).

In 1978, Koch[8] reported the first study of synthetic retinoids in oral leukoplakia, which demonstrated complete or partial remissions in 43%, 45%, and 51% of patients after treatment with all-*trans*-retinoic acid (tretinoin), 13-*cis*-retinoic acid (isotretinoin), or etretinate, respectively. This showed considerable improvement over the 15% spontaneous regression rates in oral leukoplakia. In 1986, a landmark randomized clinical trial by Hong and associates[9] clearly demonstrated the efficacy after 3 months of treatment with high-dose isotretinoin against oral leukoplakia. However, the adverse effects of high-dose isotretinoin and the observed relapse rates after discontinuation of therapy led to a follow-up trial. Lippman and associates[10] evaluated the use of high-dose isotretinoin for a 3-month induction period followed by low-dose isotretinoin for a maintenance period of 9 months compared with the use of beta carotene as maintenance. He was able to demonstrate that 92% of patients treated with low-dose isotretinoin had stable disease with minimal side effects compared with 45% response/stable disease rate in the beta carotene group. In 1990, Han and colleagues[11] reported a randomized trial using 4-hydroxyphenol retinamide (4-HPR) for 4 months in patients with oral leukoplakia. An 87% complete response rate was noted versus 17% in the placebo group. Chiesa and colleagues[12] conducted another

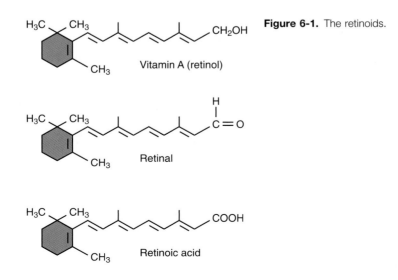

Figure 6-1. The retinoids.

Vitamin A (retinol)

Retinal

Retinoic acid

randomized trial to evaluate the effects of fenretinide (4-HPR) after surgical treatment with laser resection of oral leukoplakia. The preliminary results had suggested decreased incidence of local recurrences and minimal toxicities in the treated group. However, the long-term follow-up results were inconclusive owing to low recruitment of patients and early termination of the trial.

As a result of promising retinoid data on the effects of oral leukoplakia, Hong and associates[13,14] designed a randomized phase III clinical trial using high-dose isotretinoin for prevention of second primaries or recurrences. The long-term follow-up results indicated no significant differences in local, regional, and distant recurrences. However, the treatment group had demonstrated significantly lower rates of second primaries at 14% compared with 31% and long-lasting retinoid activity. With the compelling data reported by Hong and associates, a trial was initiated with lower doses of isotretinoin in an attempt to reduce toxicities. NCI C91-002 was a randomized trial in patients with a history of head and neck cancer treated for a 3-year period with low-dose isotretinoin versus placebo. The final analysis revealed that low-dose isotretinoin did not have an impact on second primaries but may delay recurrences.[15]

Because of the high risk of malignant transformation in advanced lesions and the resistance to single-modality therapies, the notion of combined treatment regimens emerged. Chemoprevention trials by Papadimitrakopoulou and colleagues[16] and Shin and coworkers[17] designed nonrandomized trials using interferon-α (IFN-α), alpha-tocopherol, and isotretinoin for 1 and 2 years, respectively. The trial by Papadimitrakopoulou and colleagues revealed lower response rates to treatment in patients with high p53 expression, whereas Shin and colleagues demonstrated significantly lower rates of second primary cancers with treatment. Further randomized trials are underway to validate this.

Beta Carotene

Beta carotene is a provitamin composed of two retinyl groups. It is broken down in the mucosa of the small intestine by beta carotene dioxygenase to retinal, a form of vitamin A. Beta carotene is an antioxidant that can be found in yellow, orange, and green leafy vegetables and fruits (Fig. 6-2).

Garewel and colleagues[18] conducted a phase II clinical trial to assess the response rate of beta carotene given to patients with oral leukoplakia. They reported a 71% complete or partial response. Kaugars and colleagues[19] studied the effects of 30 mg/day of beta carotene given with ascorbic acid and vitamin E (alpha-tocopherol) for 9 months to patients with oral leukoplakia. The researchers noted clinical improvement in 56% of patients. In 1994, a randomized trial was conducted to examine the effects of daily supplementation with beta carotene and alpha-tocopherol.[20] The study detected no reduction in lung cancer and suggested the possibility of harmful effects. In 1996, the Beta Carotene and Retinol Efficacy Trial (CARET), another large randomized trial to determine the effects of vitamin A and beta carotene, reported their results.[21,22] These results indicated an increased rate of lung cancer and cancer mortality, which led to a discontinuation of the trial and cessation of beta carotene in chemoprevention trials for oral leukoplakia patients. Also in 1996, the

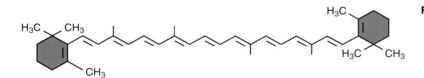

Figure 6-2. The β-carotene structure.

Alpha-Tocopherol, Beta-Carotene Cancer Prevention Study (ATBC Study), a randomized trial evaluating the effects of vitamin A and beta carotene, was terminated early because of an increased incidence of lung cancer in patients with a history of smoking or asbestos exposure.[23]

Vitamin E

Vitamin E is the collective name for a set of eight related tocopherols and tocotrienols, which are fat-soluble vitamins with antioxidant properties. Of these, alpha-tocopherol has been the most well studied for chemoprevention since it has the highest bioavailability and the body preferentially absorbs and uses this form. Vitamin E can be found in foods such as nuts, vegetable oils, avocado, and olives. Studies in animals and cell lines demonstrated inhibitory effects on growth in several cancers such as breast and prostate cancer[24] (Fig. 6-3).

Thus far, chemopreventive trials using vitamin E in oral premalignancy patients have produced disappointing results. Benner and associates[25] conducted a phase II trial in patients with oral hyperkeratosis who received alpha-tocopherol. Forty-six percent of patients demonstrated regression of the lesions with excellent compliance and tolerance. Bairati and associates[26] conducted a randomized, double-blind, placebo-controlled trial to assess the effects of alpha-tocopherol on the incidence of second primary tumors. The group who received the alpha-tocopherol demonstrated a higher rate of second primaries during the treatment period with no difference in the treatment versus control groups after 8 years of follow-up.

Selenium

Trace amounts of the trace mineral selenium are necessary for cellular function. Major dietary sources for selenium include plants that are grown or animals that are raised on food grown in selenium-rich soils. Selenium gets incorporated into proteins to make selenoproteins, which exhibit antioxidant properties by preventing cellular damage from free radicals. Free radicals, which are a natural by-product of oxygen, may contribute to the development of cancers. Selenoproteins also play a role in regulating thyroid function and the immune system. Selenium may prevent or slow tumor growth by enhancing cellular immunity and preventing tumor angiogenesis.[27]

Although large amounts of selenium are shown to be toxic, observational studies have indicated that death from cancers is lower among people who have higher levels of selenium. Yadav and associates[28] conducted a study in India that revealed that patients with lower levels of selenium had a significant increase in the incidence of cancer compared with patients with higher levels of selenium. Patients who were being treated for cancer were supplemented with 200 mg of selenium, which appeared to enhance cell-mediated immunity and enhance the cytotoxic effects on tumor cells. Similarly, Combs and associates[27] found that taking a daily supplement of selenium significantly reduced the occurrence of and death from total cancers.

On the other hand, in 1982 data from the Nurse Health Study, a prospective study of toenail clippings collected from over 60,000 nurses for selenium level analysis revealed no reduction in risk of cancer in nurses with higher levels of selenium in

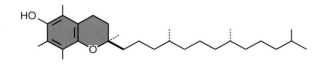

Figure 6-3. Vitamin E (alpha-tocopherol) structure.

their toenails.[29] The SU.VI.MAX study concluded that low-dose supplementation (with 120 mg ascorbic acid, 30 mg vitamin E, 6 mg beta carotene, 100 mcg selenium, and 20 mg zinc) resulted in a 31% reduction in the incidence of cancer and a 37% reduction in mortality rate from all causes in males after a sex-stratified analysis.[30] The study did not detect a significant protective effect of selenium for females. The SELECT (Selenium and Vitamin E Cancer Prevention Trial) study is a prospective trial that is currently investigating the effect of selenium and vitamin E supplementation on the incidence of prostate cancer. Further investigation is necessary to evaluate the potential chemopreventive effects of selenium.

Nonsteroidal Anti-inflammatory Drugs

Cyclooxygenase-2 Inhibitors

Chronic inflammation and carcinogenesis are believed to be intimately linked to the development of some cancers. This relationship has been studied and the pathogenesis established in colorectal cancers. Cyclooxygenase-2 (COX-2) inhibitors, such as celecoxib, have been shown to effectively prevent adenomas in patients with familial adenomatous polyposis. COX-2 overexpression has been found in several types of human cancers. More than a 100-fold increase in expression levels of COX-2 was found in head and neck squamous cell carcinoma (HNSCC) compared with normal oral mucosa.[31] Up-regulation of COX-2 and prostaglandin E_2 expression has been reported in malignant as well as premalignant head and neck lesions.[32,33] Because of its role in carcinogenesis, apoptosis, and angiogenesis, it appears to be an excellent target for an effective chemopreventive agent.

Feng and colleagues[34] reported on the dose-dependent effectiveness of celecoxib, a highly specific COX-2 inhibitor, in delaying the onset of early oral lesions and in slowing growth of the tumors in a hamster animal model. Zhang and colleagues[35] reported on the effects of targeting the epidermal growth factor receptor (EGFR) and COX-2 in human HNSCC cell lines. They concluded that the cooperative effects of targeting both pathways resulted in decreased production of phosphorylated EGFR, vascular endothelial growth factor (VEGF), and Ki-67 (important biomarkers for angiogenesis and cell proliferation). The authors advocated future trials to evaluate combination therapy.

Although animal and observational studies indicated that COX-2 inhibitors are effective agents for chemoprevention strategies, recent studies have reported increased risk of serious cardiovascular events, including heart attack and stroke. Papadimitrakopoulou and associates[36] conducted a randomized phase II pilot study to determine the effects of celecoxib on 49 patients with oral premalignant lesions. They concluded that low doses of celecoxib at 100 mg and 200 mg twice daily were not effective in controlling premalignant lesions. The potential cardiovascular toxicity and the dose-dependent efficacy of celecoxib indicated that it may be necessary to develop better methods to protect high-risk patients (Fig. 6-4).

Aspirin

Along with its anti-inflammatory and analgesic effects, aspirin is well known for its cardioprotective effects. Aspirin acts as a nonselective COX inhibitor that blocks the action of both COX-1 and COX-2. This in turn inhibits PGE_2 overexpression, which can be associated with inflammation, tumor angiogenesis, inhibition of apoptosis, and cell proliferation.[37] There is increasing evidence of the chemopreventive effects of aspirin on colorectal cancers. However, the data are limited in evaluating the role of aspirin on the risk of cancers of the upper aerodigestive tract. Researchers have

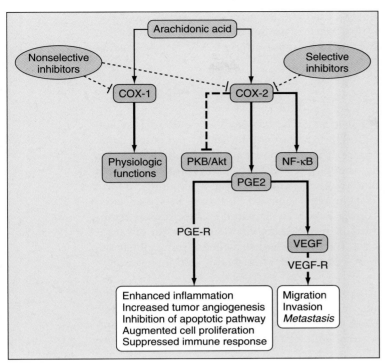

Figure 6-4. COX-PGE (cyclooxygenase-prostaglandin E) schematic demonstrates the method by which COX inhibitors exert their effects. NF-κB, nuclear (transcription) factor κB; PKB/Akt, protein kinase B; PGE-R, prostaglandin E receptor; VEGF, vascular endothelial growth factor; VEGF-R, vascular endothelial growth factor receptor.

demonstrated possible protective effects of aspirin on smoking-related cancers such as lung[38] and esophagus.[39–41]

Jayaprakash and colleagues[42] conducted a hospital-based case-control study with 529 patients in each arm. Patient characteristics were compared and analyzed. The groups were stratified into three exposure categories: never exposed, moderately exposed, and highly exposed to alcohol and tobacco. Aspirin users showed a 25% reduction in the risk of head and neck cancers at all major sites. The most significant risk reduction was noted in the moderate smoker and moderate drinker subset, and this effect was greater in women.

Future clinical trials are necessary to validate these findings and assess the potential of aspirin as a chemopreventive agent.

Targeted Therapies

The more recent interest in the multistep carcinogenesis process has led to investigations of new targets and biomarkers, which may lead to new chemopreventive agents as well as intermediate end points for trials. Molecularly targeted markers include growth factors and their receptors, tumor suppressor genes, and proto-oncogenes.

ras Gene

The *ras* proto-oncogene family includes *H-ras*, *K-ras*, and *N-ras* and is commonly found to be mutated in human tumors. Particularly, alterations in the *H-ras* gene are found in approximately one third of oral leukoplakia and squamous cell carcinomas.[43,44] Researchers have demonstrated that farnesyl transferase inhibitors (FTIs) and *S*-farnesyl thiosalicylic acid (FTS) alter the expression of this gene by inhibiting the pathway in HNSCC cell lines. FTIs have been tested in clinical trials where they exhibited some antitumor effects.[45–47] However, *K-ras* and *N-ras* remain active, thus indicating that FTIs may not effectively inhibit the *ras* gene due to other mediators that affect this pathway. Strategies that utilize a combination of *ras* inhibitors that target different points in the pathway may be more effective and require further investigation.

Epidermal Growth Factor Receptors

EGFR is a transmembrane protein that is activated by specific ligands such as epidermal growth factor, transforming growth factor-α, amphiregulin, and betacellulin. It is part of the ErbB family of receptors. It is also known as ErbB1 and Her1. Upon binding with growth factor ligands, the EGFR cell surface receptor is activated forming a homodimer. It may also bind to other members of the ErbB family to form a heterodimer. Mutations leading to the upregulation of EFGR have been associated with many cancers and are felt to correlate with an increased risk for disease recurrence. This overexpression can lead to uncontrolled cell division and result in cancer formation. The activation of EGFR tyrosine kinase and subsequent intracellular signaling events leads to cell proliferation, cell survival, angiogenesis, and metastasis[48,49] (Fig. 6-5).

A 29-fold higher level of EGFR expression was demonstrated by Grandis and colleagues[50] in patients with head and neck cancers compared with normal controls. Moreover, an increased level of EGFR expression was also noted in bronchial epithelium lesions of smokers from squamous metaplasia to dysplasia to in situ carcinoma.[51]

EGFR proto-oncogene has been a target for chemopreventive trials. Anticancer agents that are monoclonal antibody inhibitors such as cetuximab or small molecule tyrosine kinase inhibitors such as gefitinib and erlotinib are among the agents tested. Monoclonal antibodies work by blocking the extracellular ligand binding domain and kinase inhibitors inhibit the tyrosine kinase activity of EGFR, which is required for the activation of the downstream signaling cascade. EGFR inhibitors have also been shown to exert effects through antiangiogenic activity by decreasing factors such as VEGF and fibroblast growth factor. EGFR inhibitors have been well studied in lung cancers.

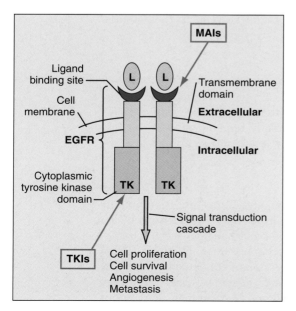

Figure 6-5. Epidermal growth factor receptor (EGFR) is a transmembrane protein with tyrosine kinase (TK) activity. The red arrows demonstrate the sites at which different EGFR inhibitors exert their effects. MAIs, monoclonal antibody inhibitors; TKIs, tyrosine kinase inhibitors.

Several studies have examined the effects of combination therapies with EGFR inhibitors, antiangiogenic agents, and radiation.[52,53] Bozec and colleagues[54] reported on the efficacy of the combination of bevacizumab, erlotinib, and radiation, showing it to have the highest tumor growth inhibition and decreased number of positive lymph nodes produced by head and neck cell lines in an animal model. In addition, agents such as gefitinib are generally well tolerated and are appealing candidates for chemoprevention trials.

EGFR inhibitors are being used in humans in combination therapy for treatment of head and neck cancer as radiosensitizing agents. Chemopreventive trials are underway to evaluate the effectiveness of these EGFR inhibitors in combination therapy for premalignant lesions in head and neck cancers.

p53 Gene

p53 is a tumor suppressor gene found on chromosome 17. Mutations in the expression of the *p53* gene have been associated with decreased apoptosis and carcinogenic progression leading to decreased survival, poor response to neoadjuvant chemotherapy, and higher risk of recurrence or second primaries. Inactivating alterations in the *p53* gene occur in 40% to 50% of HNSCC patients[55] and mutations are found in up to 45% of dysplastic lesions in the head and neck.[56]

Agents targeting the *p53* gene have shown promising results in chemopreventive trials. ONYX-015 is an adenovirus lacking the gene *E1B 55kd* that binds to and inactivates *p53*, thus allowing for viral replication and selective destruction of *p53*-mutant cells. Rudin and associates[57] conducted a phase II trial with ONYX-015 administered as a mouthwash to patients with premalignant oral lesions. They reported complete histologic resolution of dysplasia in 7 (37%) of 19 patients. It would be necessary to validate these findings by performing larger randomized trials of the efficacy of single-agent as well as combined use of ONYX-015.

Other Agents

New agents are continually being considered as chemopreventive candidates. Epidemiologic studies have found that certain dietary agents may lead to anticarcinogenic effects through the ability to regulate cellular proliferation and modulate cell cycle-associated proteins.[58] Several of these agents have been studied and remain investigational. Some of these are further discussed in the following text.

Curcumin

Curcumin is a polyphenol derived from *Curcuma longa* and is responsible for the yellow color in the Indian curry spice turmeric. Curcumin is known for its antioxidant, anti-inflammatory, antiamyloid, wound healing, and antitumor properties. The exceedingly low rates of colon and prostate cancer observed in China and India are attributed to the use of turmeric; hence its chemopreventive effects in colon and prostate cancer have been explored with promising results. Curcumin was noted to downregulate the *MDM2* oncogene, a protein associated with malignant tumor formation.[59] It has also been shown to interfere with the activity of the transcription factor NF-κB.[60] It exerts its anticancer effects by inducing apoptosis in cancer cells. Progress in the use of curcumin as a chemopreventive agent has been hindered by its low bioavailability and rapid degradation. Trials are underway to further elucidate the mechanistic role and potential as a chemopreventive agent.

Bowman-Birkman Inhibitor

In the 1940s, Bowman identified a soybean-derived serine-protease inhibitor, which was later purified by Birk in the 1960s and referred to as the Bowman-Birk inhibitor (BBI). Observational studies have alluded to the low incidence of several cancers including breast, colon, and prostate in areas such as Japan with high soy intake.[61-63] In the form of a concentrate, BBI has demonstrated anticarcinogenic activities at nanomolar concentrations and is being evaluated as a chemopreventive agent.[64]

A phase I clinical trial to evaluate the effects of oral BBI concentrate in patients with oral leukoplakia did not demonstrate any acute toxicity.[65] A follow-up phase IIa trial conducted on 31 patients with oral leukoplakia by Armstrong and associates[66] revealed a dose-dependent statistically significant decrease of 24.2% in total lesion area. The researchers were also able to demonstrate Neu staining in premalignant lesions as a possible surrogate end-point biomarker.[67] Currently, randomized, placebo-controlled trials are being performed.

Green Tea Extract

Green tea is made from the leaves of the *Camellia sinensis* plant. Epigallocatechin-3-gallate (EGCG) is the most abundant catechin and the most active phenolic constituent in green tea. EGCG has been reported to exert its antitumor effects by suppressing the phosphorylation of EGFR in numerous cancers.[68-70] EGFR is over-expressed in 80% to 90% of HNSCC, which in turn leads to enhanced tumor invasion, resistance to chemotherapy, and decreased patient survival.[71-73] Thus, agents such as EGCG offer promise of benefit.

Masuda and colleagues[68] demonstrated that EGCG inhibited cell growth by causing cell-cycle arrest and induced apoptosis in two human HNSCC cell lines. Zhang and colleagues[74] explored the effects of combining EGCG with erlotinib (an EGFR-tyrosine kinase inhibitor) in five HNSCC cell lines. They discovered that the combination of EGCG with erlotinib resulted in synergistic effects inhibiting signaling pathways and drastically augmenting induction of apoptosis.[74]

Human Papillomavirus Vaccine

Human papillomavirus (HPV) is a group of more than 100 related viruses that can affect the mucosa and epithelial tissues. An overall prevalence of HPV in HNSCC of 25.9% was reported in a worldwide review of studies.[75] Higher prevalence was observed in the oropharynx, particularly tonsil and tongue base cancers. HPV-positive oropharyngeal cancer comprises a distinct molecular, clinical, and pathologic disease entity that has a markedly improved prognosis.[76] Approximately 15% of HNSCC occur in patients who are nonsmokers and nondrinkers. A significant portion of these cancers may be related to HPV infection. HPV-16 and -18 are deemed high-risk subtypes and have the ability to promote cancer development. Approximately 90% of HPV-positive tumors show the presence of HPV-16 DNA.[77] Two bivalent and quadravalent vaccines (Gardasil and Cervarix) have been studied in cervical cancers and are FDA approved to protect against HPV-16 and -18 in young women. Assessing the effects of preventive vaccines before HPV exposure in reducing the incidence of cancers will take years. Therapeutic HPV vaccine that can enhance the immune response to eradicate or reduce already infected cells is yet to be determined.[77]

Conclusion

In spite of early detection and diagnosis of head and neck cancers, overall survival has not shown significant improvements. Patients remain at risk for developing cancers in areas of field cancerization as well as second primaries. Behavior modification to avoid known risk factors is clearly an important and effective strategy in decreasing the incidence of second primaries. Unfortunately, this is not sufficient to correct genetic alterations that have already occurred as a result of carcinogenic exposures.

The field of chemoprevention represents a promising area open to innovation in the management of head and neck cancers. Biochemoprevention and molecularly targeted agents are important potential treatment options. Clinical trials have demonstrated efficacy in the use of several chemopreventive agents and have evaluated the associated morbidities. Chemoprevention has also provided exciting results in the prevention of second primaries. Large clinical trials are necessary to evaluate newer agents and combinations of these agents in an attempt to define their role in preventing head and neck cancer in high-risk patients. In addition, ease of administration, acceptable toxicities, good patient compliance, and good bioavailability are required for successful application of a chemopreventive agent.

It is imperative to define risk stratification strategies to better tailor chemopreventive therapies. Recent studies also emphasize the need for clearly defined molecular and genomic biomarkers that can be used for risk assessment and serve as surrogate endpoints.

References

1. Vokes EE, Weichselbaum RR, Lippman SM, Hong WK: Head and neck cancer. N Engl J Med 328(3):184–194, 1993.
2. Slaughter DP, Southwick HW, Smejkal W: Field cancerization in oral stratified squamous epithelium: clinical implications of multicentric origin. Cancer 6(5):963–968, 1953.
3. Rhee JC, Khuri FR, Shin DM: Advances in chemoprevention of head and neck cancer. Oncologist 9(3):302–311, 2004.
4. Kotwall C, Razack MS, Sako K, Rao U: Multiple primary cancers in squamous cell cancer of the head and neck. J Surg Oncol 40(2):97–99, 1989.
5. Sporn MB, Dunlop NM, Newton DL, Smith JM: Prevention of chemical carcinogenesis by vitamin A and its synthetic analogs (retinoids). Fed Proc 35(6):1332–1338, 1976.
6. Fisher B, Costantino JP, Wickerham DL, et al: Tamoxifen for prevention of breast cancer: report of the National Surgical Adjuvant Breast and Bowel Project P-1 Study. J Natl Cancer Inst 90(18):1371–1388, 1998.
7. Steinbach G, Lynch PM, Phillips RK, et al: The effect of celecoxib, a cyclooxygenase-2 inhibitor, in familial adenomatous polyposis. N Engl J Med 342(26):1946–1952, 2000.
8. Koch HF: Biochemical treatment of precancerous oral lesions: the effectiveness of various analogues of retinoic acid. J Maxillofac Surg 6(1):59–63, 1978.
9. Hong WK, Endicott J, Itri LM, et al: 13-cis-retinoic acid in the treatment of oral leukoplakia. N Engl J Med 315(24):1501–1505, 1986.
10. Lippman SM, Batsakis JG, Toth BB, et al: Comparison of low-dose isotretinoin with beta carotene to prevent oral carcinogenesis. N Engl J Med 328(1):15–20, 1993.
11. Han J, Jiao L, Lu Y, et al: Evaluation of N-4-(hydroxycarbophenyl) retinamide as a cancer prevention agent and as a cancer chemotherapeutic agent. In Vivo 4(3):153–160, 1990.
12. Chiesa F, Tradati N, Marazza M, et al: Fenretinide (4-HPR) in chemoprevention of oral leukoplakia. J Cell Biochem Suppl 17F:255–261, 1993.
13. Hong WK, Lippman SM, Itri LM, et al: Prevention of second primary tumors with isotretinoin in squamous-cell carcinoma of the head and neck. N Engl J Med 323(12):795–801, 1990.
14. Benner SE, Pajak TF, Lippman SM, et al: Prevention of second primary tumors with isotretinoin in patients with squamous cell carcinoma of the head and neck: long-term follow-up. J Natl Cancer Inst 86(2):140–141, 1994.
15. Khuri FR, Lee JJ, Lippman SM, et al: Randomized phase III trial of low-dose isotretinoin for prevention of second primary tumors in stage I and II head and neck cancer patients. J Natl Cancer Inst 98(7):441–450, 2006.

16. Papadimitrakopoulou VA, Hong WK: Biomolecular markers as intermediate end points in chemoprevention trials of upper aerodigestive tract cancer. Int J Cancer 88(6):852–855, 2000.
17. Shin DM, Khuri FR, Murphy B, et al: Combined interferon-alfa, 13-cis-retinoic acid, and alpha-tocopherol in locally advanced head and neck squamous cell carcinoma: novel bioadjuvant phase II trial. J Clin Oncol 19(12):3010–3017, 2001.
18. Garewal H: Chemoprevention of oral cancer: beta-carotene and vitamin E in leukoplakia. Eur J Cancer Prev 3(2):101–107, 1994.
19. Kaugars GE, Silverman S, Jr, Lovas JG, et al: A clinical trial of antioxidant supplements in the treatment of oral leukoplakia. Oral Surg Oral Med Oral Pathol 78(4):462–468, 1994.
20. The effect of vitamin E and beta carotene on the incidence of lung cancer and other cancers in male smokers. The Alpha-Tocopherol, Beta Carotene Cancer Prevention Study Group. N Engl J Med 330(15):1029–1035, 1994.
21. Omenn GS, Goodman GE, Thornquist MD, et al: Effects of a combination of beta carotene and vitamin A on lung cancer and cardiovascular disease. N Engl J Med 334(18):1150–1155, 1996.
22. Omenn GS, Goodman GE, Thornquist MD, et al: Risk factors for lung cancer and for intervention effects in CARET, the Beta-Carotene and Retinol Efficacy Trial. J Natl Cancer Inst 88(21):1550–1559, 1996.
23. Albanes D, Heinonen OP, Taylor PR, et al: Alpha-tocopherol and beta-carotene supplements and lung cancer incidence in the alpha-tocopherol, beta-carotene cancer prevention study: effects of base-line characteristics and study compliance. J Natl Cancer Inst 88(21):1560–1570, 1996.
24. Knekt P, Aromaa A, Maatela J, et al: Vitamin E and cancer prevention. Am J Clin Nutr 53(1 Suppl):283S–286S, 1991.
25. Benner SE, Winn RJ, Lippman SM, et al: Regression of oral leukoplakia with alpha-tocopherol: a community clinical oncology program chemoprevention study. J Natl Cancer Inst 85(1):44–47, 1993.
26. Bairati I, Meyer F, Gelinas M, et al: A randomized trial of antioxidant vitamins to prevent second primary cancers in head and neck cancer patients. J Natl Cancer Inst 97(7):481–488, 2005.
27. Combs GF, Jr, Clark LC, Turnbull BW: An analysis of cancer prevention by selenium. Biofactors 14(1-4):153–159, 2001.
28. Yadav SP, Gera A, Singh I, Chanda R: Serum selenium levels in patients with head and neck cancer. J Otolaryngol 31(4):216–219, 2003.
29. Gillison ML, Koch WM, Capone RB, et al: Prospective study of toenail selenium levels and cancer among women. J Natl Cancer Inst 87(7):497–505, 1995.

30. Hercberg S, Galan P, Preziosi P, et al: The SU.VI.MAX Study: a randomized, placebo-controlled trial of the health effects of antioxidant vitamins and minerals. Arch Intern Med 164(21): 2335–2342, 2004.

31. Mestre JR, Chan G, Zhang F, et al: Inhibition of cyclooxygenase-2 expression. An approach to preventing head and neck cancer. Ann N Y Acad Sci 889:62–71, 1999.

32. Chan G, Boyle JO, Yang EK, et al: Cyclooxygenase-2 expression is up-regulated in squamous cell carcinoma of the head and neck. Cancer Res 59(5):991–994, 1999.

33. Jung TT, Berlinger NT, Juhn SKL: Prostaglandins in squamous cell carcinoma of the head and neck: a preliminary study. Laryngoscope 95(3):307–312, 1985.

34. Feng L, Wang Z: Chemopreventive effect of celecoxib in oral precancers and cancers. Laryngoscope 116(10):1842–1845, 2006.

35. Zhang X, Chen ZG, Choe MS, et al: Tumor growth inhibition by simultaneously blocking epidermal growth factor receptor and cyclooxygenase-2 in a xenograft model. Clin Cancer Res 11(17):6261–6269, 2005.

36. Papadimitrakopoulou VA, William WN, Jr, Dannenberg AJ, et al: Pilot randomized phase II study of celecoxib in oral premalignant lesions. Clin Cancer Res 14(7):2095–2101, 2008.

37. Harris RE, Beebe-Donk J, Doss H, Burr Doss D: Aspirin, ibuprofen, and other non-steroidal anti-inflammatory drugs in cancer prevention: a critical review of non-selective COX-2 blockade (review). Oncol Rep 13(4):559–583, 2005.

38. Moysich KB, Menezes RJ, Ronsani A, et al: Regular aspirin use and lung cancer risk. BMC Cancer 2:31, 2002.

39. Farrow DC, Vaughan TL, Hansten PD, et al: Use of aspirin and other nonsteroidal anti-inflammatory drugs and risk of esophageal and gastric cancer. Cancer Epidemiol Biomarkers Prev 7(2):97–102, 1998.

40. Sharp L, Chilvers CE, Cheng KK, et al: Risk factors for squamous cell carcinoma of the oesophagus in women: a case-control study. Br J Cancer 85(11):1667–1670, 2001.

41. Bosetti C, Talamini R, Franceschi S, et al: Aspirin use and cancers of the upper aerodigestive tract. Br J Cancer 88(5):672–674, 2003.

42. Jayaprakash V, Rigual NR, Moysich KB, et al: Chemoprevention of head and neck cancer with aspirin: a case-control study. Arch Otolaryngol Head Neck Surg 132(11):1231–1236, 2006.

43. Anderson JA, Irish JC, McLachlin CM, Ngan B: H-ras oncogene mutation and human papillomavirus infection in oral carcinomas. Arch Otolaryngol Head Neck Surg 120(7):755–760, 1994.

44. Oku N, Shimada K, Itoh H: Ha-ras oncogene product in human oral squamous cell carcinoma. Kobe J Med Sci 35(5-6):277–286, 1989.

45. Alsina M, Fonseca R, Wilson EF, et al: Farnesyltransferase inhibitor tipifarnib is well tolerated, induces stabilization of disease, and inhibits farnesylation and oncogenic/tumor survival pathways in patients with advanced multiple myeloma. Blood 103(9):3271–3277, 2004.

46. Cortes J, Albitar M, Thomas D, et al: Efficacy of the farnesyl transferase inhibitor R115777 in chronic myeloid leukemia and other hematologic malignancies. Blood 101(5):1692–1697, 2003.

47. Kim ES, Kies MS, Fossella FV, et al: Phase II study of the farnesyltransferase inhibitor lonafarnib with paclitaxel in patients with taxane-refractory/resistant nonsmall cell lung carcinoma. Cancer 104(3):561–569, 2005.

48. Grunwald V, Hidalgo M: The epidermal growth factor receptor: a new target for anticancer therapy. Curr Probl Cancer 26(3):109–164, 2002.

49. Albanell J, Rojo F, Baselga J: Pharmacodynamic studies with the epidermal growth factor receptor tyrosine kinase inhibitor ZD1839. Semin Oncol 28(5 Suppl 16):56–66, 2001.

50. Grandis JR, Tweardy DJ: Elevated levels of transforming growth factor alpha and epidermal growth factor receptor messenger RNA are early markers of carcinogenesis in head and neck cancer. Cancer Res 53(15):3579–3584, 1993.

51. Kurie JM, Shin HJ, Lee JS, et al: Increased epidermal growth factor receptor expression in metaplastic bronchial epithelium. Clin Cancer Res 2(10):1787–1793, 2006.

52. Jung YD, Mansfield PF, Akagi M, et al: Effects of combination anti-vascular endothelial growth factor receptor and anti-epidermal growth factor receptor therapies on the growth of gastric cancer in a nude mouse model. Eur J Cancer 38(8):1133–1140, 2002.

53. Wachsberger PR, Burd R, Marero N, et al: Effect of the tumor vascular-damaging agent, ZD6126, on the radioresponse of U87 glioblastoma. Clin Cancer Res 11(2 Pt 1):835–842, 2005.

54. Bozec A, Sudaka A, Fischel JL, et al: Combined effects of bevacizumab with erlotinib and irradiation: a preclinical study on a head and neck cancer orthotopic model. Br J Cancer 99(1):93–99, 2008.

55. Koch WM, Brennan JA, Zahurak M, et al: p53 mutation and locoregional treatment failure in head and neck squamous cell carcinoma. J Natl Cancer Inst 88(21):1580–1586. 1996.

56. Shin DM, Kim J, Ro JY, et al: Activation of p53 gene expression in premalignant lesions during head and neck tumorigenesis. Cancer Res 54(2):321–326, 1994.

57. Rudin CM, Cohen EE, Papadimitrakopoulou VA, et al: An attenuated adenovirus, ONYX-015, as mouthwash therapy for premalignant oral dysplasia. J Clin Oncol 21(24):4546–4552, 2003.

58. Meeran SM, Katiyar SK: Cell cycle control as a basis for cancer chemoprevention through dietary agents. Front Biosci 13:2191–2202, 2008.

59. Li M, Zhang Z, Hill DL, et al: Curcumin, a dietary component, has anticancer, chemosensitization, and radiosensitization effects by down-regulating the MDM2 oncogene through the PI3K/mTOR/ETS2 pathway. Cancer Res 67(5):1988–1996, 2007.

60. Aggarwal BB, Shishodia S: Suppression of the nuclear factor-kappa B activation pathway by spice-derived phytochemicals: reasoning for seasoning. Ann N Y Acad Sci 1030:434–441, 2004.

61. Messina M, Barnes S: The role of soy products in reducing risk of cancer. J Natl Cancer Inst 83(8):541–546.

62. Messina MJ, Persky V, Setchell KD, Barnes S: Soy intake and cancer risk: a review of the in vitro and in vivo data. Nutr Cancer 21(2):113–131, 1994.

63. Tominaga S: Cancer incidence in Japanese in Japan, Hawaii, and western United States. Natl Cancer Inst Monogr 69:83–92, 1985.

64. Yavelow J, Collins M, Birk Y, et al: Nanomolar concentrations of Bowman-Birk soybean protease inhibitor suppress x-ray-induced transformation in vitro. Proc Natl Acad Sci U S A 82(16):5395–5399, 1985.

65. Armstrong WB, Kennedy AR, Wan XS, et al: Single-dose administration of Bowman-Birk inhibitor concentrate in patients with oral leukoplakia. Cancer Epidemiol Biomarkers Prev 9(1):43–47, 2000.

66. Armstrong WB, Kennedy AR, Wan XS, et al: Clinical modulation of oral leukoplakia and protease activity by Bowman-Birk inhibitor concentrate in a phase IIa chemoprevention trial. Clin Cancer Res 6(12):4684–4691, 2000.

67. Armstrong WB, Wan XS, Kennedy AR, et al: Development of the Bowman-Birk inhibitor for oral cancer chemoprevention and analysis of Neu immunohistochemical staining intensity with Bowman-Birk inhibitor concentrate treatment. Laryngoscope 113(10):1687–1702, 2003.

68. Masuda M, Suzui M, Weinstein IB: Effects of epigallocatechin-3-gallate on growth, epidermal growth factor receptor signaling pathways, gene expression, and chemosensitivity in human head and neck squamous cell carcinoma cell lines. Clin Cancer Res 7(12):4220–4229, 2001.

69. Sah JF, Balasubramanian S, Eckert RL, Rorke EA: Epigallocatechin-3-gallate inhibits epidermal growth factor receptor signaling pathway. Evidence for direct inhibition of ERK1/2 and AKT kinases. J Biol Chem 279(13):12755–12762, 2004.

70. Shimizu M, Deguchi A, Lim JT, et al: (-)-Epigallocatechin gallate and polyphenon E inhibit growth and activation of the epidermal growth factor receptor and human epidermal growth factor receptor-2 signaling pathways in human colon cancer cells. Clin Cancer Res 11(7):2735–2746, 2005.

71. Chen Z, Zhang X, Li M, et al: Simultaneously targeting epidermal growth factor receptor tyrosine kinase and cyclooxygenase-2, an efficient approach to inhibition of squamous cell carcinoma of the head and neck. Clin Cancer Res 10(17):5930–5939, 2004.

72. Shin DM, Ro JY, Hong WK, Hittelman WN: Dysregulation of epidermal growth factor receptor expression in premalignant lesions during head and neck tumorigenesis. Cancer Res 54(12):3153–3159, 1994.

73. Rubin Grandis J, Melhem MF, Gooding WE, et al: Levels of TGF-alpha and EGFR protein in head and neck squamous cell carcinoma and patient survival. J Natl Cancer Inst 90(11):824–832, 1998.

74. Zhang X, Zhang H, Tighiouart M, et al: Synergistic inhibition of head and neck tumor growth by green tea (-)-epigallocatechin-3-gallate and EGFR tyrosine kinase inhibitor. Int J Cancer123(5): 1005–1014, 2008.

75. Kreimer AR, Clifford GM, Boyle P, Franceschi S: Human papillomavirus types in head and neck squamous cell carcinomas worldwide: a systematic review. Cancer Epidemiol Biomarkers Prev 14(2):467–475, 2005.

76. Gillison ML, Koch WM, Capone RB, et al: Evidence for a causal association between human papillomavirus and a subset of head and neck cancers. J Natl Cancer Inst 92(9):709–720, 2000.

77. Badaracco G, Venuti A: Human papillomavirus therapeutic vaccines in head and neck tumors. Expert Rev Anticancer Ther 7(5):753–766, 2007.

muscle, the only abductor of the vocal fold. All muscles except the cricothyroid move the arytenoid cartilage in relation to the rest of the laryngeal framework to produce vocal fold adduction or abduction. The cricothyroid muscle produces tension and elongation of the vocal folds by rocking the thyroid cartilage on the cricoid and is innervated by the ipsilateral superior laryngeal nerve, which also carries the sensory afferent fibers of the larynx above the glottis. In general, both motor and sensory innervations of the larynx are strictly lateralized; that is, there is no cross-innervation. The interaryenoid muscle may be an exception to this.

Etiology

The etiology of laryngeal cancer is generally multifactorial. Tobacco smoking and alcohol intake have a strong synergistic effect in the pathogenesis of squamous cell cancer (SCC). After cessation of smoking, the risk gradually declines, and there is almost no excess risk found after 20 years. It is interesting that a multiplicative effect has also been found for tobacco smoking and alcohol consumption.[6-13] Habitual consumption of a tea known as *mate* is associated with an increased risk of developing cancer of the larynx.[11,13] Other risk factors have been reported, such as gastroesophageal reflux disease,[14-18] dietary factors,[14-18] and exposure to asbestos, ionizing radiation, wood dust, and nitrogen mustard.[19-21] Finally, cancer of the larynx has also been reported in individuals who have never smoked or consumed alcohol.[22,23] Human papillomavirus (HPV)-associated disease, particularly in nonsmokers, represents an important category of disease that may behave in a biologically distinct manner with regard to overall aggressiveness and responsiveness to radiation. However, HPV-16 rarely is found in laryngeal lesions, and HPV-11, which causes laryngeal papillomatosis, very rarely progresses to a malignant state.

Pathology

SCC, representing 97.4% of laryngeal malignancies, is the most common histologic type. The remainder of laryngeal cancer histologic subtypes represent less than 3%.[2] Most malignant laryngeal tumors arise from the surface epithelium and therefore are SCC or one of its variants such as spindle cell or verrucous carcinoma. Sarcomas, adenocarcinomas, neuroendocrine tumors, and other unusual neoplasms make up the remainder of malignant laryngeal cancers. More than 50% of laryngeal SCCs present as localized disease, 25% present with regional metastasis, and 15% are first seen at an advanced stage with or without distant metastasis.[24,25]

Epithelial Cancers

Most laryngeal SCC results from prolonged exposure to recognized carcinogens. Some of these changes are associated with keratosis.[26] The severity of dysplasia is described as mild, moderate, or severe, depending on the extent of involvement of the surface epithelium. In general, the degree of dysplasia correlates with the likelihood of transformation to invasive carcinoma.[27,28] At best, the gross appearance of a lesion of the mucosal surface is an inconsistent indicator of malignant potential. The term *leukoplakia* describes a white lesion, usually appearing as such because of keratinization. It is strongly suggested that dysplasia leads to carcinoma in situ (CIS), which then leads to invasive carcinoma, since the CIS is usually surrounded by dysplasia. CIS is a full-thickness mucosal epithelial dysplastic change without basement membrane invasion. Tumor thickness and the depth of tumor invasion are strongly correlated with cervical lymph nodes metastasis. In addition, the degree of cellular differentiation appears to correlate with the probability of cervical metastasis and

Table 7-1. TNM Staging of Cancer of the Larynx

Tumor Stage	Characteristics
Supraglottis	
T1	Tumor limited to one subsite of supraglottis with normal vocal fold mobility
T2	Tumor invades mucosa of more than one adjacent subsite of supraglottis or glottis or region outside the supraglottis (e.g., mucosa of base of tongue, vallecula, medial wall of pyriform sinus) without fixation of the larynx
T3	Tumor limited to larynx with vocal fold fixation or invades any of the following: postcricoid area, pre-epiglottic tissues, or minor thyroid erosion (inner cortex)
T4	Tumor invades through the thyroid cartilage, or extends into soft tissues of the neck, thyroid, or esophagus
	T4a: Resectable (e.g., tumor invades trachea, soft tissues of neck, strap muscles, thyroid, or esophagus)
	T4b: Unresectable (e.g., tumor invades prevertebral space, encases carotid artery, or invades mediastinal structures)
Glottis	
T1	Tumor limited to vocal fold(s) (may involve anterior or posterior commissure) with normal mobility
	T1a: Tumor limited to one vocal fold
	T1b: Tumor involves both vocal folds
T2	Tumor extends to supraglottis or subglottis, or with impaired vocal fold mobility
T3	Tumor limited to the larynx with vocal fold fixation, or invades paraglottic space, or minor thyroid cartilage erosion (inner cortex)
T4	Tumor invades through the thyroid cartilage or to other tissues beyond the larynx (e.g., trachea, soft tissues of neck including thyroid, pharynx)
	T4a: Resectable, see above
	T4b: Unresectable, see above
Subglottis	
T1	Tumor limited to the subglottis
T2	Tumor extends to vocal fold(s) with normal or impaired mobility
T3	Tumor limited to larynx with vocal fold fixation
T4	Tumor invades through cricoid or thyroid cartilage or extends to other tissues beyond the larynx (e.g., trachea, soft tissues of neck including thyroid, esophagus)
	T4a: Resectable. Tumor invades cricoid or thyroid cartilage or invades tissues beyond the larynx (e.g., trachea, soft tissues of neck, strap muscles, thyroid, or esophagus)
	T4b: Unresectable. Tumor invades prevertebral space, encases carotid artery, or invades mediastinum

Used with the permission of the American Joint Committee on Cancer (AJCC), Chicago, Illinois. The original source for this material is the AJCC Cancer Staging Manual, Sixth Edition (2002) published by Springer Science and Business Media LLC, www.springerlink.com.

survival, although the degree of cellular differentiation is not considered the most significant factor in grading the tumor[29,30] (Table 7-1).

Other Laryngeal Cancers

Verrucous carcinoma is also of squamous origin and occurs in the oral cavity, larynx, esophagus, and sinonasal tract and on the genitalia.[24,31] Some investigators consider it a separate entity[32]; however, others believe it to be a variant of well-differentiated SCC.[33]

Diagnosing verrucous carcinoma is difficult, even when the clinical index of suspicion is high. Although these lesions often destroy cartilage, they do not tend to metastasize, and aggressiveness is characterized by local invasion. The diagnosis is largely a clinical one, achieved most effectively by a pathologist and surgeon acting in concert. The typical verrucous carcinoma is slow-growing but relentless, appears exophytic and warty, is broad-based at its interface with the mucosa, and is either tan or white. The surface often is necrotic and infected, and the associated inflammation of adjacent tissues frequently is remarkable. This tendency to cause inflammation can erroneously influence treatment planning.[34,35]

Although SCC is regarded as a radiosensitive cancer, verrucous carcinoma is regarded as radioresistant.[36] In addition, the literature suggests a potential for radiation-induced dedifferentiation of these tumors into anaplastic cancer, which may occur in 7% to 30% of verrucous carcinomas.[31,36–43] Partial laryngeal surgery generally is considered the preferred strategy for verrucous larynx cancers.[44]

Recent diagnostic techniques, such as immunohistochemical analysis, allow elucidation of more unusual laryngeal malignancies, such as neuroendocrine carcinomas.[45–47] Surgical management of neuroendocrine carcinomas does not typically enhance survival.[47,48] Despite this, for other laryngeal tumors of neuroendocrine origin such as paragangliomas and carcinoid tumors, surgical management is the preferred treatment.[49]

Other rare tumors reported to arise in the larynx are cartilaginous malignancies, plasmacytomas, sarcomas, malignant fibrous histiocytomas, adenocarcinomas, melanomas, granular cell tumors, and primary lymphomas.[49–54]

Sites of Primary Disease

Supraglottis

Supraglottic carcinomas arise most commonly from the epiglottis and less frequently from the false vocal folds and aryepiglottic folds. They can be exophytic, ulcerative, or endophytic.[55,56] The substance of the epiglottis is often destroyed by tumors on its surface.[57,58] Early supraglottic carcinomas are initially confined to the pre-epiglottic space by the ligamentous boundaries of that compartment. Once those barriers are invaded, however, tumor growth occurs more rapidly.[57,59] Modern imaging modalities, especially magnetic resonance imaging (MRI), have greatly improved the ability to recognize tumor extension into the pre-epiglottic space and base of tongue. Assessing the pre-epiglottic space and the anterior thyroid lamina is of paramount importance for patients who may be candidates for either transoral laser microsurgery or open conservation laryngeal surgery. This is not always a straightforward endeavor, since patchy ossification in the laryngeal framework may present an ambiguous radiologic and clinical picture. Typically, however, healthy, nonossified cartilage provides a fairly resistant natural barrier to cancer invasion. Finally, the quandrangular membrane within the aryepiglottic fold plays an important role in diverting the leading edge of tumors.

Supraglottic carcinomas frequently metastasize to the cervical lymph nodes owing to the rich lymphatic drainage.[60–64] The incidence of patients demonstrating clinically positive lymph nodes at the time of diagnosis is 23% to 50% for supraglottic carcinoma of all stages.[37,56,65–68] If a neck dissection is performed, a substantial number of patients with clinically negative necks are found to have histologically identifiable disease. If left untreated, this progresses to gross disease.[61,62] In supraglottic cancers, the probability of cervical metastasis and of delayed contralateral metastasis increases in direct proportion to the size of the primary (i.e., the T stage).[55,69,70] This trend may not be predictive for patients who have been previously irradiated.[5]

With clinically positive cervical nodes measuring 2 cm or more, the incidence of contralateral neck metastasis may exceed 40%.[71] Cancers of the epiglottis are par-

HARPER COLLEGE LIBRARY
PALATINE, ILLINOIS 60067

ticularly prone to produce bilateral metastasis. Even early-stage lesions may produce bilateral metastasis in more than 20%.[70]

Glottis

Glottic carcinomas are the most common type of laryngeal cancer in the United States (Fig. 7-1). Two thirds are confined to the vocal folds. Tumors arise most commonly on the anterior two thirds of the vocal fold, whereas a small percentage are isolated to the anterior commissure. The posterior commissure is rarely affected.[72]

The relatively poor lymphatic drainage of the true vocal folds (except near the posterior commissure) makes early metastasis uncommon. In addition, the conus elasticus and the thyroglottic ligament tend to divert vocal fold lesions at the free margin from continuing into the underlying vocalis muscle and paraglottic space. Likewise, the anterior commissure ligament (Broyle's ligament) serves as a barrier to cancer spread outside the level of the glottis.[73] If Broyle's ligament becomes invaded

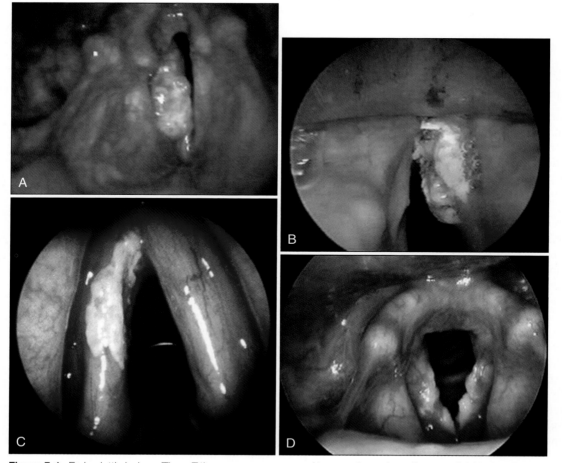

Figure 7-1. Early glottis lesions (Tis or T1) encompass a range of tumors, from plaquelike superficial lesions involving only part of one cord, to more endophytic lesions on both cords, to bulky lesions emanating from a mobile vocal fold. All of these could be treated with laser excision or radiation with a high likelihood of cure. **A,** Bulky lesion involving large portion of right true vocal fold. **B,** Similar bulky lesion of the right true vocal fold with apparent involvement of the anterior commissure. **C,** Plaque-like leukoplakia involving a large superficial area of the left true vocal fold. **D,** Multifocal bilateral ture vocal fold involvement.

with carcinoma, cartilage penetration is more likely.[74] This event is even more prevalent in the presence of thyroid cartilage ossification.[75,76]

When caudal extension does occur, extralaryngeal spread may occur into the anterior neck either into the soft tissue or the Delphian lymph node.[77] Of note, 1 centimeter of subglottic extension anteriorly or 4 to 5 mm of subglottic extension posteriorly puts the border of the tumor to the upper margin of the cricoid, which potentially limits options for conservation laryngeal surgery. In addition, when vocal ligament and thyroarytenoid muscle involvement occur, paraglottic space and thyroid cartilage involvement become more likely. Finally, the neck and thyroid gland may ultimately become involved with more aggressive lesions.

Subglottis

Subglottic cancers are unusual, constituting 1% to 8% of all laryngeal cancers.[72] They are mostly poorly differentiated and frequently demonstrate an infiltrative growth pattern. They involve the cricoid cartilage early because there is no intervening muscle layer. The incidence of cervical metastasis from subglottic cancer is reported to be 20% to 30%. The actual incidence, however, may be significantly higher because of primary spread to prelaryngeal and pretracheal nodal basins.[78,79]

Lymphatic Spread

The primary lymphatic drainage of the supraglottic larynx is to the jugulodigastric nodes. The submandibular area is rarely involved, and only a small risk of nodal involvement exists along the spinal accessory nerve. The incidence of clinically positive nodes exceeds 50% at the time of diagnosis, and bilateral nodal metastasis at diagnosis occurs in up to 16%.[60] Extension of the primary tumor to the piriform sinus, vallecula, and base of tongue increases the risk of lymph node metastases.

For glottic carcinoma, the incidence of clinically positive lymph nodes at diagnosis is negligible for Tl lesions and 1.7% for T2 lesions.[80] The incidence of cervical metastases rises to 20% to 30% for T3 and T4 tumors. Supraglottic spread is associated with metastasis to the jugulodigastric nodes. Anterior commissure and anterior subglottic invasion are associated with involvement of the Delphian node.

Pretreatment Evaluation

The preoperative workup of a patient suspected of having laryngeal cancer should serve to confirm the diagnosis through biopsy, to map the extent of the lesion, and to search for synchronous lesions and/or metastatic disease. When mapping the extent of the lesion, it is of paramount importance to focus the evaluation on findings that may indicate a worse prognosis such as anterior commissure involvement or on findings that may rule in or rule out certain laryngeal preservation procedures.

Office Examination

The preoperative evaluation starts at the initial office visit. A thorough history and physical examination should be obtained. During the physical exam, the lateral and medial compartments of the neck should be palpated carefully. Extension of the cancer through the laryngeal cartilage can sometimes be palpated. Laryngeal cancers with involvement of the subglottis may present with a Delphian node or paratracheal nodal disease. Loss of the normal crepitus palpated upon moving the larynx back and forth may indicate extension of the tumor into the postcricoid or prevertebral area. The base of tongue should be palpated to evaluate for superior extension.

Indirect mirror laryngoscopy is an invaluable tool for visualizing the larynx in the office. Most patients can be examined by this method. Limitations include an inability to visualize the subglottis, and limited visualization of the anterior commissure. In addition, a rigid 90-degree laryngoscope and a flexible fiberoptic laryngoscope may be used to further examine the larynx. By adding a stroboscopic light source, one can evaluate the mucosal wave of the true vocal folds, which may provide information regarding the depth of invasion of a glottic carcinoma. Also, the addition of a camera to the fiberoptic laryngoscope allows documentation photographically or videographically of the extent of the lesion. The rigid endoscope provides a larger, brighter picture, but patients tend to gag more often, and the larynx is not in physiologic position when examined. The flexible laryngoscope provides a more physiologic view of the larynx, and one can navigate beyond obstructing lesions to obtain a more distal view, including a view of the proximal subglottis.

Radiographic Imaging

Preoperative imaging often supplements the findings of the physical examination and can indicate subclinical involvement of the various spaces of the larynx. Computed tomography (CT) and MRI of the neck are both useful in this regard. Both can show invasion of the laryngeal framework by SCC. In addition, MRI can demonstrate involvement of the pre-epiglottic space and/or the paraglottic space that is not evident on physical exam. Radiographic delineation of the primary lesion is of critical importance when organ preservation modalities are used for treatment, since intensity-modulated radiation therapy (IMRT) techniques rely on precise anatomic details to inform the treatment protocols. In addition, several radiographic modalities, including CT, MRI, positron emission tomography (PET)-CT, and ultrasound are used in the search for regional and distant metastatic disease. PET-CT technology in particular has revolutionized the workup of distant metastatic disease. More traditional modalities used in a metastatic workup include a chest radiograph, liver function studies, and CT of the chest, abdomen, and pelvis as indicated.[81–83]

Direct Laryngoscopy and Biopsy

The latter imaging studies are not a substitute for operative assessment of the tumor with panendoscopy. Flexible or rigid esophagoscopy is performed to evaluate for synchronous primaries. A direct laryngoscopy or a suspension microlaryngoscopy is also performed to map the tumor more accurately and assess fixation of the arytenoid(s). The Dedo and Holinger laryngoscopes are used most often. The Holinger laryngoscope is particularly useful in investigating for laryngeal carcinoma because it provides excellent visualization of the anterior larynx and allows the examiner to maneuver around a larynx crowded with tumor. The Dedo laryngoscope is wider and allows the use of multiple instruments at the same time. It is more often used in suspension laryngoscopy, allowing the surgeon to have both hands free for instrumentation.

While mapping the tumor, it is important to document the anterior extent of tumor, anterior commissure involvement, involvement of the false vocal folds, ventricles, postcricoid area, hypopharyngeal mucosa, and mucosa of the arytenoids. Rigid telescopes can be used as an adjunct to examine extension of disease into the subglottis. All partial laryngeal procedures require at least one fully mobile and sensate cricoarytenoid complex and no involvement of the inter-arytenoid mucosa; therefore, this should be a focus of the laryngoscopy. Arytenoid fixation indicates involvement of the cricoarytenoid joint, or extralaryngeal spread with tumor, and may preclude conservation laryngeal surgery. True vocal fold fixation is not the same as arytenoid fixation as vocal folds may be fixed owing to the bulk of the tumor or to paraglottic space involvement, neither of which affect arytenoid mobility. Fiberoptic laryngoscopy and palpation of the vocal process of each arytenoid during operative laryngoscopy are the best ways to assess arytenoid mobility.[84,85]

Treatment Methods

Endoscopic Management of Early Larynx Cancer

The transoral laser microscopic approaches for surgically treating SCC of the larynx have improved significantly over the last 20 years with improvements in endoscopic instrumentation and laser technology. Advantages over primary radiation therapy or conservation laryngeal surgery include an abbreviated treatment time, potentially requiring only an outpatient surgical procedure. In addition, with transoral laser approaches, primary control is often attainable without necessitating the use of adjuvant radiation therapy. Early reports using transoral laser techniques validated the approach as being oncologically sound.[86] More recent reports demonstrate that both transoral laser microsurgery and primary radiation therapy provide roughly equivalent oncologic control. In their review of the existing literature comparing radiation therapy and transoral laser excision of early glottic cancers, Back and Sood[87] report a range of local control rates for early glottic cancer treated with radiation therapy from 85% to 94% for T1 lesions and from 68% to 80% for T2 lesions, whereas transoral excisions offer local control rates of 83% to 93% for T1 lesions and 73% to 89% for T2 lesions. Overall survival rates are also comparable. In addition, cost-benefit analyses argue for a transoral laser microsurgical approach. Myers and colleagues[88] demonstrated transoral laser surgery for T1 glottic lesions to be a cost-effective option compared with conservation laryngeal surgery and radiation therapy. In a later report from the same group, Smith and colleagues[89] demonstrated equivalent quality of life outcomes and functional results when comparing patients treated with endoscopic excision versus radiation therapy, but with the radiated patients experiencing increased number of work hours missed, as well as increased costs related to travel. Finally, although it has traditionally been accepted that vocal quality is superior after radiation therapy compared with transoral laser microsurgery for early glottic carcinomas, recent reports have brought this into question. Brandenburg[90] compared vocal quality in patients with T1 glottic carcinoma who received radiation therapy with those who received transoral laser microsurgery with a 63-month follow-up period. His findings demonstrated that whereas the postsurgical patient tended to have a more breathy voice, and the postradiation therapy patient tended to have a harsher, raspy voice, the overall vocal quality after laser cordotomy was comparable to voice quality after radiation therapy.

Transoral Treatment of Midcord T1 Lesions

Indications: These lesions are among the most readily accessible via a transoral endoscopic approach. Any lesion arising from the free edge of a mobile vocal fold is amenable to the transoral approach.

Contraindications: Unfavorable anatomy, includes patients with trismus or retrognathia, preventing adequate exposure for visualization and instrumentation. Also contraindicated is tumor extension to the lateral recess of the ventricle.

Technical considerations: For lesions of the midfold without evidence of vocal fold movement impairment or anterior commissure involvement, the transoral approach is fairly straightforward. A microflap technique, whereby a tissue plane is developed along the superficial lamina propria of the vocal fold, may be used to assess the depth of invasion in these lesions. Unlike the resection of a benign lesion, the microflap in this case is resected, but the approach may afford superior visualization of the depth of invasion and increased preservation of the vocal ligament. For larger lesions of the vocal fold, the CO_2 laser may aid in finesse control of the depth of dissection as well as hemostasis.

Endoscopic Cordectomy

Indications: The European Laryngological Society has developed a classification scheme addressing endoscopic excisions of vocal fold lesions, including those for endoscopic cordectomy[91] (Table 7-2). Using this classification, Gallo and colleagues[92] reviewed 156 patients with early glottic carcinoma treated with endoscopic laser surgery and stratified patients based on stage, thus advocating a specific type of cordectomy (Table 7-3).

Contraindications: Several series have demonstrated adverse outcomes in patients managed with transoral laser excisions who have anterior commissure involvement.[93] Visualization of the extent of the anterior commissure involevment may be difficult, and the anatomic attachment of the vocalis ligament to the inner aspect of the thyroid perichondrium offers little impediment to microscopic involvement of the cartilage. Other large series, however, show no difference in local control rates when comparing patients with and patients without anterior commissure involvement.[94,95] These controversies in the literature underscore the importance of thoroughly evaluating the anterior commissure with preoperative videostroboscopy, with preoperative imaging including CT and/or MRI to rule out thyroid cartilage invasion when there is any question of anterior commissure

Table 7-2. Endoscopic Cordectomy Classification by the European Laryngological Society

Subepithelial cordectomy	Type I
Subligmental cordectomy	Type II
Transmuscular cordectomy	Type III
Total or complete cordectomy	Type IV
Extended cordectomy encompassing:	
Contralateral vocal fold	Type IVa
Arytenoids	Type IVb
Ventricular fold	Type IVc
Subglottis	Type IVd

Table 7-3. Indication for Laser Resection by Stage

T Stage	Type of Cordectomy	Indication
T in situ	Type I Type II Type III	Depending on the extension of the involved area and the results of preoperative investigation (e.g., videostroboscopy)
T1a	Type III	Small (0.5–0.7 mm) superficial tumor involving middle third of TVF
T1a	Type IV	Tumor size > 0.7 mm and/or deep infiltrative pattern and/or anterior commissure involvement
T1b	Type Va	Involvement of the anterior commissure in a horseshoe pattern
	Bilateral cordectomy	Multifocal cancer

Adapted from Gallo A, de Vincentiis M, Manciocco V, et al. CO_2 laser cordectomy for early-stage glottic carcinoma: a long term follow-up of 156 cases. Laryngoscope 12:370–374, 2002.

involvement, and with the necessary endoscopic equipment requirements to ensure complete evaluation of the lesion before excision.

Technical considerations: One of the long-held principles of oncologic resection is Halstead's principle of en bloc resection. For the surgeon using transoral laser techniques, it is often not possible, nor advisable, to always attempt en bloc resection. A general principle of transoral laser techniques is that the initial incisions made with the laser are used to facilitate exposure of the tumor extent. This may include incisions through tumor, with additional laser cuts used to complete the resection with negative margins.

Endoscopic Supraglottic Laryngectomy (CO₂ Laser)

Indications: Lesions that are small and accessible are the most obvious candidates for endoscopic excision for cure, including lesions of the suprahyoid epiglottis and aryepiglottic folds. Infrahyoid epiglottic lesions and false vocal fold lesions may be more challenging to resect because of their tangential orientation to the distal end of the laryngoscope.[96]

Contraindications: As with open supraglottic laryngectomy, depending on the extent of resection, patients undergoing endoscopic laser resections are at risk for postoperative aspiration. An assessment of preoperative pulmonary function, as well as the involvement of a speech-language pathologist to assist in swallowing rehabilitation, is essential in these patients. In general, however, recovery of swallowing function in the patients who undergo endoscopic supraglottic laryngectomy is often faster and more satisfactory than those undergoing an open approach.

Technical considerations: As with glottic malignancies, en bloc resection is not essential to maintain the oncologic integrity of resection. In particular, lesions of the epiglottis may be divided by going directly through the tumor, facilitating the resection at the lateral margin. Instrumentation is particularly important when attempting endoscopic excision of supraglottic carcinomas. A variety of endoscope designs are available, including bivalved supraglottoscopes, which augment the area exposed for both visualization and instrumentation.

Endoscopic Extended Resections (CO₂ Laser)

Indications: The oncologic feasibility of CO_2 laser treatment of supraglottic carcinoma for T1 and T2 lesions is well established. For more extensive resections, transoral laser excisions may be permissible for selected patients. In their series of 124 patients treated with CO_2 laser excisions of supraglottic carcinomas, Motta and colleagues[97] stratified their patients into three categories based on T status (T1-3). For T3 patients, the investigators demonstrated acceptable 5-year local control rates of 77%. In this series, however, they stressed appropriate preoperative screening of these patients considering only those with limited pre-epiglottic space involvement.

Contraindications: CO_2 laser treatment of extensive pre-epiglottic space, tongue base or full-thickness lateral wall involvement is not recommended.

Technical considerations: Pre-epiglottic space involvement may be underestimated by standard imaging modalities necessitating re-staging based on operative findings or on final pathology. This is particularly relevant for tumors involving the laryngeal surface of the infrahyoid epiglottis. Davis and associates,[98] in their series of 46 endoscopic supraglottic laryngectomies staged as T2 preoperatively, found that 18 (39%) were upstaged based on pre-epiglottic space invasion noted on final pathology. Of note, in their series, all patients were offered planned postoperative radiation, with a 97% rate of primary control. Clearly, a thorough preoperative evaluation, including CT to rule out cartilage invasion, is essential in patients who are candidates for endoscopic extended resections.

Open Management of Early Glottic Cancer

Open management of glottic and supraglottic malignancies provides a time-tested, oncologically sound modality for the head and neck surgeon. In increasing level of complexity, the spectrum of these procedures ranges from laryngofissure with cordectomy and reconstruction, to vertical partial laryngectomy, to open supraglottic laryngectomy, and to supracricoid laryngectomy. Of paramount importance in determining whether a patient is a candidate for organ preservation surgery is the preoperative physical examination, including fiberoptic laryngoscopy. Arytenoid mobility must be carefully assessed, since arytenoid immobility secondary to cricoarytenoid joint involvement or extralaryngeal spread is a contraindication to organ preservation surgery. CT and MRI imaging modalities may aid in determining the extent of pre-epiglottic space and extralaryngeal involvement. Finally, detailed endoscopy under anesthesia using microscopic and/or endoscopic assistance to evaluate the subglottis is essential.

Cordectomy with Reconstruction

Indications: This approach is ideal for T1 glottic lesions that would otherwise be amenable to transoral laser microsurgical excision in patients with unfavorable anatomy. This includes patients with trismus or retrognathia, in whom adequate visualization of the entire larynx, particularly at the anterior commissure, is not possible.

Contraindications: Not recommended for cordectomy with reconstruction are more extensive lesions involving the contralateral vocal fold.

Technical considerations: The main advantage of cordectomy is the excellent visualization afforded by the laryngofissure. A tracheotomy is generally necessary. For simple cordectomy, healing by secondary intention is an acceptable initial strategy; however, patients are often left with a breathy voice. Several reconstruction strategies are available, aimed at improving voice and reducing aspiration. Injection medialization procedures in the setting of cordectomies are often suboptimal secondary to loss of tissue bulk, postoperative scarring, and fibrosis.[99] Alloplastic implant medialization techniques provide more consistent voice restoration. Finally, operative reconstruction based on the strap muscles to augment the neocord have shown some efficacy in voice restoration, with both open and endoscopic cordectomies.[100] Imbrication laryngoplasty may be carried out when minimal tumor involvement of the vocal fold permits resection without violation of the false fold and underlying cartilage. A horizontal strip of thyroid cartilage can then be removed allowing imbrication of the false fold to the glottic level.[101]

Vertical Partial Laryngectomy

Indications: Vertical partial laryngectomy (VPL) is most commonly used to treat T1 and select T2 lesions of the vocal fold. Local recurrence rates after vertical hemilaryngectomy for glottic carcinoma range from 0% to 11% for T1 lesions, 4% to 26% for T2 lesions, and up to 46% for T3 lesions.[102] Excellent oncologic control is generally obtained for T1 glottic carcinomas involving the mobile membranous vocal fold. Decreased oncologic control is evident with anterior commissure involvement, extension beyond the glottis, or impaired vocal fold mobility. T2

lesions with impaired vocal fold mobility may have differing degrees of thyroarytenoid invasion entering the paraglottic space, explaining decreased oncologic
control with vertical partial laryngectomy. Similarly, subglottic extension of T2
lesions may portend cricoid cartilage invasion, and extension into the supraglottis
via the ventricle may increase the risk of thyroid cartilage invasion.[103] These factors
may result in the understaging of selected T2 lesions, thus explaining the higher
local failure rates when vertical partial laryngectomy is used.

Contraindications: T3 lesions without cricoarytenoid joint involvement are better
addressed with a supracricoid laryngectomy.

Technical considerations: All vertical partial laryngectomies involve a laryngofissure
into the thyroid cartilage and paraglottic space. Placement of the thyrotomy
depends on the position of the tumor determined by endoscopy. In the standard
vertical partial laryngectomy, the resection extends from the anterior commissure
to include the full extent of one membranous vocal fold and intrinsic musculature
of the larynx to the vocal process of the arytenoid. The superior and inferior
margins of resection are from the false vocal fold to 5 mm below the level of the
true fold.[104] A variety of extensions to the basic vertical hemilaryngectomy have
been described, including the frontolateral vertical hemilaryngectomy, posterolat-
eral vertical hemilaryngectomy and extended vertical laryngectomy.[102] Of note,
when performing a vertical partial laryngectomy, it is advisable to tack the petiole
of the epiglottis back into position with a 2–0 Vicryl suture so that the epiglottis
does not prolapse posteriorly postoperatively. In addition, after the resection, the
anterior commissure of the contralateral side should be sutured to the thyroid
lamina to recreate tension of the vocal fold. As described for cordectomy with
laryngofissure, a variety of reconstructive techniques have been used to facilitate
voice restoration.

Open Supraglottic Laryngectomy

Indications: T1 and T2 lesions of the supraglottic larynx are indications for an open
supraglottic laryngectomy. Excellent local control has been reported for T1 and
T2 lesions with open supraglottic laryngectomy. T1 local control rates range from
90% to 100%, whereas T2 local control rates range from 85% to 100%. The data
on local control rates for more extensive lesions are less consistent, with T3 control
rates ranging from 0% to 75% and T4 control rates of 0% to 67%.[105–108] This dis-
crepancy in the literature may be a result of failure to appreciate extension of the
glottic level via paraglottic spread and pre-epiglottic space

Contraindications: Glottic level involvement, invasion of the cricoid or thyroid cartilage, involvement of the tongue base to within 1 cm of the circumvallate papillae,
involvement of the deep muscles of the tongue base and pre-epiglottic space are
contraindications for an open supraglottic laryngectomy.

Technical considerations: The open supraglottic laryngectomy is defined by both the
extent of the resection and the reconstruction. The typical supraglottic laryngectomy preserves both true vocal folds, both arytenoids, the tongue base, and the
hyoid bone. Pre-epiglottic space involvement necessitates resection of the hyoid,
which can otherwise be left intact. While resecting the hyoid, it is critical to preserve the superior laryngeal neurovascular pedicle, since successful swallowing
rehabilitation depends on this. The reconstruction varies among surgeons. The
approach of the senior author (R.P.T) reconstructs the neolarynx in a fashion
analogous to the reconstruction described for supracricoid laryngectomy. Three
separate, submucosal, interrupted 1-Vicryl sutures are looped around the remaining thyroid cartilage and inserted into the tongue base. In cases in which the
hyoid is preserved, the suture is looped around the hyoid as well. This creates an

impaction of the tongue base, with or without the hyoid bone, onto the remaining thyroid cartilage.

Supracricoid Laryngectomy

Indications: T1b, T2, T3, and selected T4 supraglottic and glottic carcinomas with decreased vocal fold motion or fixation, pre-epiglottic space invasion, glottic level involvement at the anterior commissure or ventricle, and limited thyroid cartilage invasion without frank extralaryngeal spread are indications for supracricoid laryngectomy. Excellent local control and actuarial 5-year survival rates have been reported for both early glottic lesions (T1b-T2) and more advanced lesions.[109] Chevalier and coworkers[110] reported a 5-year actuarial survival rate of 84.7% and local control rates of 97.3% in 112 patients with either vocal fold fixation or impaired motion on presentation.

Contraindications: Fixation of the arytenoid secondary to cricoarytenoid joint fixation, extrinsic laryngeal muscle involvement, or recurrent laryngeal nerve involvement, subglottic extension to the level beyond 1 cm or direct invasion of the cricoid, posterior commissure involvement, extralaryngeal spread, or extension to the outer perichondrium of the thyroid cartilage constitute contraindications to supracricoid laryngectomy.

Technical considerations: The supracricoid laryngectomy is likewise defined by both the extent of the resection and reconstruction. The surgical excision is en bloc and includes both true vocal folds, both false vocal folds, both paraglottic spaces, ± epiglottis, the entire thyroid cartilage and may include one partial or full arytenoid resection.

Some key surgical points include:

1. The disarticulation of the cricothyroid joint is of critical importance and should be performed carefully to prevent recurrent laryngeal nerve damage.
2. The cricothyroid membrane should be incised along the superior border of the cricoid cartilage, and the subglottic region should be inspected to rule out subglottic extension of the tumor.
3. The arytenoid cartilage (or posterior arytenoid mucosa if the arytenoid is resected) must be gently pulled forward so that it will remain in proper position postoperatively. This is achieved by placing a 4–0 Vicryl suture just above the vocal process or into the arytenoid mucosa and secured anteriorly with an air knot.
4. The reconstruction is predicated upon impacting the hyoid bone and tongue base ± the epiglottis to the cricoid cartilage using three symmetric 1-Vicryl submucosal sutures.
5. The tracheotomy should be placed at the level of the skin incision line, but the superior skin flap should be closed to the strap muscles to separate the tracheostoma from the remainder of the neck contents.

Radiation Therapy for Early Larynx Cancer

Part of the multidisciplinary evaluation of the patient with glottic carcinoma includes an assessment by a radiation oncologist. Early glottic malignancies are notable for low incidence of occult nodal metastasis, and, as such, single-modality treatment with curative radiation therapy is an acceptable option for many patients. Radiation therapy has several advantages, including its noninvasive nature, acceptable voice outcome, and excellent local control rates. For early-stage lesions, functional outcomes are generally good, with most patients experiencing only self-limited symptoms of mucositis, xerostomia, dysphagia, odynophagia, and local soft tissue reactions. Vocal quality has been demonstrated to change after radiation therapy, but most patients regain near-normal phonation after 1 year. Harrison and colleagues[111] prospectively examined patients treated with early glottic cancer through computer-assisted voice analysis and determined that the majority of irradiated patients with early glottic cancer demonstrated a decrease in breathiness and increased strain after primary radiation therapy, but enjoyed normal phonation 9 months after treatment.

Primary radiation therapy of glottic carcinoma results in excellent local control rates. In his review of patients treated with primary radiation therapy for T1 glottic carcinoma among a series from a single institution, Lee[112] reported local control rates between 81% to 93%. Local control rates for T2 glottic lesions ranged from 65% to 78%. Prognostic factors, such as involvement of the anterior commissure, tumor bulk, and the technical aspects of radiation biology have been evaluated in the literature. In several series, patients with involvement of the anterior commissure who were treated with primary radiation therapy fared worse in terms of local control, particularly for T1 lesions.[113,114] In a published 30-year experience of T1 glottic cancers treated with primary radiation therapy, Reddy and colleagues[115] examined the effects of tumor bulk, T stage, anterior commissure involvement, treatment duration, and fraction size on local control. Although anterior commissure involvement was not prognostic in this series, tumor bulk proved to be a significant prognostic factor on multivariate analysis, since patients with bulky tumors had lower local control and disease-free survival rates and shorter duration to recurrence than those with small tumors. Finally, technical aspects of radiation therapy, including total dose, fraction size, and overall treatment duration have been demonstrated to be significant prognostic factors for local control of T2, but not T1 carcinomas.[113]

Primary radiation therapy of early supraglottic malignancies likewise results in excellent local control rates. In contrast to glottic level malignancies, supraglottic carcinomas have extensive lymphatic networks bilaterally, resulting in a high incidence of occult jugulodigastric nodal metastasis at diagnosis. Local control after radiation therapy for early-stage supraglottic carcinoma ranges from 88% to 100% for T1 lesions and from 65% to 89% for T2 lesions.[116–121] Because of the concern for regional nodal metastasis, the treatment volume for carcinoma of the supraglottis includes both the primary lesion and the regional nodal basin.[122] The specifics of the radiation techniques vary, ranging from single fractionated once-daily treatments to twice-daily hyperfractionation and accelerated hyperfraction schedules.

Surgical Salvage of Early Cancer of the Larynx

Although total laryngectomy traditionally has been standard of care for surgical salvage of radiation failure laryngeal cancer, transoral laser microsurgical and open conservation laryngeal surgery approaches are gaining acceptance for selected patients who present with recurrence. Steiner and colleagues[123] have advocated transoral laser microsurgery as a surgical modality in the salvage setting for patients with recurrent glottic carcinoma after radiation. In their series of 34 patients with early and advanced recurrent glottic carcinoma after full-course radiation therapy, they demonstrated a 71% cure rate with one or more laser procedures, with only one patient requiring total laryngectomy (because of chondroradionecrosis).

Conservation laryngeal surgical approaches have also been used in the salvage setting with success. In their 20-year review of the MD Anderson Cancer Center experience of treating radiation failures with salvage surgery, Holsinger and associates[124] reported adherence to well-established contraindications for conservation laryngeal surgery approaches including arytenoid fixation, extensive pre-epiglottic space invasion, subglottic extension, and extralaryngeal spread to exclude patients who were inappropriate candidates. For patients who were good candidates, a conservation laryngeal surgical approach rather than total laryngectomy did not cause a demonstrable change in locoregional control or disease-free survival. Other groups have reported similar results. In their review of 15 patients treated with supracricoid partial laryngectomy for surgical salvage, Spriano and colleagues[125] reported excellent long-term oncologic control. Laccourreye and colleagues[126] demonstrated a 75% long-term larynx preservation rate with 100% local control for patients initially treated with supracricoid laryngectomy after failed radiation therapy. Motamed and colleagues[127] investigated open versus endolaryngeal approaches for surgical salvage in a review of the literature. In their meta-analysis of all published literature on surgical salvage in laryngeal cancer, they found a preponderance of evidence to support the role of conservation laryngeal surgery in the treatment of recurrent localized disease after radiation therapy. However, the researchers exhibited a modest benefit of open versus endolaryngeal approaches in overall local control.

Complications in the postoperative setting are higher in patients who have previously received radiation therapy. In radiation-naïve patients, supracricoid partial laryngectomy can be performed with low morbidity and mortality. In one of the largest series published of radiation-naïve patients undergoing supracricoid partial laryngectomy, Naudo and associates[128] demonstrated a 1% mortality rate and 12% local complication rate. Previously radiated patients seem to fare worse, however. In a series of 23 patients managed with supracricoid laryngectomy for surgical salvage over a 14-year period, Makeieff and colleagues[129] found that 17 of 23 patients experienced rapid recovery of swallowing; however, a significant percentage (17.4%) developed long-term swallowing impairments, with two patients dying from aspiration complications. Several series have demonstrated markedly elevated early and late complication rates in previously radiated patients. In their series, Laccourreye and colleagues[126] had a major complication rate of 42%. Spriano and associates[125] described a similarly high major complication rate in previously radiated patients. A subsequent series by the same group demonstrated that swallowing problems were the most common challenge in the previously radiated patient.[130] Likewise, in their meta-analysis, Marioni and colleagues[138] found prolonged dysphagia and aspiration to be more common in radiated patients, with aspiration pneumonia and neolaryngeal edema to be the most frequently reported postoperative complications overall. Several groups have advocated early gastrostomy tube placement for this reason.

Management of the Neck in Early Larynx Cancer

Factors influencing management of the neck in early glottic cancer include the TNM staging of the primary lesion, the subsite of the larynx involved, and the modality chosen to treat the primary lesion. As discussed previously, early-stage lesions of the glottic larynx have low rates of regional lymph node metastasis because of the relative paucity of lymphatic drainage from this area. For early-stage lesions of the glottis in the N0 neck, close observation is an acceptable management strategy. The supraglottic larynx, on the other hand, has an extensive bilateral network of lymphatics along the jugulodigastric nodal basin. Lutz and colleagues[132] at the University of Pittsburgh, in a retrospective review of 202 patients with supraglottic SCC treated with surgery or combined therapy, demonstrated a locoregional failure rate of 23%. In those treatment failures, 83% occurred in the neck with 90% of neck failures occurring in the undissected, contralateral side. A subsequent report by the same group showed a reduction in cervical recurrence from 20% to 9% by performing routine bilateral neck dissections in these patients.[133] In their most recent report advocating routine bilateral neck dissections in all patients with T2 to T4 lesions and selected patients with T1 lesions, this approach demonstrated a further risk reduction for cervical recurrence to 7.8%.[134] These data documenting such a significant risk reduction in locoregional failure in the neck provide a compelling argument for routine bilateral neck dissection in the management of supraglottic cancer. Steiner and colleagues,[135] in their 24-year series of patients treated with transoral laser resection of supraglottic carcinomas, advocate management of the neck by either neck dissection or postoperative radiation therapy. Observation of the neck in patients with selected T1 lesions treated with primary transoral laser mircrosurgery may be an acceptable management strategy in the N0 neck, although this remains controversial in the literature.

Management strategies of the neck in patients undergoing salvage laryngeal surgery for recurrent/persistent laryngeal cancer are highly variable. Yao and associates,[136] because of the risk of occult disease, advocate bilateral neck dissections for T3 and T4 recurrent glottic lesions, and bilateral neck dissections for all recurrent supraglottic lesions. In the institution of the senior author (R.P.T.), patients undergoing salvage total or supracricoid laryngectomy for laryngeal cancer recurrence/persistence after primary radiation therapy are staged by a preoperative CT scan. In patients staged N0, the neck is managed expectantly. We have previously reported no increased risk of recurrence in these patients with long-term follow-up.[137] The addition of PET-CT in both the preoperative staging and postoperative surveillance period could potentially aid the head and neck surgeon in assessing the risk of occult disease and treating the neck appropriately.

References

1. Jemal A, Siegel R, Ward E, et al: Cancer statistics, 2007. CA Cancer J Clin 57(1):43–66, 2007.
2. Davies L, Welch HG: Epidemiology of head and neck cancer in the United States. Otolaryngol Head Neck Surg 135(3):451–457, 2006.
3. Farrag TY, Koch WM, Cummings CW, et al: Supracricoid laryngectomy outcomes: the Johns Hopkins experience. Laryngoscope 117(1):129–132.
4. Farrag TY, Lin FR, Cummings CW, et al: Importance of routine evaluation of the thyroid gland prior to open partial laryngectomy. Arch Otolaryngol Head Neck Surg 132(10):1047–1051, 2006.
5. Farrag TY, Lin FR, Cummings CW, et al. Neck management in patients undergoing postradiotherapy salvage laryngeal surgery for recurrent/persistent laryngeal cancer. Laryngoscope 116(10):1864–1866, 2006.
6. Lewin F, Norell SE, Johansson H, et al: Smoking tobacco, oral snuff, and alcohol in the etiology of squamous cell carcinoma of the head and neck: a population-based case-referent study in Sweden. Cancer 82(7):1367–1375, 1998.
7. Maier H, Dietz A, Gewelke U, et al: Tobacco and alcohol and the risk of head and neck cancer. Clin Invest 70(3–4):320–327, 1992.
8. Maier H, Tisch M, Conradt C, et al: Alcohol drinking and cancer of the upper aerodigestive tract in women (abstract). Dtsch Med Wochenschr 124(28–29):851–854, 1999.
9. Russo A, Crosignani P, Berrino F: Tobacco smoking, alcohol drinking and dietary factors as determinants of new primaries among male laryngeal cancer patients: a case-cohort study. Tumori 82(6):519–525, 1996.
10. Crosignani P, Russo A, Tagliabue G, Berrino F: Tobacco and diet as determinants of survival in male laryngeal cancer patients. Int J Cancer 65(3):308–313, 1996.
11. De Stefani E, Correa P, Oreggia F, et al: Risk factors for laryngeal cancer. Cancer 60(12):3087–3091, 1987.
12. Freudenheim JL, Graham S, Byers TE, et al: Diet, smoking, and alcohol in cancer of the larynx: a case-control study. Nutr Cancer 17(1):43–45, 1992.
13. Goldenberg D, Lee J, Koch WM, et al: Habitual risk factors for head and neck cancer. Otolaryngol Head Neck Surg 131(6):986–993, 2004.
14. Galli J, Cammarota G, Volante M, et al: Laryngeal carcinoma and laryngo-pharyngeal reflux disease. Acta Otorhinolaryngol Ital 26(5)260–263, 2006.
15. Mercante G, Bacciu A, Ferri T, Bacciu S: Gastroesophageal reflux as a possible co-promoting factor in the development of the squamous-cell carcinoma of the oral cavity, of the larynx and of the pharynx. Acta Otorhinolaryngol Belg 57(2):113–117, 2003.
16. Galli J, Cammarota G, Calo L, et al: The role of acid and alkaline reflux in laryngeal squamous cell carcinoma. Laryngoscope 112(10):1861–1865, 2002.
17. Chen MY, Ott DJ, Casolo BJ, et al: Correlation of laryngeal and pharyngeal carcinomas and 24-hour pH monitoring of the esophagus and pharynx. Otolaryngol Head Neck Surg 119(5):460–462, 1998.
18. Galli J, Frenguelli A, Calo L, et al: Role of gastroesophageal reflux in precancerous conditions and in squamous cell carcinoma of the larynx: our experience. Acta Otorhinolaryngol Ital 21(6):350–355, 2001.
19. Kurozumi S, Harada Y, Sugimoto Y, et al: Airway malignancy in poisonous gas workers. J Laryngol Otol 91:217–225, 1997.
20. Morgan R, Shettigara P: Occupational asbestos exposure, smoking, and laryngeal carcinoma. Ann N Y Acad Sci 271:308–310, 1976.
21. Goolden A: Radiation cancer of the pharynx. Br Med J 2:1110–1112, 1951.
22. Wight R, Paleri V, Arullendran P: Current theories for the development of nonsmoking and nondrinking laryngeal carcinoma. Curr Opin Otolaryngol Head Neck Surg 11(2):73–77, 2003.
23. Leon X, Rinaldo A, Saffiotti U, Ferlito A: Laryngeal cancer in non-smoking and nondrinking patients. Acta Otolaryngol 124(6):664–669, 2004.
24. Luna MA, Tortoledo ME: Verrucous carcinoma. In Gnepp DR (ed): Pathology of the Head and Neck. New York: Churchill Livingstone, 1988, p 497.
25. Mansel RH, Vemeersch H: Panendoscopies for second primaries in head and neck cancer. Presented at: American Laryngological Society Meeting, May 1981, Vancouver, BC.
26. Crissman J: Laryngeal keratosis preceding laryngeal carcinoma. Arch Otolaryngol 108:445–448, 1982.

27. Sllamniku B, Bauer W, Painter C, et al: The transformation of laryngeal keratosis into invasive carcinoma. Am J Otolaryngol l0:42–54, 1989.

28. Hojslet PE, Nielsen VM, Palvio D: Premalignant lesions of the larynx. Acta Otolaryngol 107;150–155, 1989.

29. Kashima H: The characteristics of laryngeal cancer correlating with cervical lymph node metastasis. In Alberti P, Bryce D (eds): Workshops from the Centennial Conference on Laryngeal Cancer. East Norwalk, CT: Appleton-Century-Crofts, 1976, p 855.

30. Spiro RH, Alfonso AE, Parr HW, Strong EW: Cervical node metastases for epidermal carcinoma: a critical assessment of current staging. Am J Surg 128:562–567, 1974.

31. Biller HF, Ogura JH, Bauer WC: Verrucous cancer of the larynx. Laryngoscope 81:1323–1329, 1971.

32. Abramson AL, Brandsma J, Steinberg B, et al: Verrucous carcinoma of the larynx: possible human papillomavirus etiology. Acta Otolaryngol (Stockh) 111:709–715, 1985.

33. Glanz H, Kleinsasser O: Verrucous carcinoma of the larynx-a misnomer. Arch Otorhinolaryngol 244:108–111, 1987.

34. Medina JE, Dichtel W, Luna MA: Verrucous-squamous carcinomas of the oral cavity. A clinicopathologic study of 104 cases. Arch Otolaryngol 110:437–440, 1984.

35. Vidyasagar MS, Fernandes DJ, Kasturi D, et al: Radiotherapy and verrucous carcinoma of the oral cavity. A study of 107 cases. Acta Oncol 31:43–47, 1992.

36. Kraus FT, Perezmesa C: Verrucous carcinoma: clinical and pathological study of 105 cases involving oral cavity, larynx, and genitalia. Cancer 19:26–38, 1966.

37. Kirchner JA, Owen JR:. Five hundred cancers of the larynx and pyriform sinus. Laryngoscope 87:1288–1303, 1977.

38. Fonts EA, Greenlaw RH, Rush BF, et al: Verrucous squamous cell carcinoma of the oral cavity. Cancer 23:152–160, 1969.

39. Perez CA, Kraus FT, Evans JC, et al: Anaplastic transformation in verrucous carcinoma of the oral cavity after radiation therapy. Radiology 26:108–115, 1966.

40. Elliot GB, Macdougall JA, Elliot JD: Problems of verrucous squamous carcinoma. Ann Surg 177:21–29, 1973.

41. Hagen P, Lyons GD, Haindel C: Verrucous carcinoma of the larynx: role of human papillomavirus, radiation and surgery. Laryngoscope 103:253–257, 1993.

42. Demian SD, Bushkin FL, Echevarria RA: Perineural invasion and anaplastic transformation of verrucous carcinoma. Cancer 32:395–401, 1973

43. Tharp ME II, Shidnia H: Radiotherapy in the treatment of verrucous carcinoma of the head and neck. Laryngoscope 105:391–396, 1995.

44. Burns HP, van Nostrand AW, Bryce DP: Verrucous carcinoma of the larynx; management by radiotherapy and surgery. Ann Otol Rhinol Laryngol 85:538–543, 1976.

45. Hong W, O'Donoghue G, Sheetz S: Sequential response patterns to chemotherapy and radiotherapy in head and neck cancer. In Wagener D, Bligham G, Sweets V, et al (eds): Primary Chemotherapy in Cancer Medicine, vol. 201. New York: Alan R. Liss, 1985, p 191.

46. Myerowitz R, Barnes EL, Myers E: Small cell anaplastic (oat cell) carcinoma of the larynx. Laryngoscope 88:1697–1702, 1978.

47. Gould VE, Linnoila RI, Memoli VA, Warren W: Neuroendocrine components of the bronchopulmonary tract. Lab Invest 49:519–537, 1983.

48. Mullins JD, Newman RK, Coltman CA, Jr: Primary oat cell carcinoma of the larynx. Cancer 43:711–717, 1979.

49. Goldman NC, Hood CI, Singleton GG: Carcinoid of the larynx. Arch Otolaryngol 90:64–67, 1969.

50. Huizenga C, Balogh K: Cartilaginous tumors of the larynx. Cancer 36:201–210, 1970.

51. Blitzer A, Lawson W, Biller H: Malignant fibrous histiocytoma of the head and neck. Laryngoscope 87:1479–1499, 1977.

52. Maniglia AJ, Xue JW: Plasmacytoma of the larynx. Laryngoscope 93:741–744, 1983.

53. Booth JB, Osborn DA: Granular cell myoblastoma of the larynx. Acta Otolaryngol 70:279–293, 1970.

54. Anderson HA, Maisel RH, Cantrell RW: Isolated laryngeal lymphoma. Laryngoscope 86:1251–1257, 1976.

55. McGavran MH, Bauer WC, Ogura HJ: The incidence of cervical lymph node metastases from epidermoid carcinoma of the larynx and their relationship to certain characteristics of the primary tumor. Cancer l4:55–66, 1961.

56. Kirchner JA, Comog JL, Jr, Holmes RE: Transglottic cancer: its growth and spread within the larynx. Arch Otolaryngol 99:247–251, 1974.

57. Kirchner JA: One hundred laryngeal cancer studies by serial section. Ann Otol Rhinol Laryngol 78:689–709, 1969.

58. Olofsson J, Lord IJ, van Nostrand AW: Vocal cord fixation in laryngeal carcinoma. Acta Otolaryngol (Stockh) 75:496–510, 1973.

59. Micheau C, Luboinski B, Sancho H, et al: Modes of invasion of cancer of the larynx; a statistical, histological and radioclinical analysis of 120 cases. Cancer 38:346–360, 1976.

60. Lindberg R: Distribution of cervical lymph node metastases from squamous cell carcinoma of upper respiratory and digestive tracts. Cancer 29:1446–1449, 1972.

61. Ogura J, Biller H, Wette R: Elective neck dissection for pharyngeal and laryngeal cancers. Ann Otol Laryngol 60:646–650, 1971.

62. Putney FJ: Elective versus delayed neck dissection in cancer of the larynx. Surg Gynecol Obstet 112:736–742, 1961.

63. Fletcher GH: Elective irradiation of subclinical disease in cancers of the head and neck. Cancer 29:1450–1454, 1972.

64. Levendag P, Vikram B: The problem of neck relapse in early-stage supraglottic cancer—results of different treatment modalities for the clinically negative neck. Int J Radial Oncol Biol Phys 13:1621–1624, 1987.

65. Ogura JH, Sessions DG, Specter GJ: Conservation surgery for epidermoid carcinoma of the supraglottic larynx. Laryngoscope 85:1808–1815, 1975.

66. Fayos JV: Carcinoma of the endolarynx: results of irradiation. Cancer 35:1525–1532, 1975.

67. Hansen HS: Supraglottic carcinoma of the aryepiglottis fold. Laryngoscope 85:1667–1681, 1975.

68. Shah J, Tollefsen H: Epidermoid carcinoma of the supraglottic larynx. Am J Surg 128:494–499, 1974.

69. Ogura JH, Spector GJ, Sessions DG: Conservation surgery for carcinoma of the marginal area. Laryngoscope 85:1801–1807, 1975.

70. Biller HF, Davis WH, Ogura JH: Delayed contralateral cervical metastasis with laryngeal and laryngopharyngeal cancers. Laryngoscope 81:1499–1502, 1971.

71. Som ML: Conservation surgery for carcinoma of the supraglottis. J Laryngol Otol 84:655–678, 1970.

72. Lawson W, Biller H, Suen J: Cancer of the larynx. In Myers G, Suen J (eds): Cancer of the Head and Neck, 2nd ed. New York: Churchill Livingstone,1989, p 533.

73. Kirchner JA: Staging as seen in serial sections. Laryngoscope 85:1816–1821, 1975.

74. Fischer JJ: Anterior commissure cancer. In Alberti P, Bryce D (eds): Workshops from the Centennial Conference on Laryngeal Cancer. East Norwalk, CT: Appleton-Century-Crofts, 1976, p 679.

75. Jesse RH, Lindberg RD, Horiot JC: Vocal cord cancer with anterior commissure extension; choice of treatment. Am J Surg 122:437–439, 1971.

76. Sessions D, Ogura, J, Fried M: Laryngeal carcinoma involving anterior commissure and subglottis. In Alberti P, Bryce D (eds): Workshops from the Centennial Conference on Laryngeal Cancer. East Norwalk, CT: Appleton-Century-Crofts, 1976, pp 674–678.

77. Olofsson J, van Nostrand AWP: Growth and spread of laryngeal and hypopharyngeal carcinoma with reflections on the effect of preoperative irradiation: 139 cases studied by whole organ serial sectioning. Acta Otolaryngol Suppl (Stockh) 308:1–84, 1973.

78. Stell P: The subglottic space. In Alberti P, Bryce D (eds): Workshops from the Centennial Conference on Laryngeal Cancer. East Norwalk, CT: Appleton-Century-Crofts, 1976, p 682.

79. Harrison DE: The pathology and management of subglottic cancer. Ann Otol Rhinol Laryngol 80:6–12, 1971.

80. Mendenhall WM, Parsons IT, Stringer SP, et al: T1-T2 vocal cord carcinoma: a basis for comparing the results of radiotherapy and surgery. Head Neck Surg 10:373–377, 1988.

81. Mancuso AA: Imaging in patients with head and neck cancer. In Million RR, Cassisi NJ (eds): Management of Head and Neck Cancer: A Multidisciplinary Approach, 2nd ed. Philadelphia: JB Lippincott, 1994, pp 43–59.

82. McLaughlin MP, Mendenhall WM, Mancuso AA, et al: Retropharyngeal adenopathy as a predictor of outcome in squamous

cell carcinoma of the head and neck. Head Neck 17:190–198, 1995.

83. Mancuso AA. Hanafee WN: Computed Tomography and Magnetic Resonance Imaging of the Head and Neck, 2nd ed. Baltimore: Williams & Wilkins, 1985.

84. Verdonck-de Leeuw IM, Hilgers FJM, Keus RB, et al: Multidimensional assessment of voice characteristics after radiotherapy for early glottic cancer. Laryngoscope 109:241–248, 1999.

85. Benninger MS, Gillen J, Thieme P, et al: Factors associated with recurrence and voice quality following radiation therapy for T1 and T2 glottic carcinomas. Laryngoscope 104:294–298, 1994.

86. Casiano RR, Cooper JD, Lundy DS, et al: Laser cordectomy for T1 glottic carcinoma: a 10-year experience and videostroboscopic findings. Otolaryngol Head Neck Surg 104:831–837, 1991.

87. Back G, Sood S: The management of early laryngeal cancer: options for patients and therapists. Curr Opin Otolaryngol Head Neck Surg 13:85–91, 2005.

88. Myers EN, Wagner RL, Johnson JT: Microlaryngoscopic surgery for T1 glottic lesions: a cost-effective option. Ann Otol Rhinol Laryngol 103:28–30, 1994.

89. Smith JC, Johnson JT, Cognetti DM, et al: Quality of life, functional outcome and costs of early glottic cancer. Laryngoscope 113:68–76, 2003.

90. Brandenburg JH: Laser cordotomy versus radiotherapy: an objective cost analysis. Ann Otol Rhinol Laryngol 110:312–318, 2001.

91. Remacle M, Eckel HE, Antonelli A, et al: Endoscopic cordectomy: a proposal for a classification by the working committee: European Laryngological Society. Eur Arch Otorhinolaryngol 257:227–231, 2000.

92. Gallo A, de Vincentiis M, Manciocco V, et al: CO_2 laser cordectomy for early-stage glottic carcinoma: a long term follow-up of 156 cases. Laryngoscope 12:370–374, 2002.

93. Chen MF, Chang JT, Tsang NM, et al: Radiotherapy of early-stage glottic cancer: analysis of factors affecting prognosis. Ann Otol Rhinol Laryngol 112:904–911, 2003.

94. Zeitels SM, Hillman RE, Franco RA, et al: Voice and treatment outcome from phonosurgical management of early glottic cancer. Ann Otol Rhinol Laryngol Suppl 190:3–20, 2002.

95. Steiner W, Ambrosch P, Rodel RM, et al: Impact of anterior commissure involvement on local control of early glottic carcinoma treated by laser microresection. Laryngoscope 114:1485–1491, 2004.

96. Zeitels SM: Surgical management of early supraglottic cancer. Otolaryngol Clin North Am 30:59–78, 1997.

97. Motta G, Esposito E, Testa D, et al: CO2 laser treatment of supraglottic cancer. Head Neck 26:442–446, 2004.

98. Davis RK, Kriskovich MD, Galloway EB, et al: Endoscopic supraglottic laryngectomy with postoperative irradiation. Ann Otol Rhinol Laryngol 113:132–138, 2004.

99. Hsiung MW, Woo P, Minasian A, et al: Fat augmentation for glottic insufficiency. Laryngoscope 110:1026–1033, 2000.

100. Su CY, Chuang HC, Tsai SS, Chiu JF: Bipedicled strap muscle transposition for vocal fold defect after laser cordectomy in early glottic cancer patients. Laryngoscope 115:528–533, 2005.

101. Liu C, Ward PH, Pleet L: Imbrication reconstruction following partial laryngectomy. Ann Otol Rhinol Laryngol 195:567–571, 1986.

102. Tufano RP, Laccourreye O, Rassekh C, et al: Conservation laryngeal surgery. In Cummings' Otolaryngology—Head and Neck Surgery, 4th ed. Philadelphia: Elsevier Mosby, 2005, pp 2357–2358.

103. Mohr RM, Quenelle J, Shumrick DA: Vertico-frontolateral laryngectomy (hemilaryngectomy). Arch Otolaryngol 109:384–395, 1983.

104. Shah H: A view of partial laryngectomy in the treatment of laryngeal cancer. J Laryngol Otol 101:143–154, 1987.

105. Lee NK, Goepfert H, Wendt CD: Supraglottic laryngectomy for intermediate stage cancer: UT MD Anderson Cancer Center experience with combined therapy. Laryngoscope 100:831–836, 1990.

106. Burstein FD, Calcaterra TC: Supraglottic laryngectomy: series report and analysis of results. Laryngoscope 95:833–836, 1985.

107. Alonso Regules JE, Blasiak J, de Vilaseca BA: End results of partial horizontal (functional) laryngectomy in Uruguay. Can J Otolaryngol 4:397–399, 1975.

108. Spaulding CA, Constable WC, Levine PA, et al: Partial laryngectomy and radiotherapy for supraglottic cancer: a conservative approach. Ann Otol Rhinol Laryngol 98:125–129, 1988.

109. Laccourreye O, Muscatello L, Laccourreye L, et al: Supracricoid partial laryngectomy with cricohyoidoepiglottopexy for "early" glottic carcinoma classified as T1-T2N0 invading the anterior commissure. Am J Otolaryngol 18:385–390, 1997.

110. Chevalier D, Laccourreye O, Brasnu D, et al: Cricohyoidoepiglottopexy for glottic carcinoma with fixation or impaired motion of the true vocal cord: 5-year oncologic results with 112 patients. Ann Otol Rhinol Laryngol 106:364–369, 1997.

111. Harrison LB, Solomon B, Miller S, et al: Prospective computer-assisted voice analysis for patients with early stage glottic cancer: a preliminary report of the functional result of laryngeal irradiation. Int J Radiat Oncol Biol Phys 19:123–127, 1990.

112. Lee DJ: Definitive radiotherapy for squamous cell carcinoma of the larynx. Otolaryngol Clin North Am 35:1013–1033, 2002.

113. Le QT, Fu KK, Kroll S, et al: Influence of fraction size, total dose and overall time on local control of T1-T2 glottic carcinoma. Int J Radiat Oncol Biol Phys 39:115–126, 1997.

114. Nozaki M, Furata M, Murakami Y, et al: Radiation therapy for T1 glottic cancer: involvement of the anterior commissure. Anticancer Res 20:1121–1124, 2000.

115. Reddy SP, Hong RL, Naqda S, et al: Effect of tumor bulk on local control and survival of patients with T1 glottic cancer: a 30-year experience. Int J Radiat Oncol Biol Phys 69(5):1389–1394, 2007.

116. Ghossein NA, Bataini JP, Ennuyer A, et al: Local control and site of failure in radically irradiated supraglottic laryngeal cancer. Radiology 112:187–192, 1974.

117. Wall TJ, Peters LJ, Brown BW, et al: Relationship between lymph node status and primary tumor control probability in tumors of the supraglottic larynx. Int J Radiat Oncol Biol Phys 11:1895–1902, 1985.

118. Wang CC, Montgomery WW: Deciding on optimal management of supraglottic carcinoma. Oncology 5:41–46, 1991.

119. Nakfoor BM, Spiro IJ, Wang CC, et al: Results of accelerated radiotherapy for supraglottic carcinoma: a Massachusetts General Hospital and Massachusetts Eye and Ear Infirmary experience. Head Neck 20:379–384, 1998.

120. Sykes AJ, Slevin NJ, Gupta NK, et al: 331 cases of clinically node-negative supraglottic carcinoma of the larynx: a study of modest size fixed field radiotherapy approach. Int J Radiat Oncol Biol Phys 46:1109–1115, 2000.

121. Hinerman RW, Mendenhall WM, Amdur RJ, et al: Carcinoma of the supraglottic larynx: treatment results with radiotherapy alone or with planned neck dissection. Head Neck 24:456–467, 2002.

122. Kumar P: Radiation therapy for the larynx and hypopharynx. In Cummings Otolaryngology and Head and Neck Surgery, 4th ed. Philadelphia: Elsevier Mosby, 2005, pp 2401–2419.

123. Steiner W, Vogt P, Ambrosch P, et al: Transoral carbon dioxide laser microsurgery for recurrent glottic carcinoma after radiotherapy. Head Neck 26:477–484, 2004.

124. Holsinger FC, Funk E, Roberts DB, et al: Conservation laryngeal surgery versus total laryngectomy for radiation failure in laryngeal cancer. Head Neck 28:779–784, 2006.

125. Spriano G, Pellini R, Romano G, et al: Supracricoid partial laryngectomy as salvage surgery after radiation failure. Head Neck 24:759–765, 2002.

126. Laccourreye O, Weinstein G, Naudo P, et al: Supracricoid partial laryngectomy after failed laryngeal radiation therapy. Laryngoscope 106:495–498, 1996.

127. Motamed M, Laccourreye O, Bradley BJ: Salvage conservation laryngeal surgery after irradiation failure for early laryngeal cancer. Laryngoscope 116:451–455, 2006.

128. Naudo P, Laccourreye O, Weinstein G, et al: Functional outcome and prognosis factors after supracricoid partial laryngectomy with cricohyoidopexy. Ann Otol Rhinol Laryngol 106:291–295, 1997.

129. Makeieff M, Venegoni D, Mercante G, et al: Supracricoid partial laryngectomies after failure of radiation therapy. Laryngoscope 115:353–357, 2005.

130. Pellini R, Manciocco V, Spriano G: Functional outcome of supracricoid partial laryngectomy with cricohyoidopexy. Arch Otolaryngol Head Neck Surg 132:1221–1225, 2006.

131. Clark J, Morgan G, Veness M: Salvage with supracricoid partial laryngectomy after radiation failure. ANZ J Surg 75:958–962, 2005.

132. Lutz CK, Johnson JT, Wagner RL, et al: Supraglottic carcinoma: patterns of recurrence. Ann Otol Rhinol Laryngol 99:12–17, 1990.

133. Weber PC, Johnson JT, Myers EN: The impact of bilateral neck dissection on pattern of recurrence and survival in supraglottic carcinoma. Arch Otolaryngol Head Neck Surg 120:703–706, 1994.

134. Chiu RJ, Myers EN, Johnson JT: Efficacy of routine bilateral neck dissection in the management of supraglottic cancer. Otolaryngol Head Neck Surg 131:485–488, 2004.

135. Iro H, Waldfahrer F, Altendorf-Hofmann A, et al: Transoral laser surgery of supraglottic cancer: follow-up of 141 patients. Arch Otolaryngol Head Neck Surg 124:1245–1250, 1998.

136. Yao M, Roebuck JC, Holsinger FC, et al: Elective neck dissection during salvage laryngectomy. Am J Otolaryngol 26:388–392, 2005.

137. Farrag TY, Lin FR, Cummings CW, et al: Neck management in patients undergoing postradiotherapy salvage laryngeal surgery for recurrent/persistent laryngeal cancer. Laryngoscope 116:1864–1866, 2006.

138. Marioni G, Marchese-Ragona R, Pastore A, et al: The role of supracricoid laryngectomy for glottic carcinoma recurrence after radiotherapy failure: a critical review. Acta Otolaryngol 126:1245–1251.

8

Surgical Treatment of Early Oral Cavity and Oropharyngeal Cancers

David Goldenberg and Wayne M. Koch

KEY POINTS

- The accessible location of the oral cavity makes it an ideal site for early detection of epithelial malignancy.
- The less accessible nature of the oropharynx, together with a topography of deep crypts and mucosal folds, and prominent gag reflex which impedes examination of many patients makes the oropharyngeal a challenging site for early detection of cancer.
- Prolonged exposure to tobacco and alcohol is the principle risk factor for oral cancer, while human papillomavirus (HPV)-16 infection is responsible for most cases of oropharyngeal cancer.
- Metastasis to nodal basins in levels I and II correlates with primary lesion thickness in the oral cavity, whereas (more frequently) bilateral metastasis to levels II and III characterizes oropharyngeal cancers.
- Field precancerous change is common in cases of oral cavity cancer with associated recurrences and second primary lesions.
- Primary surgical extirpation is the mainstay of oral cavity cancer treatment. Combined chemotherapy and radiation therapy have taken ascendancy as preferred first-line treatment for all but the smallest oropharyngeal lesions.
- Advances in microvascular reconstruction and the advent of transoral laser and robotic surgery extend the surgical options available for oral cavity and oropharyngeal lesions.

Epidemiology

Each year 30,000 Americans are diagnosed with oral or oropharyngeal cancer. These entities cause over 8000 deaths, roughly one person every hour. Of the 30,000 newly diagnosed individuals, only 50% will be alive in 5 years. These statistics have not improved significantly over recent decades. In the United States, 36% of oral cavity/oropharyngeal cancer patients have localized disease at the time of diagnosis.[1] It is generally agreed that the stage of oral cavity/oropharyngeal cancer at the time of diagnosis is one of the most important prognostic factors. Small localized oral cancers are readily curable with single-modality therapy, with control rates approaching or exceeding 90%. Unfortunately, most oral cavity squamous cell carcinomas and oropharyngeal squamous cell carcinomas are detected only after they become symptomatic and are typically no longer early stage.

Anatomy

The oral cavity extends from the skin-vermilion junctions of the anterior lips to the junction of the hard and soft palates above and to the line of the circumvallate papillae below and is divided into the following specific areas: lip, anterior two thirds of tongue, buccal mucosa, floor of mouth, lower gingiva, retromolar trigone, upper gingival, and hard palate (Fig. 8-1). The oropharynx is located between the soft palate

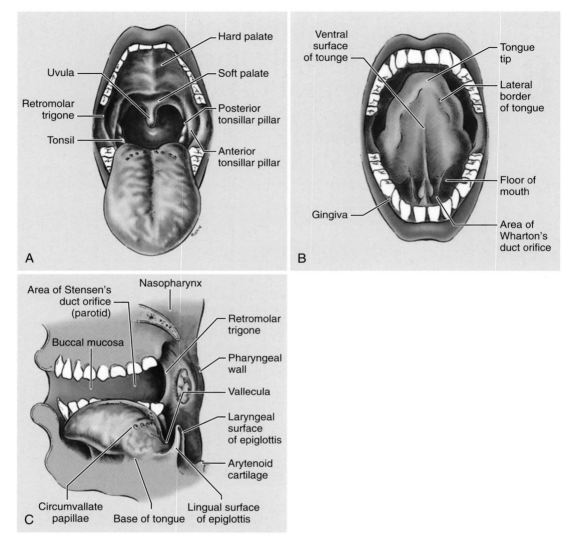

Figure 8-1. Anatomy of the oral cavity and oropharynx.   A, Open-mouth view. **B,** Tongue elevated, showing floor of mouth. **C,** Sagittal view. (From Abeloff MD, Armitage JO, Niederhuber JE, et al: Abeloff's Clincal Oncology, 4th ed. Philadelphia: Churchill Livingstone, 2008, Figure 72-18.)

superiorly and the vallecula inferiorly; it is continuous with the oral cavity anteriorly, the nasopharynx superiorly, and the supraglottic larynx and hypopharynx inferiorly. It contains the base of tongue, soft palate, palatine tonsils, uvula, and lateral and posterior oropharyngeal walls.

Etiology

Although this chapter discusses the treatment of both oral cavity and oropharyngeal carcinoma, it is important to recognize that these are two very distinct tumors with different risk factors, clinical behavior, treatment response, and outcomes. Oral cavity cancer (excluding lip cancer) is caused primarily by tobacco and alcohol abuse in the Western world. In Asia, where oral cancer is far more prevalent, chewing betel nuts with or without tobacco is a primary etiologic risk factor. Other known risk factors throughout the world include yerba mate, marijuana, and khat[2] (Fig. 8-2).

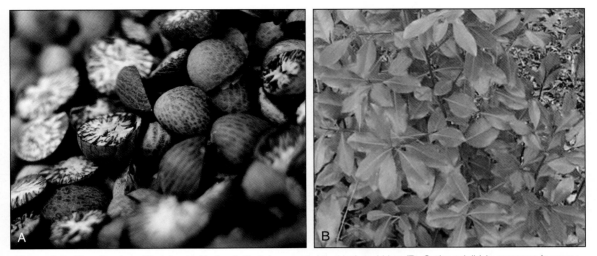

Figure 8-2. The chewing of betel nuts (**A,** the fruit of *Areca catechu Linn*) and khat (**B,** *Catha edulis*) is common in many parts of the world. Betel nuts are either crushed or sliced very thin; the fresh leaves of khat are chewed. Often tobacco is added to the ground nuts or leaves. (Photo A © iStockphoto.com. Photo B from www.tradewindsfruti.com.)

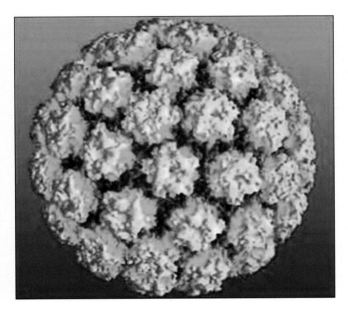

Figure 8-3. The molecular surface of the atomic model of human papillomavirus generated by researchers at the Harrison Laboratory of the Howard Hughes Medical Institute. (Courtesy of the Harrison Laboratory.)

Although oropharyngeal carcinoma is often caused by tobacco and alcohol abuse, there is a growing trend toward the development of oropharyngeal tumors in younger nonsmoking nondrinking persons. The human papillomavirus (HPV) is increasingly being recognized as an etiologic factor in oropharyngeal tumors of the palatine and lingual tonsils[3-5] (Fig. 8-3). HPV-16 is identified in most HPV-positive tumors, which have molecular-genetic alterations indicative of viral oncogene function.

Another distinct difference between oral cavity and oropharangeal carcinoma is the time course and tumor size at diagnosis. Cancers of the oral cavity are often readily visible on inspection by dental or medical primary care providers, or even by alert patients. Furthermore, because these lesions may be painful, they are amenable

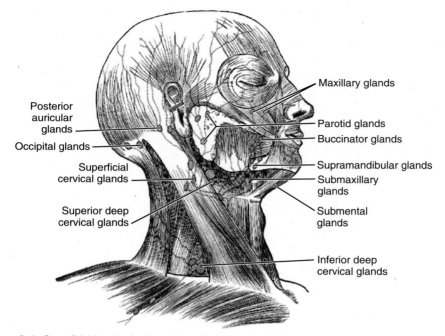

Figure 8-4. Superficial lymph glands and lymphatic vessels of the head and neck. (From Gray H: Anatomy of the Human Body, 20th ed. Philadelphia: Lea & Febiger, 1918, Fig. 602.)

to early detection. On the other hand, although oropharyngeal tumors may be small at diagnosis, lymph node metastasis is common because of the rich lymphatic drainage of the base of tongue and tonsillar region (Fig. 8-4). Approximately 70% of the patients have ipsilateral cervical nodal metastases; 30% or fewer have bilateral cervical lymph node metastases at diagnosis. Cervical lymph node metastases from oropharyngeal cancers may be cystic, mimicking benign cystic diseases.[6] Thus, although the primary tumor may be small, it is rare to detect oropharyngeal cancers at an early stage.

Diagnostic Workup

Lesions of the oral cavity are often detected by visual inspection. Certain subsites of the oral cavity are more likely to spawn lesions, particularly the lateral tongue, floor of mouth, alveolar surfaces, and buccal mucosa. The tongue dorsum and hard palate are uncommon locations for oral cancer.[7] These sites may occasionally manifest tumors of minor salivary gland origin. Lesions have several characteristic appearance patterns including leukoplakia (Fig. 8-5), erythroplakia (Fig. 8-6), ulceration, or exophytic growth. Palpable thickness and firmness as well as "friability," the tendency to blush or bleed with manipulation, are important features raising suspicion of cancer. Lesion surface extent and thickness should be estimated, as well as the presence of regional nodal metastases by palpation. Bimanual palpation of the submental and submandibular regions is important for the detection of small but firm nodes (Fig. 8-7). Radiologic imaging may contribute to the diagnostic evaluation through visualization of regional nodes and cortical bone erosion. Biopsy of oral lesions can often be accomplished in the outpatient clinic.

Oropharyngeal lesions are more difficult to detect because of their more posterior position exacerbated by the often overactive gag reflex of many individuals (Fig. 8-8). Furthermore, the deeply involuted and irregular surface of the palatine and lingual

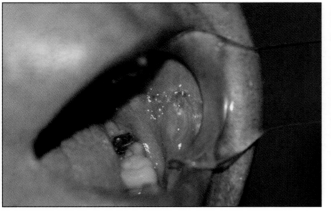

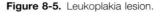

Figure 8-5. Leukoplakia lesion.

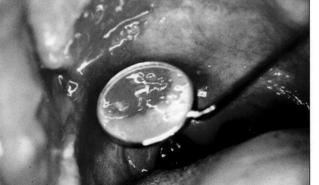

Figure 8-6. Erythroplakia lesion.

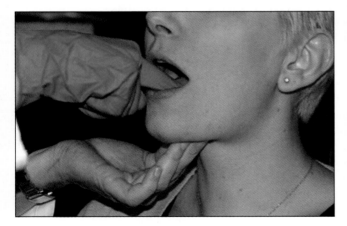

Figure 8-7. Bimanual examination of the submental and submandibular regions of oral cavity.

tonsils hinders visualization of small lesions. Palpation of tonsil and tongue base, though causing gagging, is actually reasonably well tolerated in the office setting and is the best method of detection of small tongue-base cancers. The presence of a firm, raised area may be detected. However, the relative difficulty of detection of oropharyngeal mucosal lesions and the early dissemination of these tumors into the rich lymphatic system results in many cases presenting as regional nodal metastasis without obvious primary source. Computed tomography (CT), magnetic resonance imaging

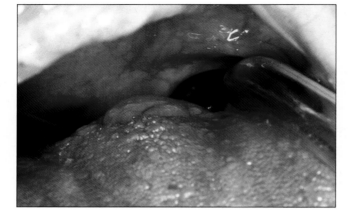

Figure 8-8. Tongue base tumor.

(MRI), or positron emission tomography (PET) may help identify the occult primary site in some cases, but in others, panendoscopy with biopsy of common primary site candidates is needed.

Bilateral tonsillectomy is recommended in a patient presenting with nodal metastasis of unknown primary when the palatine tonsils are in place.[8] The presence of HPV DNA in fine-needle aspirate samples of occult nodal metastasis further increases suspicion of an oropharyngeal tonsillar primary cancer.[9]

Prognostic Factors in Early Oral Cavity and Oropharyngeal Cancer

At surgery, the adequacy of resection is important. A positive pathologic resection margin conveys a higher risk of local recurrence, probably indicative of a more aggressive growth pattern that eludes physical judgment of disease extent.[10] Patients with microscopically clear margins at initial resection have a significantly better prognosis than those with positive margins even when repeated excision with subsequent negative margins is achieved or adjuvant postoperative radiation is given.[11] The determination of the tumor-free resection margin is highly dependent on the serial sectioning and fixation techniques. However, most authors agree that an adequate margin should be at least 5 mm wide in the resection specimen after ethanol fixation.

Tumor Thickness and Depth

Clinical staging takes into account the two-dimensional surface extent of an oral cancer, but does not consider the depth of invasion until there is evidence of bone or deep muscle invasion (T4). Many authors have reported tumor thickness of even small lesions to be a significant prognostic factor for the risk of occult nodal metastasis and hence higher stage and poorer outcome.[12,13] Kurokawa[14] found that tumor thickness was the only factor that had significant predictive value for subclinical nodal metastasis, local recurrence, and survival. They concluded that tumor thickness should be considered in the management planning of patients with early oral tongue carcinoma. Lim and colleagues[15] reported that tumor thickness greater than 4 mm (Fig. 8-9) and low immunohistochemical expression of E-cadherin predicted poorer outcome in early tongue cancers. Some authors report that the depth of invasion (and not thickness) of the oral tumor is key. Jones and associates[16] reported that a tumor depth over 5 mm significantly increases the risk of local recurrence in stage I and stage II oral squamous cell cancer and suggested that combined-modality treatment may be beneficial in these patients. Kane and colleagues[17] also concluded that depth is the most significant predictor of cervical node metastasis in early squamous

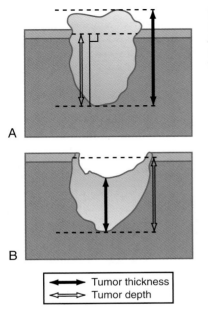

Figure 8-9. Graphic representation of tumor thickness and depth. Exophytic (**A**) and endophytic (**B**) tumors. (From Kane SV, Gupta M, Kakane AC, et al: Depth of invasion is the most significant histological predictor of subclinical cervical lymph node metastasis in early squamous carcinomas of the oral cavity. Eur J Surg Oncol 32(7):2006, Fig. 1.)

cell carcinomas of the oral cavity. Other important histologic prognostic parameters include grade of differentiation and lymphovascular and perineural invasion.[18]

Patients with HPV-positive oropharyngeal tumors reportedly have an improved prognosis when compared with patients with HPV-negative tumors in several published studies. Patients with HPV-positive tumors may have as much as a 60% to 80% reduction in risk of dying from cancer when compared with the HPV-negative patient.[4]

Treatment

Oropharyngeal and oral cavity cancer are best managed by a multidisciplinary team of health care professionals (Box 8-1). The relative infrequency of these cancers and the technical nature of oral cavity/oropharyngeal cancer treatment suggest that treatment of all but the simplest cases should be managed at cancer centers with experienced staff. All cases should be reviewed by a tumor board, consisting of pathologists, radiologists, head and neck surgeons, radiation oncologists, and medical oncologists. Other key team members include oral surgeons, primary dentists, and prosthodontists, speech-language pathologists, nutritionists, and social service professionals. At the multidisciplinary conference, the participants discuss each case in depth to optimize treatment planning.

The Primary Tumor

Depending on the site and extent of the primary tumor and the status of the lymph nodes, the treatment of lip and oral cavity cancer may be surgery alone, radiation therapy alone, or a combination of both modalities.

Surgical excision is typically the treatment of choice for early-stage primary disease (T1-T2) of the lip, floor of mouth, oral tongue, alveolar ridge, retromolar trigone, hard palate, or buccal mucosa. Surgery must adequately encompass all the gross as well as the presumed microscopic extent of disease. In most cases, local excision of the tumor with a margin of clinically uninvolved tissue of 1.0 to 1.5 cm in all dimensions including depth yields optimal 5-year survival rates.[19]

Box 8-1. The Multidisciplinary Team

Core Team Members
Pathologists

Radiologists

Head and neck surgeons

Radiation oncologists

Medical oncologists

Other Disciplines
Oral surgeons

Primary dentists and prosthodontists

Speech-language pathologists

Nutritionists

Social service professionals

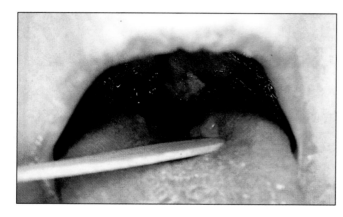

Figure 8-10. Squamous cell carcinoma of the oropharynx. (From Skarin AT (ed): Atlas of Diagnostic Oncology, 3rd ed. Philadelphia: Mosby, 2003, Fig. 3.50.)

Many small oral tumors can be surgically extirpated via the oral cavity with no need for lip or mandible split. If regional nodes are positive or if high risk of occult disease exists, cervical node dissection is usually performed at the same time.

The Oropharynx

The main goals in treating patients with oropharyngeal cancer are achieving a cure and preserving both speech and swallowing functions. Squamous cell cancer of the base of tongue is readily treated by surgery or radiation therapy (Fig. 8-10). Results are equivalent with respect to survival and locoregional control. Surgical treatment of early primary lesions has been associated with local control rates of 74% to 100%.[20]

However, surgery of the tongue base often causes speech and swallowing difficulty, which is not always fully compensated despite reconstructive procedures. If undertaken, surgery for early unilateral tongue base lesions entails resection of the base of tongue with primary closure. Surgical approach can be transoral, or it can be transcervical entering the pharynx above the hyoid or via a mandibulotomy, depending on the location of the tumor and the preference of the surgeon. Transoral resection of small tongue base lesions using the laser with or without robotic assistance is getting increasing attention and may permit adequate extirpation with minimal functional deficit.[21]

Tonsillectomy is often performed for diagnosis of tonsil cancer.[22] In the setting of very early occult disease, simple tonsillectomy may result in extirpation with adequate tumor margins. However, it does not achieve adequate surgical treatment in many cases. Before 1990, most tonsil cancers were treated definitively with surgery. Over the last decade, however, a number of reports have suggested that primary radiation therapy may offer a therapeutic and functional advantage for the treatment of early disease.[23] The phenomenon of nodal metastasis from palatine tonsils to the retropharyngeal nodal basin not included in standard neck dissection is often cited as a reason to treat patients with early oropharyngeal cancer with radiation even after surgical excision with adequate margins.

Treatment of the Neck in Early Oral and Oropharyngeal Malignancy

The patient with no clinical neck disease or very limited neck disease (N1) may be treated electively by radiation therapy or neck dissection. Because cure rates are generally comparable, the neck is generally treated with the same modality selected for the primary site. Regardless of the site of the primary tumor, a single lymph node found in either the ipsilateral or the contralateral side of the neck with extracapsular spread reduces the 5-year survival rate by 50%. The rate of metastasis reflects the aggressiveness of the primary tumor and is an important prognostic indicator. Modified and selective neck dissections clearly have been demonstrated as oncologically equal to the radical neck dissection in treating N0 neck disease.

Sentinel lymph node biopsy is proposed by some for evaluation of early oral cavity and oropharyngeal patients with clinically negative necks. Authors state that sentinel node technique has the potential to decrease the number of neck dissections performed in clinically negative necks.[24]

Transoral Laser Microsurgery

Laser excision of carcinomas of the upper aerodigestive tract has been advocated for several decades. The most widely used lasers are Nd:YAG and the CO_2 lasers. Transoral laser microsurgery (TLM) offers an alternative organ and function sparing surgical therapy to the primary tumor site. The benefits of TLM to patients include safety, shorter periods of hospitalization, organ preservation, and improved functional and cosmetic results.[25] TLM has been used in both oral cavity and oropharyngeal lesions. In one study, CO_2 laser microsurgery was found to be highly effective for accurate excision of early oral tongue cancers.[26]

Laser surgical treatment of cancer of the base of tongue presents a challenge even for experienced surgeons. A number of factors complicate the laser resection of carcinomas of the tongue base, including adequate exposure with identification of tumor borders and more pronounced carbonization encountered as a result of the increased vascularization and the glandular tissue present in the tongue.[27] The evidence base for long-term survival and functional outcomes for tongue base cancer have yet to be established, but preliminary results are encouraging.[28]

Transoral Robotic Surgery

The last decade has seen a tremendous growth in the field of robotic surgery with an increasing number of procedures performed each year. Several attributes of this technology may offer advantages in oropharyngeal surgery in that it allows for exceptional visualization of the operative field, precise handling of soft tissues, and multiplanar transection of tissues.[29]

Robot-assisted technology may overcome surgical limitations (such as line-of-sight obstruction and limited operative field). In one study, O'Malley and associates[21] concluded that transoral robotic surgery provides excellent three-dimensional visualization and instrument access that allowed excellent manipulation of the tongue base and shortened procedure time.

One of the disadvantages of robotic surgery is the large initial capital investment.

Photodynamic Therapy

Even in the treatment of small oral and oropharyngeal tumors, surgery and radiation therapy can cause considerable morbidity, such as xerostomia, disfiguration, and impairment of swallowing, mastication, and speech.[30] The method of photodynamic therapy (PDT) involves the use of a photosensitizing agent that is selectively concentrated in abnormal or neoplastic cells (Table 8-1). Depending on the type of photosensitizer, it may be injected intravenously, ingested orally, or applied topically.[31] After application of the photosensitizer, it is selectively retained by tumor cells so that after several hours to days (determined by the kinetics of the compound's distribution) there is more sensitizer in the neoplastic tissue than in the normal tissue. The photosensitizer is then activated with a specific wavelength of light matching the absorption characteristics that are unique to that specific photosensitizer, usually using a laser or other light source.

Initially, photodynamic therapy was considered experimental and had only limited applications for some superficially spreading tumors.[32] New powerful photosensitizing agents with reduced skin phototoxic effects and improvements in light sources have led to photodynamic therapy being regarded as a viable clinical alternative to more conventional treatment modalities. Within the last decade, numerous clinical investigations have demonstrated the effectiveness of photodynamic therapy with dihematoporphyrin ether (PHOTOFRIN), 5-aminolevulinic acid (ALA), and meta-tetrahydroxyphenylchlorin(mTHPC) in the treatment of minimally invasive early head and neck squamous cell carcinoma.[33-37]

The most extensively studied first-generation photosensitizer is PHOTOFRIN, which is photoactivated at 630 nm, penetrating tissues to a depth of 0.5 ± 1.0 cm (Fig. 8-11). Dihematoporphyrin ether (DHE) concentrates in malignant tissue, is activated by penetrating light (630 nm), produces fluorescence, and is photochemically efficient. The molecular and cellular mechanisms of PHOTOFRIN-mediated photodynamic therapy include two prominent theories or mode of action: (1) irreversible oxidation of cellular components via an energy transfer process from the light-activated or excited triplet state of the photosensitizing drug to oxygen-producing singlet oxygen, resulting in mitochondrial insult and apoptosis; and (2) vascular endothelial damage with erythrocyte leakage and ischemic tumor necrosis.[38]

Table 8-1. Commonly Used Photosensitizers in Head and Neck PDT					
Drug	**Dose (mg/kg)**	**Light (J/cm²)**	**DLI (hr)**	**Wavelength (nm)**	**Photosensitivity (days)**
PHOTOFRIN	2.0	80	48	630	28
Foscan	0.15	20	96	652	14
ALA	30–60[a]	80	6	630	1

[a]Also used as a topical cream with 10–20% ALA, with only local photosensitivity.
DLI, drug injection-light irradiation interval. From Allison RR, Cuenca RE, Downie GH, et al: Clinical photodynamic therapy of head and neck cancers: a review of applications and outcomes. Photodiag Photodyn Ther 2:205–222, 2005, Table 1.

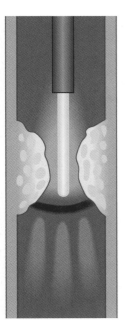

Figure 8-11. PHOTOFRIN by itself is inactive. After it is injected into tissues, it is activated by a laser, and together the PHOTOFRIN and laser destroy cancer cells.

A recent study has suggested that photodynamic therapy causes the suppression of factors responsible for tumor invasion (MMP-2 and MMP-9) and that this may play a role in the therapeutic value of photodynamic therapy.[39]

Reconstructive Options

Small surgical defects in the floor of mouth, buccal and hard palate mucosa may be left to heal by granulation and re-epithelialization. Lesions of the lateral tongue can often be closed primarily, although it is necessary to be sure that deep margins are clear, since primary closure will involute the deep surface farther into the tongue structure. Split-thickness skin grafts (STSG) provide epithelial lining that maintains tongue mobility and are particularly useful for lesions involving the ventral surface of the tongue and floor of mouth.[40] Meticulous attention to proper immobilization of the graft with a gauze bolster is a key feature in successful reconstruction using this approach. However, with early lesions that can be excised transorally, split-thickness skin grafts provide adequate reconstruction with far less time, expense, hospitalization, and donor site morbidity than more advanced reconstructive options, such as radial forearm free tissue transfer.

Conclusion

Of all sites in the head and neck, oral cavity lesions should be amenable to early detection because the mucosa is accessible for viewing by both the patient and general health care provider. Furthermore, the rich innervation of oral mucosa ensures that even small lesions are likely to elicit tenderness or pain. Early diagnosis is also facilitated by the accessibility to biopsy without general anesthesia. Lesions of the oropharynx are more challenging on both counts. Oral cavity lesions arise in typical smoker-drinkers, but also with an alarmingly increased frequency along the lateral tongue in young nonsmokers, making the selection of subjects for screening efforts more problematic.

Early detection is the first step toward the overall goal of early treatment, which holds the promise of greater efficacy (more likely, cure) with lesser morbidity, since single-modality treatment is sufficient in many cases. Typically, in the oral cavity that treatment is simple surgical extirpation.

Although standard surgery remains the mainstay of treatment, the oral cavity provides an ideal location for application of alternative approaches such as photodynamic therapy, whereas oropharyngeal lesions, typically treated with radiation, are increasingly the focus of attention of the newly developing programs using flexible laser fiberoptics and robotics. Whether these modalities will maintain high disease control with reduced morbidity remains to be demonstrated.

A second aim that should be feasible for many patients who present with an early oral lesion is maintenance of oral function, particularly articulation and deglutition. Treatments ideally should not unduly disrupt tongue motion, oral sensation, salivary function and dental health.

References

1. Wallner PE, Hanks GE, Kramer S, McClean CJ: Patterns of Care Study. Analysis of outcome survey data—anterior two-thirds of tongue and floor of mouth. Am J Clin Oncol 9(1):50–57, 1986.
2. Goldenberg D, Lee J, Koch WM, et al: Habitual risk factors for head and neck cancer. Otolaryngol Head Neck Surg 131(6):986–993, 2004.
3. Mork J, Lie AK, Glattre E, et al: Human papillomavirus infection as a risk factor for squamous-cell carcinoma of the head and neck. N Engl J Med 344(15):1125–1131, 2001.
4. Gillison ML, Koch WM, Capone RB, et al: Evidence for a causal association between human papillomavirus and a subset of head and neck cancers. J Natl Cancer Inst 92(9):709–720, 2000.
5. Gillison ML, Koch WM, Shah KV: Human papillomavirus in head and neck squamous cell carcinoma: are some head and neck cancers a sexually transmitted disease? Curr Opin Oncol 11(3):191–199, 1999.
6. Goldenberg D, Sciubba J, Koch W: Cystic metastasis from head and neck squamous cell cancer: a distinct disease variant? Head Neck 28(7):633–638, 2006.
7. Goldenberg D, Ardekian L, Rachmiel A, et al: Carcinoma of the dorsum of the tongue. Head Neck 22(2):190–194, 2000.
8. McQuone SJ, Eisele DW, Lee DJ, et al: Occult tonsillar carcinoma in the unknown primary. Laryngoscope 108:1605–1610, 1998.
9. Begum S, Gillison ML, Nicol TL, Westra WH: Detection of human papillomavirus-16 in fine-needle aspirates to determine tumor origin in patients with metastatic squamous cell carcinoma of the head and neck. Clin Cancer Res 13(4):1186–1191, 2007. [PMID: 17317828.]
10. Al-Rajhi N, Khafaga Y, El-Husseiny J, et al: Early stage carcinoma of oral tongue: prognostic factors for local control and survival. Oral Oncol 36(6):508–514, 2000.
11. Scholl P, Byers RM, Batsakis JG, et al: Microscopic cut-through of cancer in the surgical treatment of squamous carcinoma of the tongue. Prognostic and therapeutic implications. Am J Surg 152(4):354–360, 1986.
12. Moore C, Kuhns JG, Greenberg RA: Thickness as prognostic aid in upper aerodigestive tract cancer. Arch Surg 121(12): 1410–1414, 1986.
13. Ambrosch P, Kron M, Fischer JG, Brinck U: Micrometastases in carcinoma of the upper aerodigestive tract: detection, risk of metastasizing, and prognostic value of depth of invasion. Head Neck 17(6):473–479, 1995.
14. Kurokawa H, Yamashita Y, Takeda S, et al: Risk factors for late cervical lymph node metastases in patients with stage I or II carcinoma of the tongue. Head Neck 24(8):731–736, 2002. [PMID: 12203797.]
15. Lim SC, Zhang S, Ishii G, et al: Predictive markers for late cervical metastasis in stage I and II invasive squamous cell carcinoma of the oral tongue. Clin Cancer Res 10(1 Pt 1):166–172, 2004. [PMID: 14734465.]
16. Jones KR, Lodge-Regal LD, Reddick RL, et al: Prognostic factors in the recurrence of stage I and II squamous cell cancer of the oral cavity. Arch Otolaryngol Head Neck Surg 118(5):483–485, 1992.
17. Kane SV, Gupta M, Kakane AC, D'Cruz A: Depth of invasion is the most significant histological predictor of subclinical cervical lymph node metastasis in early squamous carcinomas of the oral cavity. Eur J Surg Oncol 32(7):795–803, 2006.
18. Martinez-Gimeno C, Rodriguez EM, Vila CN, Varela CL: Squamous cell carcinoma of the oral cavity: a clinicopathologic scoring system for evaluating risk of cervical lymph node metastasis. Laryngoscope 105(7 Pt 1):728–733, 1995.
19. Mashberg A, Samit A: Early diagnosis of asymptomatic oral and oropharyngeal squamous cancers. CA Cancer J Clin 45(6):328–351, 1995.
20. Gourin CG, Johnson JT: Surgical treatment of squamous cell carcinoma of the base of tongue. Head Neck 23(8):653–660, 2001.
21. O'Malley BW, Jr, Weinstein GS, Snyder W, Hockstein NG: Transoral robotic surgery (TORS) for base of tongue neoplasms. Laryngoscope 116(8):1465–1472, 2006.
22. Koch WM, Bhatti M, Williams MF, Eisele DW: Oncologic rationale for bilateral tonsillectomy in head and neck squamous cell carcinoma of unknown primary source. Otolaryngol Head Neck Surg 124(3):331–333, 2001.
23. Moose BD, Kelly MD, Levine PA, et al: Definitive radiotherapy for T1 and T2 squamous cell carcinoma of the tonsil. Head Neck 17(4):334–338, 1995.
24. Tschopp L, Nuyens M, Stauffer E, et al: The value of frozen section analysis of the sentinel lymph node in clinically N0 squamous cell carcinoma of the oral cavity and oropharynx. Otolaryngol Head Neck Surg 132(1):99–102, 2005. [PMID: 15632917.]
25. Grant DG, Salassa JR, Hinni ML, et al: Carcinoma of the tongue base treated by transoral laser microsurgery, part one: untreated tumors, a prospective analysis of oncologic and functional outcomes. Laryngoscope 116(12):2150–2155, 2006.
26. Wang CP, Chang SY, Wu JD, Tai SK: Carbon dioxide laser microsurgery for tongue cancer: surgical techniques and long-term results. J Otolaryngol 30(1):19–23, 2001.
27. Werner JA, Dunne AA, Foltz BJ, Lippert BM: Transoral laser microsurgery in carcinomas of the oral cavity, pharynx, and larynx. Cancer Control 9(5):379–386, 2002.
28. Steiner W, Fierek O, Ambrosch P, et al: Transoral laser microsurgery for squamous cell carcinoma of the base of the tongue. Arch Otolaryngol Head Neck Surg 129(1):36–43, 2003.
29. Hockstein NG, O'Malley BW, Jr, Weinstein GS: Assessment of intraoperative safety in transoral robotic surgery. Laryngoscope 116(2):165–168, 2006.
30. Sciubba J, Goldenberg D: Oral complications of radiotherapy. Lancet Oncol 7(2):175–183, 2006.
31. Biel M: Advances in photodynamic therapy for the treatment of head and neck cancers. Lasers Surg Med 38(5):349–355, 2006.
32. Schweitzer VG: Photodynamic therapy for treatment of head and neck cancer. Otolaryngol Head Neck Surg 102(3):225–232, 1990.

33. Biel MA: Photodynamic therapy and the treatment of head and neck cancers. J Clin Laser Med Surg 14(5):239–244, 1996.

34. Gluckman JL: Hematoporphyrin photodynamic therapy: is there truly a future in head and neck oncology? Reflections on a 5-year experience. Laryngoscope 101(1 Pt 1):36–42, 1991.

35. Gluckman JL: Photodynamic therapy for head and neck neoplasms. Otolaryngol Clin North Am 24(6):1559–1567, 1991.

36. Grossweiner LI, Hill JH, Lobraico RV: Photodynamic therapy of head and neck squamous cell carcinoma: optical dosimetry and clinical trial. Photochem Photobiol 46(5):911–917, 1987.

37. Wenig BL, Kurtzman DM, Grossweiner LI, et al: Photodynamic therapy in the treatment of squamous cell carcinoma of the head and neck. Arch Otolaryngol Head Neck Surg 116(11):1267–1270, 1990.

38. Schweitzer VG: PHOTOFRIN-mediated photodynamic therapy for treatment of early stage oral cavity and laryngeal malignancies. Lasers Surg Med 29(4):305–313, 2001.

39. Sharwani A, Jerjes W, Hopper C, et al: Photodynamic therapy down-regulates the invasion promoting factors in human oral cancer. Arch Oral Biol 51(12):1104–1111, 2006.

40. Schramm VL, Johnson JT, Myers EN: Skin grafts and flaps in oral cavity reconstruction. Arch Otolaryngol 109(3):175–177, 1983.

9

Early Treatment with Radiation and Chemotherapy

Boris Hristov, Michael K. Gibson, and Gopal Bajaj

KEY POINTS

- Head and neck squamous cell carcinoma (HNSCC) develops in a stepwise progression from early premalignancy to invasive cancer.
- On a molecular level, this progression involves a "field effect," in which carcinogen exposure can cause premalignant changes to cells throughout the mucosal area.
- Radiation therapy and surgery are currently the two preferred treatments. Chemotherapy shows great promise in addressing the challenges of early treatment of HNSCC, especially with patients who are at high risk for progressing to invasive cancer; however, more study is needed to improve delivery and prove effectiveness.
- Radiation therapy derives its main therapeutic advantage from the differential response of normal and cancerous cells to radiation as defined by radiobiologic principles of repair, repopulation, reassortment, and reoxygenation. Altered fractionation regimens and recent technologic advances in the field hold the promise of further widening this therapeutic window.
- Premalignant lesions (e.g., carcinoma in situ [CIS]) are amenable to definitive radiation therapy and may be treated with small opposed lateral fields with minimal toxicity. Recent evidence supports the use of higher doses per fraction for these slower-growing preinvasive entities.
- T1 and T2N0 laryngeal cancer can be effectively treated with radiation therapy alone; small opposed lateral fields are generally used unless the lesion is supraglottic or invading the supraglottis/subglottis, in which case elective nodal irradiation is carried out. Although functional outcome comparisons between surgery and radiation are scant, the effectiveness of both modalities in terms of local control is similar.
- The preferred treatment for patients with early oropharyngeal cancer is definitive radiation therapy; parotid-sparing techniques (e.g., intensity-modulated radiation therapy [IMRT]) should be used to reduce the incidence of late complications, particularly xerostomia.
- The preferred initial treatment for early cancer of the oral cavity is surgery, followed by radiation therapy as indicated. Selected lesions and tumors at certain sites are, however, quite amenable to definitive radiation therapy; tumor thickness/depth of invasion are important predictors of outcomes after treatment.
- Brachytherapy is a way of delivering dose through radioactive sources to a very localized area in an attempt to spare normal tissues; this technique has been successfully used, either alone or in conjunction with external-beam radiation therapy, in selected early cancers of the oropharynx and the oral cavity.
- Adverse effects from radiation can be either acute or late in manifestation, and their magnitude depends on a variety of factors. When compared with early-stage laryngeal cancer, lesions of the oral cavity and oropharynx carry a relatively higher risk of adverse effects from radiation owing to their close proximity to some important normal structures (i.e., parotid glands, mandible, etc) and to their general requirement for elective nodal treatment.
- Current research efforts in chemotherapy are pursuing approaches that target the epidermal growth factor receptor (EGFR). EGFR is expressed in virtually all preinvasive and invasive HNSCC, and, when combined with radiation therapy, targeting EGFR contributes to the control of advanced disease. These factors have prompted the investigation of drugs that target this protein for use in early treatment of HNSCC.

Introduction

Head and neck squamous cell cancer (HNSCC) remains a significant cause of morbidity worldwide, with approximately 400,000 new cases per year. At diagnosis, more than 50% of patients present with advanced locoregional disease.[1,2] Of these, less than 30% are alive at 5 years after conventional surgery plus radiation therapy. Although ongoing advances in combined modality therapy (CMT) continue to improve locoregional control, 60% to 70% of patients still experience recurrence within 2 years, and 20% to 30% develop distant metastases.[3]

Treatment of early cancer or even preneoplasia offers a chance at a higher rate of cure. Specific aspects of HNSCC make this early treatment challenging. For example, one common attribute is field cancerization, in which exposure to a carcinogen can cause precancerous changes to cells throughout the entire mucosal landscape. Because of this, treatment in one area may not prevent cancer from arising in other mucosal areas.

There are three approaches for dealing with early HNSCC: surgery, radiation, and chemotherapy. Surgery and radiation therapy are currently the dominant approaches. These approaches are well understood, and oncologists continue to fine-tune the exact combination of surgery and radiation and the order and dosages that result in higher rates of cure and better quality of life after treatment. The first section of this chapter provides a detailed summary of the current use of radiation therapy (often combined with or used instead of surgery) in managing early HNSCC.

Chemotherapy is the least studied of the three approaches, although early studies show that it has great promise in its ability to address field cancerization and the role that epidermal growth factor receptor (EGFR) plays in the growth of HNSCC. The second section of this chapter explores the potential of chemotherapy in early treatment of HNSCC.

Radiation Therapy

General Radiotherapeutic Principles

Radiation therapy has played a long and prominent role in the management of head and neck malignancies. Just like surgery, it is an important way of achieving locoregional control and of potentially affecting long-term cure, especially in patients with early carcinomas of the head and neck. Radiation exerts its effects by the planned and targeted deposition of large amounts of energy in tissues. As a matter of fact, the gray (Gy), which is the principal unit of dose in radiation therapy, represents energy delivered per unit mass and is quantified in joules per kilogram (J/kg). Radiation exerts its deleterious effect primarily by ionizing atoms and molecules, which in turn leads to the formation of highly unstable and reactive chemical moieties that interact with tissues. The biologic changes that result from these ionization events occur at the cellular level and result primarily from damage to critical molecules, such as DNA. Depending on the type of radiation delivered, the effect can be either direct or indirect and can result in either single-stranded or double-stranded DNA breaks. Direct damage is common with heavy charged particles (e.g., protons), whereas indirect damage predominates with electromagnetic radiation (e.g., photon irradiation). The latter effect is called indirect because the energy deposited affects the water molecules in tissues first, causing the creation of highly reactive hydroxide radicals that then go on to directly damage the DNA strands. Since photon irradiation is the most common way of delivering radiation today, the indirect effect is the principal mechanism by which radiation exerts its effects on cancerous and normal cells alike.

By disrupting the genomic integrity of tumor cells in a way that they cannot effectively repair, radiation preferentially eradicates cancerous cells. Normal tissues, though receiving substantial amounts of radiation as well, have intact repair mechanisms that enable them to eventually recover from the insult of radiation. An important reason for this response differential is the fact that normal tissues undergo a coordinated cell-cycle arrest when exposed to excessive amounts of radiation, which allows for repair mechanisms to be activated and for the incurred genomic damage to be fixed. This ability of normal cells to "pause" and to effectively repair minimal to moderate DNA damage allows radiation its main therapeutic advantage. Tumor cells cannot undergo such an arrest and as a result do not undergo adequate repair. In addition, the repair mechanisms of tumor cells are often flawed, and the inflicted damage cannot be repaired as effectively as in normal cells. This overall lack of repair leads to a propagation of errors as these cancerous cells continue to divide, leading ultimately to so many irreversible chromosomal aberrations that the cells cannot continue their basic functions and eventually die.

The inherent ability of normal tissues to repair DNA is also one important reason why the total radiation dosage delivered is usually divided or fractionated into smaller daily portions. Early in the history of radiation therapy, investigators noted that normal tissues recovered very well and without many long-term side effects if the dose was divided into smaller daily fractions and given over a longer period of time. Only later did it become clear that delivering radiation in such a fashion allows additional time not only for normal cells to recover and repair any damage (sublethal damage repair), but also for these normal cells to undergo a few divisions and to repopulate the injured tissues. Fractionation can in addition enhance tumor sensitivity to radiation through reassortment and reoxygenation. Because cells are more susceptible to radiation during mitosis and because not all tumor cells are undergoing active division during a particular radiation session, fractionation allows for redistribution of these cells into a more sensitive cycle and thereby for continued cell kill with each successive treatment.

Reoxygenation, on the other hand, occurs when well-oxygenated tumor cells die between fractions, creating an environment in which previously hypoxic cells are exposed to greater amounts of oxygen. Oxygen is necessary for radiation damage to be "fixed," since in its absence the damaged and highly reactive DNA molecule can be quickly reconstituted through the recruitment of hydrogen atoms from other molecules (i.e., water).

However, as far as head and neck cancer is concerned, locoregional control can be suboptimal when radiation therapy alone is used on a once-daily schedule. For this reason, altered fractionation regimens have been developed in which two and sometimes three doses of radiation are delivered every day. The time interval between fractions needs to be at least 6 hours to minimize normal tissue toxicity. Hyperfractionation usually refers to twice-daily radiation therapy delivery. For example, instead of delivering 2 Gy per day in one fraction, 1.25 Gy can be delivered twice per day for a total daily dose of 2.5 Gy. Accelerated fractionation, on the other hand, uses a total dose and fraction size similar to conventional treatment but achieves a shorter overall treatment time by giving two to three doses daily. Accelerated hyperfractionation uses features of both accelerated fractionation and hyperfractionation. This regimen has been used as a way of increasing tumor kill while minimizing late complications. Yet another approach is delivering once-daily treatments for the first few weeks and then twice-daily treatments for the remainder of the treatment course, a technique called *concomitant boost*. A final approach is hypofractionation, a method defined by the administration of less than five fractions per week, generally in higher doses per fraction as in the treatment of cutaneous melanomas of the head and neck (e.g., two 6 Gy fractions/week for a total dose of 30 Gy).

Through many years of both clinical experience and experimentation, radiation oncologists have established dose and fractionation regimens for a variety of tumors and conditions that achieve adequate tumor control while minimizing the collateral damage to normal tissues. More recently, the therapeutic advantage of radiation has been further increased by modern technologic advances such as three-dimensional planning and intensity-modulated radiation therapy (IMRT). These new ways of delivering radiation, along with new immobilization and image guidance techniques, allow for a much more precise and reproducible way of delivering dose. This has enabled clinicians to achieve ever greater normal tissue sparing and to further minimize the adverse effects and complications from radiation therapy.

Carcinoma in Situ and Preinvasive Disease

Radiation therapy has been successfully used for many years as a primary treatment for premalignant lesions of the head and neck. These lesions range from premalignant atypia or dysplasia to carcinoma in situ (CIS) and superficially invasive carcinoma, and they almost always arise from the squamous epithelium lining the mucosa of the head and neck. Actually, these lesions are believed to give rise to invasive carcinoma through a multistep process of molecular and genetic derangements as described for other cancers.[4,5] They are most commonly encountered in the glottic larynx and the oral cavity, where they are most likely to be symptomatic and hence detected at these sites. As a matter of fact, the largest experience of treating such lesions with radiation has been accumulated from patients with laryngeal lesions because they often present with hoarseness even when the true vocal cords are minimally involved by these preinvasive entities. CIS is the most common of these entities and represents on pathology investigation carcinomatous changes that are confined to the epithelium without a breach of the lamina propria. Its clinical appearance is that of a white or grayish thickening of the affected mucosa of the affected vocal cord. The management of CIS of the glottis is controversial, with treatment practices ranging from primary radiation or surgery (vocal cord stripping, microexcision, cordectomy, or partial laryngectomy) to observation after biopsy. A few studies on the latter approach, however, have documented high rates of progression to invasive squamous cell carcinoma that is often no longer amenable to voice-preserving therapy.[6] In addition, some series have shown that, owing to limited biopsy sampling, many patients with CIS actually harbor invasive disease.[7] Therefore, most physicians advocate treatment, either with minimally invasive surgery or radiation.

Complete stripping of the mucosa of the cord is often curative for early dysplastic lesions (leukoplakia, erythroplakia, and hyperkeratosis). However, the disadvantage of this method is that patients need careful observation and frequently require repeat procedures that may eventually scar the cords, thus obscuring new lesions and leading to hoarseness. Furthermore, many radiation oncologists believe that surgical techniques tend to be more operator-dependent than the well-established approaches and treatment paradigms with radiation, and that, unless patients are undergoing these procedures at high-volume head and neck cancer centers, they should preferentially be steered toward radiation. These considerations favor radiation therapy, which has traditionally conferred excellent local control rates in the range of 85% to 100%[8–14] (Table 9-1). In addition, surgical salvage rates after recurrence are excellent, ranging from 90% to 100%, whereas the salvage potential of radiation after surgery in early glottic lesions has not been as extensively investigated. The main disadvantages of radiation therapy are the acute adverse effects from treatment and the duration of treatment. Also, radiation for early disease limits the options available in the rare event of treatment failure or the more common development of a second primary cancer within the radiation field. Reirradiation is fraught with difficulties and is used uncommonly. This leaves surgery as the principle means of salvage treatment.

Table 9-1. Local Control Results From Large Recent Studies of Radiation Therapy for Early Glottic Cancer

Study	Year	N	% Five-Year Local Control
Tis			
Wang[8]	1997	60	92
Spayne et al[9]	2001	67	98
Garcia-Serra et al[10]	2002	30	88
Cellai et al[11]	2006	89	84
T1			
Wang[8]	1997	665	93
Warde et al[12]	1998	449	91 (T1a)
			82 (T1b)
Mendenhall et al[13]	2001	291	94 (T1a)
			93 (T1b)
Cellai et al[11]	2006	831	84
T2			
Wang[8]	1997	237	71–77
Warde et al[12]	1998	230	69
Frata et al[14]	2006	256	73

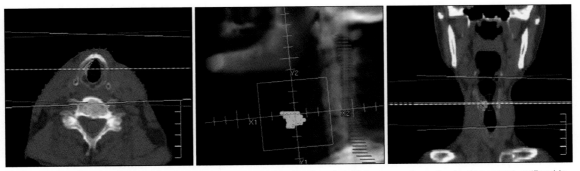

Figure 9-1. Fields for a patient with extensive carcinoma in situ of right true vocal cord. Lesion extent outlined in yellow. Total dose given was 66 Gy in 2 Gy per fraction.

Furthermore, some critics point out that most patients salvaged with surgery after recurrence require total laryngectomy and that initial treatment with surgery tends to be more cost-effective.[15,16]

The radiation techniques for CIS lesions are pretty standard, and setup is quite simple. Patients are usually treated with two 5 × 5 cm opposed lateral fields that cover the glottic larynx with a 1- to 2-cm margin. The superior border of the field is placed at the top of the thyroid cartilage, and the inferior border is extended to the bottom of the cricoid. Anteriorly, the field extends 1 to 2 cm past the skin surface, and posteriorly it stops at the anterior edge of the cervical vertebral bodies (Fig. 9-1). Occasionally, the fields are turned (collimated) slightly to match the prevertebral line posteriorly and tilted inferiorly by 5 to 10 degrees to avoid the shoulders, especially in patients with short necks. Both cobalt-60 and 4 to 6 megavoltage (MV) photons can provide adequate coverage of the glottis, whereas higher energy beams are generally avoided because of a greater risk of underdosing the anterior commissure. This consideration arises from a phenomenon called *dose buildup*, which

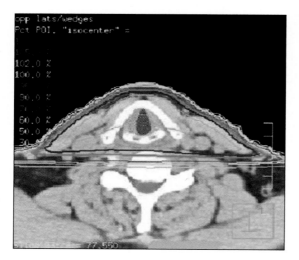

Figure 9-2. Isodose lines (dose distribution as percentages of prescribed total dose) for a patient with CIS of the glottis.

essentially means that higher energy beams deposit most of their energy deeper into tissues while sparing/underdosing superficial structures. Even with 6 MV, there is some risk of underdosing anterior tumors, especially in very thin patients, thus necessitating tissue equivalent bolus material to allow for adequate buildup.

Bolus is a general term used in radiation oncology that defines various ways of simulating additional tissue in the patient so that the dose can be effectively modified to cover more superficial structures (i.e., skin, subcutaneous structures). Computed tomography (CT)-based planning is generally recommended to better assess dose distribution and to determine whether wedges should be used. Wedges are beam modifiers that when placed in front of the beam allow for a varying dose distribution in tissue, depending on the angle of the wedges used. With laryngeal lesions, two 15-degree wedges are usually used to improve homogeneity and dose distribution to the mid and posterior portions of the vocal cords (Fig. 9-2). Treating without wedges, on the other hand, is recommended for anterior lesions, since small hot spots in areas of disease are generally acceptable. Radiation doses of 66 Gy in 2 Gy per fraction have been traditionally used. However, recent data from Japan have substantiated the use of larger doses per fraction for these early and slower-growing lesions.[17] As a result, some centers now irradiate with fractions of 2.25 Gy, administering total doses of 56.25 to 58.5 Gy for CIS.

Early Laryngeal Cancer

Laryngeal Anatomy and General Treatment Considerations

Laryngeal cancer is the most common head and neck cancer, affecting approximately 10,000 Americans per year and accounting for almost one third of all head and neck malignancies.[18] The larynx is divided into three anatomic regions: supraglottic, glottic, and subglottic. The supraglottic larynx comprises the supra- and infrahyoid epiglottis, the aryepiglottic folds, the arytenoids, and the false vocal cords. The glottic larynx encompasses the true vocal cords (including anterior and posterior commissures), and the subglottic larynx extends from the lower edge of the glottis to the inferior aspect of the cricoid cartilage.

Because of its early manifestation of disease by hoarseness of voice, most glottic carcinoma is often discovered early and is therefore a highly curable malignant tumor. Supraglottic lesions, on the other hand, are less likely to present early and often

Box 9-1. T-Staging for Early Laryngeal, Oropharyngeal, and Oral Cavity Carcinoma

Larynx

Tis: Carcinoma in situ

T1: Supraglottis: Tumor limited to one subsite of supraglottis with normal cord mobility
    Glottis: T1a, tumor limited to one vocal cord or T1b, tumor limited to both vocal cords with
        normal cord mobility
    Subglottis: Tumor limited to subglottis

T2: Supraglottis: Tumor invades more than one supraglottic subsite or glottis or region outside
        supraglottis without larynx fixation
    Glottis: Tumor extends to supra- or subglottis and/or with impaired cord mobility
    Subglottis: Tumor extends to glottis with normal or impaired cord mobility

Oropharynx and Oral Cavity

Tis: Carcinoma in situ

T1: Tumor 2 cm or less in greatest dimension

T2: Tumor more than 2 cm but not more than 4 cm in greatest dimension

Used with the permission of the American Joint Committee on Cancer (AJCC), Chicago, Illinois. The original source for this material is the AJCC Cancer Staging Manual, Sixth Edition (2002) published by Springer Science and Business Media LLC, www.springerlink.com.

present with locoregional lymph node involvement. In contrast to the supraglottis, the glottis has virtually no lymphatic drainage, and therefore a very small risk of lymph node metastasis with T1 or small T2 lesions[19] (Box 9-1). For example, the incidence of lymphadenopathy at diagnosis is about 5% for early glottic lesions and 20% for the more extensive T3/4 tumors.[20] In addition, according to Byers and colleagues,[21] the rate of occult nodal involvement is approximately 16% in patients with T3-4N0 disease at the time of elective nodal dissection, with the most frequently involved nodes being the upper and mid-jugular nodes. As smaller tumors grow, however, they begin to involve the supraglottic or subglottic structures, which have more extensive lymphatic networks, thus significantly increasing the risk of nodal involvement. For example, older studies have shown that 55% of patients with supraglottic cancers have clinically involved lymph nodes and that up to 50% of the remaining clinically node-negative patients have pathologic nodal involvement upon further evaluation.[22,23]

Subglottic tumors have a similarly high rate of lymph node involvement, but in contrast to supraglottic cancers, which tend to preferentially involve the upper and mid-jugular nodes, they tend to spread to the lower jugular, pretracheal, and prelaryngeal (*Delphian*) nodes first. Based on these and other studies, it is generally accepted that patients with T1/2 glottic tumors do not require elective nodal irradiation, whereas patients with early supraglottic and subglottic tumors merit a comprehensive treatment of the nodal chains in addition to the primary tumor.

Early Glottic Cancer

Both radiation therapy and voice-preserving surgery (excision, cordectomy, or hemilaryngectomy) are accepted treatment modalities for early invasive lesions (T1-2N0) of the glottis. Even though large individual series have demonstrated comparable local control rates, there has been no direct comparison of these two treatment modalities in a prospective trial. A recent Cochrane review tried to compare the effectiveness of radiation therapy and surgery in early laryngeal cancer but concluded that there is not enough evidence to establish a clear superiority.[24] In addition, there are no randomized data on functional outcomes after either treatment to help guide clinicians in their recommendations. In general, the choice of therapy is dictated by both the need for tumor control and the desire to preserve phonation after therapy, which in turn depend on a variety of factors, such as tumor location, volume of disease, extent of invasion, anterior commissure involvement, and nodal status. In addition, socioeconomic considerations, such as patient age, occupation, and likelihood of compliance, can also inform the physician as to what treatment method may be most appropriate for a particular patient.

Regardless of the choice of therapy, both surgery and radiation offer excellent local control rates in patients with T1 glottic cancer. For example, in one of the largest surgical series reported to date, the 3-year local control rates for patients with T1a and T2b lesions undergoing laser cordectomy were 94% and 91%, respectively.[25] In another large study using radiation as the treatment of choice, the 5-year local control rates were comparable at 94% for T1a and 93% for T1b tumors.[13] Because T1 lesions can be so diverse in terms of presentation, many clinicians base their treatment recommendations on ancillary criteria, such as lesion size, shape, location, and anterior commissure involvement. Some of these criteria, such as involvement of the anterior commissure, are thought to be poor prognostic factors that have a negative impact on the likelihood of local control and voice preservation after therapy.[26] The largest retrospective study on outcomes in radiation therapy in T1 glottic cancer recently published by Cellai and colleagues[11] from Italy lends further support to these findings. A total of 831 patients with T1N0 glottic tumors were analyzed and a 5-year local control rate of 84% was reported (see Table 9-1). This compares favorably with local control rates from other published series, but more important, in this study lesion extent and anterior commissure involvement were shown to predict in a statistically significant way for local or locoregional failure on both univariate and multivariate analyses.[11] In addition, some investigators have reported significantly lower actuarial local control rates after radiation therapy for bulky versus small T1 lesions, lending some credence to the approach of laser excision followed by radiation for more extensive T1 tumors.[27] In general, however, either radiation therapy or surgery alone is used, and both are given equal consideration if the lesion is small, is limited to one vocal cord (T1a), and has no extension to the arytenoids or the anterior commissure.

Occasionally endoscopic laser resection is recommended over radiation therapy for the well-defined superficial lesion located in the middle third of the vocal cord, particularly when it is along the cord's free edge, because radiation therapy takes much longer to administer. This recommendation is also supported by studies that have shown very similar voice quality measures in patients with mid cord tumors undergoing limited excision as well as those receiving definitive radiation therapy for such early glottic lesions.[28] In contrast, because the surgical management of larger (especially T1b) lesions requires the removal of greater amounts of tissue with an increasing potential for poor voice quality as a result, radiation is usually the preferred initial treatment for those tumors.

Even though many clinicians take into consideration the potential for dysphonia after either mode of therapy, there are really very few good studies comparing voice quality after radiation with voice quality after laser excision. In fact, most studies are retrospective single-institution series, which, when taken together, yield conflicting impressions. On the one hand, Hirano and colleagues[29] concluded in the 1980s that hoarseness and poor approximation of the vocal cords were more frequently observed in patients treated with laser excision. Similarly, data from our institution suggested a few years later that a higher proportion of patients treated with radiation for T1 glottic carcinoma retain normal to near-normal voice quality when compared with patients treated with laser excision.[30] However, more recent evidence seems to contradict these findings, perhaps reflecting improvements in endoscopic microsurgical techniques. A study from Canada, for example, suggests that even though vocal cord function (as assessed by videostroboscopy) was superior in the patients who received radiation, the patients who underwent endoscopic resection of their tumors actually scored higher on subjective and objective voice assessments (Voice Handicap Index questionnaire and Visi-Pitch parameters).[16] In addition, a recent meta-analysis of almost 300 patients with T1 glottic tumors treated either with laser excision or radiation concluded that both treatment methods result in comparable levels of voice handicap.[31]

Other investigators have attempted to single out specific patient- or treatment-related characteristics that predict poor voice quality after treatment. For instance, McGuirt and colleagues[28] observed that the greater the amount of vocalis muscle resected during laser excision, the greater the decline of voice quality post-treatment. As far as radiation is concerned, continued heavy tobacco exposure during radiation therapy and extensive vocal cord stripping or multiple biopsies before radiation therapy have been postulated by some to adversely affect postirradiation voice quality.[32] Others have suggested that voice overuse during radiation may also degrade one's voice after treatment.[33]

In summation, it is very challenging to discern any significant benefit of one treatment versus another in patients with T1 lesions of the glottis. Radiation therapy continues to be one standard approach in treating these patients. Endoscopic laser excision can provide comparable local control rates and post-treatment voice quality in selected patients and has the main advantage of brevity at a potentially lower cost, being in most cases a single outpatient procedure.

Given that T2 lesions are by definition larger, extending beyond the glottis or causing some impairment of vocal cord mobility, it is not surprising that these tumors are somewhat more difficult to control with either surgery or radiation. Local control rates with radiation alone range from 65% to 80%, ultimately reaching 70% to 90% after surgical salvage[8,12,14] (see Table 9-1). As far as surgery is concerned, both a vertical partial laryngectomy or a partial supracricoid laryngectomy are acceptable options for bulkier and more invasive T2 lesions, especially since local control rates are excellent and preservation of vocal cord function is somewhat less of an issue once phonation has been compromised by tumor invasion. Endoscopic resection is also an option, particularly in selected patients with T2 glottic tumors that are discrete, superficial, and with normal vocal cord mobility. Nonetheless, radiation alone is still the preferred treatment approach at many institutions because of the somewhat better functional outcomes. Some investigators have even shown improved rates of disease control (92% versus 72%, 5-year disease-free survival) and better voice preservation rates (89% versus 61%) for T2N0 tumors treated with concurrent chemoradiation. However, given the low incidence of distant dissemination in these patients and the greater toxicity, this approach should not be routinely recommended without further validation.[34]

The wide range in local control rates for T2 glottic cancer is in part due to the heterogeneity of presentations within this stage of disease. The second largest experience to date on T2 lesions treated with radiation alone was recently reported by Frata and colleagues,[14] who attempted to single out features associated with a poor outcome. Over 250 cases were analyzed retrospectively, and a cumulative local control probability of 73% was reported at 5 years. The main determinants of inferior local control on both univariate and multivariate analyses in this study were tumor extent and impaired cord mobility. Other investigators have looked for prognostic factors in this group of patients as well and found very similar results. For example, patients with T2 lesions treated with radiation at the Massachusetts General Hospital (MGH)were found to have a slightly better local control at 5 years if they did not have impaired vocal cord mobility (77% versus 71%).[5] In contrast, studies from M.D. Anderson Cancer Center (MDACC) did not show a clear relationship between cord mobility and outcomes after radiation therapy.[35,36] Furthermore, the influence of impaired cord mobility on surgical salvage rates after radiation is far from clear, and anterior commissure involvement has failed to emerge as an independent prognostic factor in this group of patients. If anything, many investigators believe nowadays that the latter is simply a marker of more extensive disease, which is the actual and more significant determinant of outcome.[37] What has more clearly emerged as a predictor of local control in T2 glottic cancer is the way in which radiation is delivered—namely over what period of time and to what total dose. For example, investigators recently reiterated that treatment duration of 54 days and radiation doses of 67 Gy correlate with significantly better 5-year local control rates (87% versus 71%, P = .023 and 91% versus 60%, P = .0013).[38]

Radiation doses for T1 and T2 glottic cancer have traditionally ranged from 60 to 70 Gy administered in 2-Gy fractions. This approach is based on results from various studies demonstrating superior local control with fraction doses larger than 1.8 Gy[39,40] (Table 9-2). Usually, a dose of 60 Gy is administered after surgery when there is no evidence of gross disease. For intact T1 lesions, a dose of 66 Gy has been used, whereas T2 lesions have traditionally received 70 Gy. More recently, however, several studies, including a prospective randomized study from Japan, have convincingly shown that fraction doses of more than 2 Gy are even more effective in controlling early glottic cancer than conventional fraction sizes without much added toxicity[17,35,41] (see Table 9-2). For example, the Japanese study by Yamazaki and colleagues[17] demonstrated a 5-year local control rate of 92% for patients with T1 lesions receiving 2.25 Gy per fraction (total 56.25 to 63 Gy) and 77% for those receiving 2 Gy per fraction (total 60 to 66 Gy). This difference in local control was statistically significant with a P value of .004.[14] As a result of this and other studies, some centers now irradiate with fractions of 2.25 Gy, administering total doses of 63 Gy for T1N0 and 65.25 Gy for T2N0 lesions.

In addition, hyperfractionation and accelerated fractionation schemes have also been extensively investigated in early glottic cancer. Garden and coinvestigators[35] reported on 230 patients with T2 glottic cancer more than a third of which were treated with twice-daily fractionation. The 5-year local control rate was 79% for patients treated with the twice-daily regimen and 67% for those receiving once-daily treatments. A more recent study from Japan suggests that hyperfractionation, when compared with conventional radiation dosing, may improve the 5-year laryngeal preservation rate in patients with T2 glottic lesions (95.3% versus 52% to 60%,

Table 9-2. Impact of Fraction Size on Local Control from Large Recent Series of Radiation Therapy (RT) for Early Glottic Cancer

Study	Year	N	Stage	Radiation, Gy (Dose/Fraction)	% Five-Year Local Control		P Value
Schwaibold et al[39]	1988	56	T1	1.8	75		<.01
				2	100		
Le et al[40]	1997	398	T1, T2	<1.8	79 (T1)	44 (T2)	NS for T1
				≥1.8–2.24	81–92 (T1)	73–79 (T2)	.003 for T2
				>2.25	94 (T1)	100 (T2)	
Burke et al[41]	1997	100	T1, T2	<2	44		<.01
				≥2	92		
Garden et al[35]	2003	146	T2	2	59		<.001
				2.06–2.26	80		
Yamazaki et al[17]	2006	180	T1	2	77		.004
			T1	2.25	92		

$P < .05$).[42] Furthermore, hyperfractionation and accelerated fractionation schemes have also been validated through a few randomized trials in more advanced head and neck cancers.[43–47] For example, two of the more recent trials, Radiation Therapy Oncology Group (RTOG) 90-03 and the Continuous Hyperfractionated Accelerated Radiotherapy (CHART) trials, demonstrated a benefit to altered fractionation for locally advanced squamous cell cancers of the head and neck but did so at the expense of added toxicity. RTOG 95-12, which randomized patients with T2 glottic tumors to a standard course of 70 Gy in 2 Gy per fraction or to 79.2 Gy in twice-daily 1.2-Gy fractions, recently completed accrual and is hoped to add more to our knowledge of hyperfractionation in early head and neck cancer.

The fields for T1 lesions are virtually identical in setup to those for CIS (Fig. 9-3). The fields for T2 lesions are generally slightly larger to account for the greater extent of disease and the potential for supra- or subglottic involvement. They usually measure 6 × 6 cm and encompass at least one tracheal ring below the cricoid, especially when there is subglottic extension. Posteriorly, the field covers the anterior one third to one half of the cervical vertebral bodies. At our institution, we also extend the superior border to 2 cm above the angle of the mandible to cover the upper jugular nodes, particularly when there is clear evidence of supraglottic extension (Fig. 9-4). In addition, some radiation oncologists bring in the posterior edges of their T1 and T2 fields by 1 and 1.5 cm, respectively, for the last few fractions as a

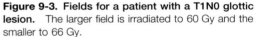

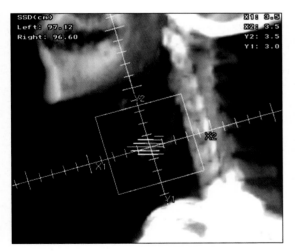

Figure 9-3. Fields for a patient with a T1N0 glottic lesion. The larger field is irradiated to 60 Gy and the smaller to 66 Gy.

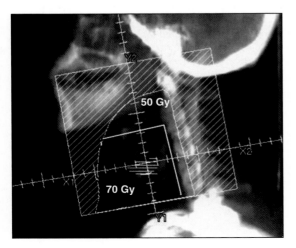

Figure 9-4. Lateral fields for a patient with a T2N0 glottic lesion with supraglottic extension.

way of reducing some of the dose to the pharynx. However, caution must be exercised with this technique so as not to underdose lesions that extend to the posterior glottis.

Early Supraglottic Cancer

Supraglottic carcinoma is second in incidence after glottic cancer and carries a somewhat poorer prognosis. The treatment options for early supraglottic lesions (T1-2N0) include laser endoscopic excision; supracricoid (subtotal), supraglottic, or total laryngectomy; or definitive radiation therapy, with the latter two being voice-preserving and therefore preferred. Surgical control rates range from 80% to 90%, whereas most radiation therapy series cite local control rates between 76% and 100%, depending on T stage and various other prognostic factors.[48] Traditionally, local control rates for radiation have been somewhat lower than for surgery; however, direct comparisons of the two treatment modalities are complicated by the fact that many patients undergoing partial laryngectomy subsequently receive adjuvant radiation. Also, because the leading complication of surgery is aspiration, most surgical candidates tend to be younger and more fit medically (e.g., without evidence of chronic obstructive pulmonary disease). Confounding the issue even more is the higher incidence of nodal involvement, even with early stages of disease, and the resultant need for managing the neck.

Comparative studies of these early lesions have noted similar rates of local control. However, they have also concluded that radiation therapy is generally associated with less complications and that morbidity due to chronic aspiration as a result of surgery can be quite high. For example, Robbins and colleagues[49] reported a 16% incidence of significant aspiration and an 8% rate of permanent tracheostomy in patients treated with supraglottic laryngectomy. Therefore, the general recommendation is to irradiate or laser excise tumor in patients with T1 and small exophytic T2 lesions, as well as in patients who are medically unfit (e.g., those with poor pulmonary function). All other patients with early-stage disease are usually amenable to partial laryngectomy, with adjuvant radiation therapy or chemoradiation as indicated for positive/close margins, multiple positive nodes, or positive nodes with extracapsular extension.

The traditional radiation therapy approach uses opposed lateral fields that extend inferiorly to the bottom of the cricoid or at least 2 cm past the lowest extent of disease. Superiorly, they encompass the larynx as well as the upper and mid-jugular nodes (Fig. 9-5). CT-based planning is preferred. Furthermore, to reduce the

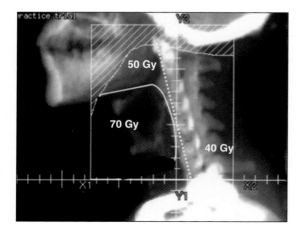

Figure 9-5. Shrinking field technique for a patient with a T2N0 supraglottic tumor. Posterior low-risk neck nodes are usually boosted to 50 Gy with electrons after a dose of 40 Gy is delivered with photons.

likelihood of setup errors, the patient's head and neck are immobilized during the treatment sessions with a plastiform mask (or equivalent device), which is applied and custom-fitted at the time of simulation. Also, out of consideration for spinal cord tolerance, a shrinking field technique is used, which delivers the last 13 to 15 fractions to the tumor by excluding the posterior neck and underlying cord. This is acceptable because the posterior cervical nodes are at a very low risk of involvement with T1-2N0 tumors. This smaller field still includes the upper jugular nodes and is carried to doses sufficient to eradicate microscopic disease. Finally, the superior edge of this field is brought down by a few centimeters to the angle of the mandible, and this smaller field, which includes the lesion and the area at highest risk for locoregional failure, is then irradiated to its definitive dose (see Fig. 9-5).

Patients with T1 tumors usually receive 66 to 68 Gy in 2 Gy per fraction or 63 Gy when a 2.25-Gy fractionation scheme is used. T2 lesions are given 2-Gy fractions for a total dose of 70 Gy. Nodal basins at risk are irradiated to 50 Gy using the shrinking field technique, with the off-spinal reduction occurring earlier in the treatment course at 40 to 42 Gy. Alternatively, some clinicians advocate using a hyperfractionated twice-daily regimen, whereas others suggest an accelerated schedule with a concomitant boost. Investigators at MGH analyzed 566 patients with supraglottic carcinoma, most of them with T1-3N0 disease. The patients (n = 244) received once-daily radiation, and 322 received twice-daily treatments. At 5 years, a statistically significant difference favoring hyperfractionation was observed in terms of both local control and disease specific survival.[8] However, these approaches merit further investigation as they have been shown by some to confer added toxicity.[50]

In summation, even though a clear survival advantage has not been demonstrated with either larynx-preserving surgery or radiation over total laryngectomy, most patients with T1 or T2 laryngeal cancer are nowadays routinely being offered larynx-preserving treatments, since these are associated with significantly better functional outcomes and a better overall quality of life. Most current evidence supports larynx-preserving techniques, either with surgery or radiation, and this approach has recently been reinforced by the American Society of Clinical Oncology (ASCO), which recommended in a 2006 consensus statement that all patients with T1 or T2 laryngeal lesions be treated initially with the intent to preserve the larynx.[51]

Early Oropharyngeal Cancer

The oropharynx is second only to the larynx in head and neck cancer incidence. It consists of the base of tongue, the palatine tonsillar region, the soft palate, and the posterior/lateral oropharyngeal walls. A clear association between human papillomavirus (HPV)-16 and oropharyngeal cancer has recently been established, and it has been shown convincingly that HPV-related tumors of this site respond much better to chemotherapy and radiation as reflected by markedly superior survival outcomes.[52] Since this region of the head and neck is indispensable for proper speech and swallowing and since certain treatments such as surgery can lead to further functional deterioration (e.g., base-of-tongue lesions), radiation alone is generally the preferred treatment for early oropharyngeal tumors.[53] A possible exception may be made for very small palatine tonsillar cancers fully excised at diagnostic tonsillectomy. An additional advantage of radiation therapy is that it can provide coverage of the retropharyngeal nodes, which are at greater risk of involvement with increasing tumor size and which cannot be easily removed with surgery. Occasionally, radiation can also be administered postoperatively for these tumors, especially with evidence of positive margins or perineural/perivascular invasion.

The extent of radiation (i.e., of elective nodal irradiation) is dependent on the likelihood of occult nodal involvement, which in turn depends on the primary lesion's site of origin. For example, even early-stage (T1-2N0) base-of-tongue lesions carry a very high risk of both ipsilateral and contralateral subclinical nodal disease, thus necessitating elective irradiation of both necks. Early lesions of the palatine tonsils carry a somewhat lower risk of contralateral neck disease, thus obviating the need for widespread nodal irradiation.[54] Only when these lesions involve the soft palate or the base of tongue and gain access to these structures' rich lymphatic networks are they likely to spread to the contralateral nodal stations and require radiation of those regions. Because even early-stage oropharyngeal tumors require at least ipsilateral neck irradiation and because the adverse effects from radiation (particularly xerostomia) are more pronounced with larger fields, IMRT (intensity-modulated radiation therapy) is the preferred technique for delivering external-beam radiation.

This form of radiation has been greatly refined over the last few years and has, as a result, experienced an exponential growth in utilization. In contrast to the traditional approach, which achieves a homogeneous dose throughout the entire volume treated, IMRT allows for greater conformality by delivering significantly lower doses to structures that are at low risk for disease but critical in terms of head-and-neck–related quality of life (e.g., the parotid glands). This type of treatment requires a computer-controlled multi-leaf collimator (MLC) at the head of the machine, which conforms the radiation beam to various shapes (i.e., segments or subfields) throughout the course of a single treatment session. Even though there are a few different techniques to execute an IMRT plan, the ultimate goal is to create one continuous area that is made up of many smaller areas of varying intensities of radiation. In other words, this technique allows for the modulation of dose over very small distances in tissue, thus allowing for greater sparing of adjacent normal tissues (Fig. 9-6).

The tissue-sparing effects of IMRT have been studied extensively in head and neck cancer patients, and many series have demonstrated excellent efficacy in terms of tumor control with a concomitant reduction in late toxicities, particularly xerostomia. For example, Li and Jabbari from the University of Michigan have shown repeatedly that saliva production is significantly affected by radiation doses over 25 to 30 Gy and that the use of IMRT techniques results in much less xerostomia and better long-term quality of life.[55,56] As far as outcomes are concerned, recent data from MDACC indicate excellent locoregional control for small (less than 4 cm) oropharyngeal tumors treated with IMRT. The 2-year locoregional control, recurrence-free, and overall survival rates in that study were 94%, 88%, and 94%, respectively.[57]

Another advantage of IMRT is the fact that one continuous area of tissue can be treated and that no field matching is required. Field matching can be problematic because of over- and underdosed areas (hot or cold spots), which can arise from daily variations in setup and which may ultimately compromise normal tissues and tumor coverage. With IMRT, most anatomic constraints, such as short necks, low-lying lesions, and stoma location, are no longer an issue and the need for field matching, with all of its inherent risks of over- and underdosing critical structures, can be eliminated. With great conformality, however, comes great responsibility and as a prerequisite, IMRT requires a proper selection and a much more precise delineation of target volumes. Instead of shrinking fields to deliver varying doses of radiation, areas of high, intermediate, and low risk for disease are first delineated based on the presence of macroscopic disease and the likelihood for microscopic extension of tumor cells. Macroscopic disease usually encompasses the primary tumor and involved nodes and is irradiated to a total dose of 70 Gy in 2-Gy fractions. Intermediate- and low-risk areas are carried to 60 and 50 Gy, respectively, using the same fractionation schedule. Alternatively, some have successfully used a simultaneous integrated boost

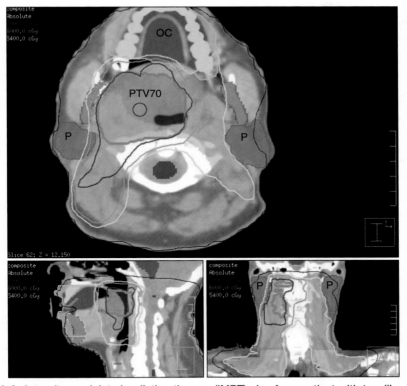

Figure 9-6. Intensity-modulated radiation therapy (IMRT) plan for a patient with tonsillar cancer. Note the conformal shape of isodose lines (dose coverage regions) and the relative sparing of the parotid glands (P) and oral cavity (OC). PTV70 designates area around the tumor that should be receiving the maximum prescribed dose (70 Gy).

approach that delivers similar total doses to each area but uses different fractionation schemes, depending on the area at risk, and thus obviating the need for a separate final boost and enabling the patient to finish treatment sooner.

Radiation therapy is the preferred treatment for T1 and T2 tonsillar cancers at most institutions. Surgery is usually an option only for small or superficial tumors when the procedure can be performed transorally and when the likelihood of a positive resection margin is low. Early studies from MDACC and MGH reported excellent local control and disease-specific control rates for T1 and T2 lesions treated with radiation therapy alone[8,57,58–60] (Table 9-3). Local control rates with radiation range from 89% to 94% and 79% to 84% for T1 and T2 lesions, depending on the series. In addition, several investigators have identified subsites of the tonsillar region that are associated with inferior local control rates when involved by disease. For example, Mendenhall and colleagues[60] noted improved local control rates with lesions originating in the tonsillar fossa or posterior pillar. Similarly, Bataini and colleagues[59] noted that tonsillar fossa tumors have a significantly higher likelihood of locoregional control after radiation when compared with that for lesions originating at other sites ($P = .01$). These findings are not only relevant prognostically, however, since they may occasionally influence the dose or fractionation scheme used by the clinician as a way of achieving better locoregional control. As a matter of fact, several investigators have reported outcomes on twice-daily fractionation for lesions of the tonsil and have documented significantly higher rates of both local control and disease-specific survival in patients with larger (primarily T2 and T3) lesions.[8]

Table 9-3. Outcomes of Radiation Therapy (RT) for Early Tonsillar Cancer

Study	Year	N	Stage	RT Dose (Gy)	% Five-Year Local Control
Wong et al[58]	1986	76	T1	64	94
			T2	68	79
Bataini et al[59]	1989	465	T1	65	89
			T2		84
Wang[8]	1997	138	T1	65–73	81
			T2		79
Mendenhall et al[60]	2000	400	T1	76.8 (H in 60%)	83
			T2		81
Garden et al[57]	2007	51	T1	66.8–73.9	100
			T2	(IMRT)	88

H, Hyperfractionated regimen; IMRT, intensity-modulated radiation therapy.

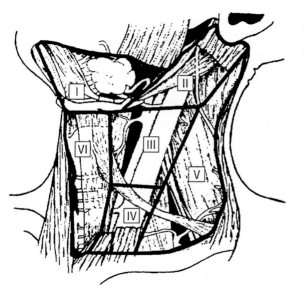

Figure 9-7. Head and neck lymph node regions. (From Robbins TK, Clayman G, Levine PA, et al: Neck dissection classification update. Arch Otolaryngol 128:751–758, 2002, Figure 1).

Early-stage cancer of the tonsillar region is treated with fields encompassing the primary tumor with a margin (usually 1 to 2 cm) and the ipsilateral nodes, particularly levels IB, II, and III (Fig. 9-7). IMRT planning is typically used, and doses of 70 Gy and 50 to 54 Gy are delivered to the primary and the elective (clinically uninvolved) neck, respectively. This approach of unilateral irradiation is based primarily on studies documenting rather low rates of contralateral nodal involvement with early-stage tonsillar lesions, particularly those not involving the soft palate or the base of tongue. For example, O'Sullivan and colleagues[54] from the Princess Margaret Hospital (PMH) cited a combined contralateral failure rate of 3.25% for patients with T1-2N0 tumors. Furthermore, a surgical series from the Mayo Clinic reported a contralateral neck failure rate of 11% after surgery for T1 and T2 lesions.[61] Given these findings, it is reasonable to consider unilateral irradiation for small (T1) lesions of the tonsil that arise in the tonsillar fossa and do not involve the soft palate or the base of tongue. However, since it is often difficult to exclude such involvement with larger T2 lesions and since IMRT provides for greater sparing of parotid function, many radiation oncologists favor bilateral irradiation for these tumors.

In contrast to that seen with tonsillar lesions, patients with base-of-tongue tumors are more likely to present with bilateral cervical lymphadenopathy. Almost two thirds of patients with T1 lesions have clinically involved nodes, and the risk of occult metastases approaches 50%.[21,62,63] Therefore, treatments should always include both sides of the neck, preferably with IMRT to achieve parotid sparing. Both surgery and radiation therapy have been successfully used in the treatment of these tumors, and both modalities provide similar rates of local control and disease-specific survival. However, surgery tends to be quite debilitating, often requiring either partial or total glossectomy and flap reconstruction. For this reason, functional outcomes are usually better with radiation therapy, making it the treatment of choice at most institutions. This approach in favor of radiation has also been substantiated by a few studies assessing quality-of-life parameters in these patients. In one study, for example, most patients who received radiation achieved and maintained excellent functional status after therapy and scored consistently higher in terms of performance and quality-of-life status than their surgical counterparts.[53]

Outcomes with radiation treatment alone for base-of-tongue carcinoma are good with 5-year local control rates ranging from 89% to 100% for T1 and 71% to 98% for T2 tumors[8,64-66] (Table 9-4).The dose per fraction and fractionation schedules vary between and within studies, with some showing no statistically significant differences between daily and twice-daily regimens,[8] while others show slightly better local control rates with hyperfractionation or concomitant boost techniques.[65-66] Most of these studies used traditional fields to include base of tongue, suprahyoid epiglottis, pre-epiglottic space, and the bilateral upper and lower neck nodes. Two opposed lateral upper fields are usually matched to a single anterior lower field just above the arytenoids at the thyroid notch, unless the lesion extends into the vallecula, in which case the match is placed lower. Nowadays, many institutions use IMRT with the goal of minimizing adverse effects even for these early lesions and even though there is some paucity of site-specific and mature data on its use. Outcomes, however, appear to be largely unaffected, with recent data showing 5-year locoregional control rates over 90% with IMRT for small (less than 4 cm) oropharyngeal lesions.[57] Regardless of the method used, a dose of 70 Gy is usually administered to the primary lesion, whereas the elective nodal areas receive 50 to 54 Gy. In addition, with IMRT, patients with early-stage disease can potentially be treated per RTOG protocol 0022 with 66 Gy to regions of gross disease, 60 Gy to intermediate-risk regions, and 54 Gy to elective nodal areas (all in 30 fractions).

Unlike base-of-tongue cancer, early-stage tumors of the soft palate behave in a relatively indolent manner and are less likely to involve adjacent lymph nodes. However, the rate of occult nodal involvement remains high enough to justify bilat-

Table 9-4. Outcomes of Radiation Therapy (RT) for Early Base-of-Tongue Cancer

Study	Year	N	Stage	RT Dose, Gy	% Five-Year Local Control
Spanos et al[64]	1976	175	T1	60–65	91
			T2	65–75	71
Mak et al[65]	1995	31	T1	66–74	100
			T2		98
Wang[8]	1997	109	T1	65–73	89
			T2		79
Mendenhall et al[66]	2000	105	T1	56.6–80	96
			T2		91

Table 9-5. Outcomes of Radiation Therapy (RT) for Early Soft Palate Cancer					
Study	**Year**	**N**	**Stage**	**RT Dose (Gy)**	**% Local Control**
Keus et al[70]	1988	76	T1	68	92 (3 yr)
			T2		70
Wang[8]	1997	33	T1	65–70	96 (5 yr)
		54	T2		85
Erkal et al[71]	2001	17	T1	65	86 (5 yr)
		48	T2	76.8 (H in 47%)	91

CSS, cause-specific survival; H, hyperfractionated regimen.

eral elective neck treatment in most cases. These tumors are not associated with the HPV as are those arising in lymphoepithelial tonsillar tissue. Since HPV-related tumors appear to be more responsive to radiation and chemotherapy, knowing the HPV status of an oropharyngeal tumor may be an important factor for treatment selection in the near future. Tumor thickness appears to be particularly related to the likelihood of nodal involvement. For example, one study noted that no lesions thicker than 2.86 mm were associated with cervical adenopathy, whereas all lesions thicker than 3.12 mm had palpable neck disease. In addition, patients with the thicker tumors had a worse overall prognosis.[67] Also, surgical resection results in marginal recurrences in up to 50% of these patients with early-stage tumors, justifying adjuvant radiation therapy in many cases.[68] Only small lesions of the uvula are typically amenable to full resection without the need for further intervention. Therefore, most patients with early cancer of the soft palate can be initially treated with radiation alone. Even though prophylactic neck irradiation remains controversial in these patients, we generally recommend bilateral neck irradiation, preferably with IMRT.

Local control rates with primary external-beam radiation therapy are excellent, ranging from 81% to 100% for T1 and 67% to 91% for T2 lesions[8,69-71] (Table 9-5). For example, Wang documented 5-year local control rates of 96% and 85% for T1 and T2 lesions without nodal involvement and reported a 17% neck failure rate in those who received partial or no neck irradiation. Since half of the patients who failed were successfully salvaged with a neck dissection, the author concluded that elective neck irradiation may not be justified routinely for early (T1) well-differentiated N0 lesions.[8] In addition, some investigators have reported good results with an intraoral applicator for these tumors, either before the external-beam phase or thereafter as a boost.[70] Because the intraoral applicator can deliver dose more locally at the affected site, this technique allows for increased sparing of normal tissues, thereby decreasing normal tissue complications. Researchers from the University of Florida have also tried a hyperfractionated approach for these tumors and demonstrated excellent results, particularly for T2 lesions. In addition, they established in their study that a protracted treatment course was associated with significantly inferior local control ($P = .0002$).[71]

In conclusion, early-stage oropharyngeal carcinoma can be treated effectively with radiation alone. Since most of these lesions require bilateral neck irradiation and since they are often in close anatomic proximity to the parotid glands, IMRT can be effectively used to minimize the dose to these and other normal structures.

Early Oral Cavity Cancer

The oral cavity extends from the inner surface of the lips to the hard-soft palate junction and the circumvallate papillae of the tongue posteriorly. Radiation therapy and surgery are both standard treatments for early lesions at this site. In general, however, surgery is the initial treatment of choice for most lesions, with radiation being reserved for certain sites (lip commissure, retromolar trigone) or for the adjuvant clearance of suspected microscopic disease.

The lip is the most common primary site affected within the oral cavity with most lesions occurring in the lower lip. Most of these lesions are small and well differentiated at presentation with the risk of lymph node dissemination being associated primarily with the depth of invasion, the degree of differentiation, and the size of the primary lesion. In addition, investigators from the Mayo Clinic have demonstrated a substantially higher rate of nodal metastasis (19%) for lesions involving the lip commissure.[72] Therefore, elective treatment of the nodal regions is generally not recommended for T1 lesions that are well differentiated and that don't involve the commissure. Results with surgery are excellent, particularly for such early lesions. For example, de Visscher and colleagues[73] reported a local control rate of 95% for surgically treated T1 lesions of the lower lip. Mohs and colleagues[74] demonstrated a similarly high 5-year local control rate of 94% for T1 tumors excised with Mohs microsurgical techniques.

Radiation therapy is usually reserved for lesions that are close to or involve the commissure, since surgical resection of these tumors compromises overall cosmesis. Moreover, radiation is preferred for the rare T1 lesion that is poorly differentiated because the radiation field can encompass a more generous treatment volume, including the level IA and IB lymph nodes. If such lesions involve the commissure, level II lymph nodes are included in the treatment volume. T2 lesions are also preferentially addressed with radiation therapy, since removing more than one half of the lip produces poor cosmetic and functional outcomes. For example, Stranc and colleagues[75] compared functional outcomes after surgery or radiation and concluded that radiation produced better preservation of lip sensation and elasticity.

Outcomes with external-beam radiation are similar to if not better than those of surgery alone. For example, in one study of over 100 patients with T1 and T2 squamous cell carcinomas of the lower lip, local control rates were 99% and 77%, respectively.[76] Furthermore, radiation therapy is typically used in the adjuvant setting when resection margins are close/positive or when there is evidence of perineural/perivascular invasion. This approach has been substantiated by various investigators, who report significantly higher local recurrence rates for tumors resected to positive or close (2 mm) margins.[77]

External-beam radiation for carcinoma of the lips is usually administered with either orthovoltage photons or electron beams, since these modalities allow for a more superficial delivery of dose due to a relatively shorter dose build-up distance. This allows for greater sparing of the mandible and oral cavity as well as for better coverage of the skin surface that is usually involved by cancer. In addition, a lead shield is generally placed behind the lip to further reduce the dose to the posterior structures. Margins of 1 to 1.5 cm around the palpable lesion are used if photons are used, whereas 2- to 2.5-cm margins are required with electrons. Doses of 66 Gy and 70 Gy are typically administered for T1 and T2 tumors, respectively.

The second most common cancer of the oral cavity is cancer of the oral tongue. Nearly all tumors arise on the lateral or ventral surface of the tongue and nearly 50% of patients have clinical evidence of nodal dissemination at diagnosis.[19] In addition, Byers and colleagues have documented a 19% incidence of occult disease in T1N0 and T2N0 lesions, emphasizing the need for adequately addressing the neck, even in early-stage disease.[21] The incidence of nodal involvement rises sharply with depth of invasion/tumor thickness over 2–5 mm (varying by study) and the degree of de-differentiation, both of which are especially important factors when considering elective treatment of the neck.[78,79] Therefore, elective radiation to the level I and

Table 9-6. Outcomes of Radiation Therapy (RT) for Early Oral Tongue Cancer

Study	Year	Treatment	Stage	% Local Control (CSS)
Fein et al[82]	1994	RT	T1/T2	79/72 (2 years)
		S ± RT	T1/T2	76/76 (2 years)
Wang[8]	1997	RT	T1/T2	85/69 (5 years)
Sessions et al[83]	2002	RT	T1/T2	75/59 (5-year CSS)
		S	T1/T2	71/87 (5-year CSS)
		S + RT	T1/T2	81/50 (5-year CSS)

CSS, cause-specific survival; S, surgery.

II lymph nodes is recommended for well- to moderately differentiated T1 lesions, whereas the entire neck should be irradiated for T2 and/or poorly differentiated tumors. Some clinicians even advocate the routine inclusion of the ipsilateral level III and IV neck nodes, since some data show significant rates of skip metastases (15.8%), even in patients with early-stage disease.[80] Most well-lateralized and superficial T1 and T2 lesions can be resected to negative margins via a partial glossectomy without any long-term sequelae, making surgery the initial treatment of choice. In contrast, radiation therapy is the primary treatment modality for central tumors or tumors resected to close or positive margins. As a matter of fact, Hicks and colleagues[81] documented a recurrence rate of only 9% in patients resected to adequate (over 1 cm) margins versus a rate of 15% for those with negative but close (less than 1 cm) margins, emphasizing yet again the need for adjuvant therapy in this latter group of patients. Where feasible and appropriate, outcomes of definitive radiation therapy are generally excellent and compare favorably with those of surgery alone or surgery followed by radiation[8,82,83] (Table 9-6). Furthermore, early studies by Wang and colleagues at the MGH suggested a statistically significant benefit to hyperfractionation, particularly in T2 tumors of the oral tongue. For example, 5-year local control rates of 91% versus 82% for T1 ($P = .04$) and 82% versus 43% for T2 ($P = .0001$) lesions were established with twice-daily versus once-daily fractionation.

These same investigators also showed that various boost techniques (e.g., interstitial implant, intraoral cone, or external-beam) could be used to dose-escalate while minimizing the exposure to normal tissues. They demonstrated superior 5-year local control rates with the use of an intraoral cone boost when compared with brachytherapy or external-beam boosts (90% versus 70% versus 66% for T1 and 81% versus 38% versus 52% for T2 lesions). This difference between intraoral cone and other boost techniques was particularly pronounced for T2 tumors ($P = .0001$).[8]

As far as field design is concerned, parallel opposed fields are used to treat the primary tumor and the cervical lymph node regions (Fig. 9-8). If an intraoral cone is used, this portion of the treatment is usually administered before external-beam radiation because the lesion can be more clearly defined at the beginning of the course of radiation and before the onset of mucositis. An external-beam dose of 50 Gy is generally used in conjunction with an intraoral cone dose of 20 Gy or an interstitial brachytherapy dose of 30 Gy, for a total dose of 70 Gy or greater. Doses of 66 Gy and 60 Gy to the surgical bed are generally deemed sufficient in the adjuvant setting for tumors resected to positive and negative margins, respectively. In addition, various devices and techniques can be made use of to reliably and reproducibly position the oral tongue for radiation.

Early-stage carcinomas of the floor of mouth are treated in a similar fashion to cancers of the oral tongue in that surgery is the preferred initial treatment modality. Of particular concern with these tumors is the high risk of osteonecrosis of the

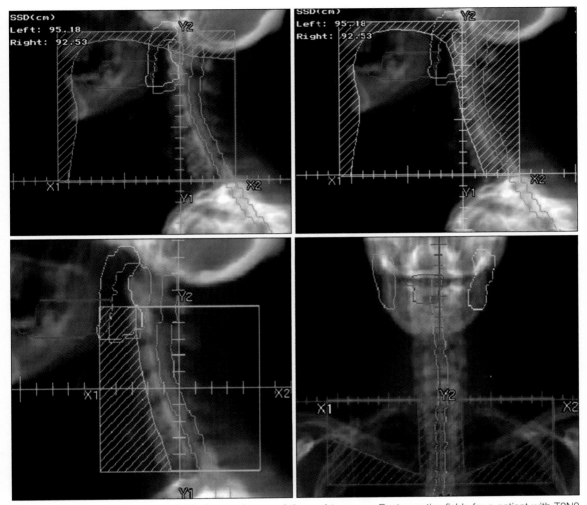

Figure 9-8. Radiation treatment fields for carcinoma of the oral tongue. Postoperative fields for a patient with T2N0 multifocal carcinoma of the oral tongue (postoperative high-risk region in red). The initial field (green) is treated to 40Gy, followed by a cone-down boost (yellow field) to 60 Gy (50 Gy, followed by intraoral cone to 70 Gy for definitive cases). Posterior neck region (blue field) is irradiated with electrons to an additional 10 Gy for a total dose of 50 Gy. The anterior supraclavicular field also receives a total dose of 50 Gy.

mandible from radiation, particularly with interstitial brachytherapy. These oral cavity lesions also carry an increasing risk of nodal involvement with increasing tumor thickness, and therefore the general recommendation is to address the neck, either surgically or with radiation, especially in T2 disease or when the depth of invasion is greater than 2 to 3 mm.[84] Again, with small well-lateralized/posterior lesions, ipsilateral elective neck treatment is sufficient, whereas more anterior/central lesions require bilateral cervical management.

Most series report a somewhat inferior local control with radiation when compared with surgery or surgery and radiation[8,83,85] (Table 9-7). However, Wang[8] reported excellent 5-year local control rates with definitive radiation therapy for T1 and T2 lesions (92% and 71%). Unlike the series reported by this group on oral tongue cancers, local control did not differ significantly by type of boost delivered, and complications were noted to be significantly higher in patients receiving the brachytherapy boost (25% versus 5%, $P = .0016$). Also, hyperfractionation did not seem to significantly improve local control in these early lesions when compared with

Table 9-7. Outcomes of Radiation Therapy (RT) for Early Floor-of-Mouth Cancer

Study	Year	Treatment	Stage	% Local Control (CSS)
Rodgers et al[85]	1993	RT	T1/T2	86/69 (2 years)
		S	T1/T2	90/75 (2 years)
		S + RT	T1/T2	100/100 (2 years)
Wang[8]	1997	RT	T1/T2	92/71 (5 years)
Sessions et al[83]	2002	RT	T1/T2	42/33 (5-year CSS)
		S	T1/T2	81/50 (5-year CSS)
		S + RT	T1/T2	75/42 (5-year CSS)

CSS, cause-specific survival; S, surgery.

once-daily treatments. Based on these and other retrospective series, T1 tumors may in fact be quite amenable to primary radiotherapeutic management. Of these, superficial (4 mm thick) and well-differentiated lesions may be treated either with brachytherapy alone (if far enough from mandible) or local intraoral cone irradiation with orthovoltage x-rays or electrons. All other early lesions carry a significantly higher risk of nodal involvement and are best treated with higher-energy external-beam irradiation to extended fields (see Fig. 9-8). The junction between the upper fields and the low neck/supraclavicular field is typically placed at the thyroid notch, and the larynx is shielded with a midline block. Doses are virtually identical with those used in the treatment of early oral tongue lesions, and radiation can be similarly used postoperatively in the presence of positive or close margins, bone erosion, and perivascular/perineural invasion.

Early lesions of the buccal mucosa, gingiva, hard palate, and retromolar trigone are relatively rare, accounting for a minority of oral cavity cancers. Surgery is again the preferred treatment modality for T1 and superficial T2 lesions, with radiation being reserved for bulky T2 tumors, buccal lesions involving the commissure, and retromolar lesions invading the tonsillar pillar, soft palate, or buccal mucosa. Also, radiation therapy can be used in the adjuvant setting for lesions with adverse pathologic features on resection (e.g., involved/close margins, perineural invasion, increasing tumor thickness/depth of invasion). Early lesions at these sites have a moderately high rate of both overt and occult involvement of the first echelon nodes, necessitating at least ipsilateral irradiation or dissection of the upper neck.[86,87]

Outcomes with definitive radiation therapy are good for early tumors at these sites. For example, Lo and colleagues[88] documented rather satisfactory local control rates in the range of 70% to 71% for T1 and T2 retromolar trigone tumors, with ultimate local control rates rising to 100% and 94%, respectively, after surgical salvage. Similarly, Wang[8] reported local control rates of 89% and 70% for T1 and T2 lesions at this site, whereas Byers and colleagues[87] reported very similar failure rates between surgery and radiation alone (12% versus 16%). Early tumors of the buccal mucosa are also responsive to primary radiation therapy, with local control rates ranging from 70% to 100%, depending on the series.

Nair and colleagues[89] reported their experience with radiation in over 240 patients from southern India, where buccal tumors constitute the majority of oral cavity malignancies owing to the habitual chewing of betel and areca nuts. Of these patients, the majority was treated with varying fractionation regimens of external-beam radiation, and about 25% had early-stage (I or II) disease. Local control rates at 3 years were 100% and 73%, whereas 3-year disease-free survival was 85% and 63% for patients with T1 and T2 lesions, respectively. Radiation therapy results for carcinoma of the hard palate, which is typically of adenoid cystic or mucoepidermoid rather than of squamous cell histology, are equally encouraging, with 5-year local control rates near 80% for early-stage disease.[90] On the other hand, mostly because of the relatively low tolerance of the mandible to radiation, very few retrospective series have addressed the use of radiation as a definitive treatment for carcinoma of the gingiva. One report from MGH cites 5-year local control rates of 65% and 67% for T1 and T2 gingival lesions treated with radiation therapy alone, whereas most other series document significantly better outcomes when radiation is used postoperatively for close margins, nerve involvement, or extensive nodal metastases.[8,86]

Techniques of irradiation and immobilization for gingival lesions vary, depending on the region involved; however, most tumors that are treated definitively are irradiated by intraoral cone in combination with external-beam radiation therapy. Interstitial brachytherapy has a very limited role in the management of tumors of the oral cavity because of the anatomic proximity of the oral cavity to bone and the associated risk for osteoradionecrosis. Small superficial tumors are typically treated with either a "wedged pair" of two 6-MV photon fields or a combination of an ipsilateral en face photon and electron field. The former field arrangement is usually preferred because it allows for better variation of the dose at depth and, as a result, for better coverage of the medial portion of the tumor (Fig 9-9). The fields should encompass the primary lesion with a 2-cm margin and the first echelon lymph nodes. Traditional opposed fields are used with the rare T1 or T2 lesion that is extending to involve more central structures, such as the soft palate or the tongue. In these cases, the beam ipsilateral to the lesion is weighted more heavily than its contralateral counterpart (i.e., it delivers a greater portion of the total dose, such as in a 3:2 weighting). Total doses of 66 Gy and 70 Gy are delivered over 6 to 7 weeks for T1 and T2 lesions, respectively, with the last 6 to 10 fractions being typically delivered by an intraoral cone or through a smaller cone-down external-beam field. Alternatively, a hyperfractionated schedule (e.g., 1.2 Gy per fraction, administered twice daily to 74 to 76 Gy) is preferred by some clinicians.[91]

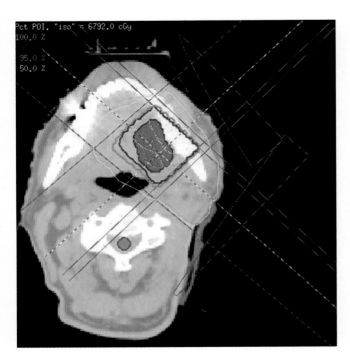

Figure 9-9. Wedge pair technique for selected lesions of the oral cavity. Note coverage of postoperative tumor bed volume at risk for residual disease (red) by 95% and 97% isodose lines.

Brachytherapy

Brachytherapy involves the placement of various small radioactive sources in close proximity to the tumor as a way of delivering high-dose radiation over very short distances in tissues (hence *brachy*, from Greek meaning short). This is a particularly appealing way of delivering dose to tumors located next to critical structures, since the dose falls off rapidly within a few centimeters (Fig. 9-10). The most common approach in head and neck cancer is to use an interstitial treatment, meaning that the sources are implanted in tissues directly or placed for some duration within catheters that are pre-implanted in the target volume. The greatest experience with brachytherapy for early lesions of the head and neck has been accumulated in patients with early cancers of the oropharynx and the oral cavity because these lesions typically require relatively high doses of radiation for local control and because they are most commonly located near normal structures with dose-tolerance limitations at or below doses required for adequate local control. Since the area irradiated by the implant is generally limited, the typical approach is to use interstitial brachytherapy (IB) as a supplement (i.e., a boost) to the dose delivered through external-beam radiation. This brachytherapy boost phase is typically initiated once the tolerance of normal tissues in the area is reached through external-beam techniques (usually at 45 to 55 Gy).

Most series with brachytherapy in oropharyngeal cancer cite excellent locoregional control rates[92-98] (Table 9-8). For example, Harrison and associates[95] reported on nearly 50 patients with early-stage lesions of the base of tongue treated with external-beam radiation therapy to 50 to 54 Gy followed by a 20- to 30-Gy boost to the primary using an iridium-192 implant. The 5-year local control rates were 87% and 93% for T1 and T2 tumors respectively. Similarly, several investigators from France have explored a similar approach for patients with tonsillar cancer. For example, Mazeron and colleagues[94] treated over 100 patients with cancer of the tonsillar region with external-beam radiation therapy (median 47 Gy) followed by interstitial brachytherapy (median 31 Gy). Five-year local control rates ranged from 91% to 94%, depending on the time period of treatment and the techniques used.

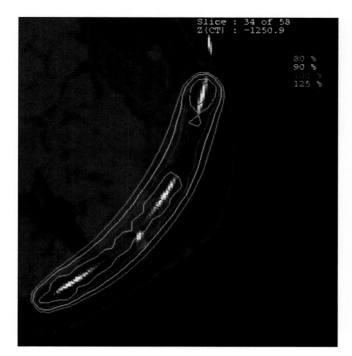

Figure 9-10. Interstitial brachytherapy. Note catheter in white running through the muscles/ tissues. The radioactive source "dwells" at different predetermined positions for predetermined periods of time to allow for optimal cumulative dose coverage (illustrated by isodose lines). Also, note rapid dose fall-off within a few centimeters as depicted by the relative proximity of the isodose lines to each other.

Table 9-8. Outcomes of Brachytherapy for Select Early Oropharyngeal/Oral Cavity Cancers

Study	Year	Site	Treatment	Stage	% Five-Year Local Control
Jorgensen et al[92]	1973	Lip	IB	T1	93
				T2	87
Esche et al[93]	1988	Soft palate	IB ± EBRT	T1	100
				T2	57
Mazeron et al[94]	1996	Tonsil	EBRT + IB	T1/2	91
Harrison et al[95]	1998	BOT	EBRT + IB	T1	87
				T2	93
Tombolini et al[96]	1998	Lip	IB	T1/2 (82%)	90
Fujita et al[97]	1999	Oral tongue	IB ± EBRT	T1	93
				T2a	82
				T2b	72
Marsiglia et al[98]	2002	Floor of mouth	IB	T1	93
				T2	88

BOT, base of tongue; EBRT, external beam radiation therapy; IB, interstitial brachytherapy, T2a, 2–3 cm; T2b, 3–4 cm.

Even though these techniques have been clearly validated in early oropharyngeal cancer, they are extremely operator-dependent and require a surgical intervention for catheter implantation that may predispose to infections and other complications related to wound healing. For this reason and because IMRT allows for adequate dose distribution and normal tissue sparing in many patients, brachytherapy, a method of combined irradiation, has slowly fallen out of favor, with most centers preferring conformal external-beam techniques alone.

Brachytherapy is used somewhat more frequently in early cancers of the oral cavity, given that these lesions are often in close proximity to the mandible and given that adequate coverage, dose inhomogeneity, and setup reproducibility are somewhat more of an issue with external-beam planning at this site. Multiple retrospective experiences with interstitial brachytherapy alone or in combination with external-beam radiation have been published (see Table 9-8). Both low dose rate (less than 1 to 2 Gy/h) and high dose rate (more than 10 Gy/h) interstitial techniques have been used with 5-year local control rates higher than 90% for early-stage lesions. For example, Jorgensen and colleagues[92] investigated the use of interstitial radium implants in patients with early carcinoma of the lip and documented impressive 5-year local control rates of 92.6% and 87.3% for T1 and T2 tumors respectively. Furthermore, a recent pattern of care analysis performed by the European Society for Therapeutic Radiology and Oncology (ESTRO) showed that brachytherapy can be offered as an exclusive treatment in most patients with early (T1/2) stage cancers.[99] This modality is most appropriate for patients with small (less than 5 cm) lesions, whereas tumors larger than 5 cm should generally be treated with external-beam irradiation followed by a brachytherapy boost. Moreover, brachytherapy is contraindicated in cases with bone involvement and in cases with a significant loss of tissue as a result of surgery.

Brachytherapy has been studied as a definitive or supplemental treatment modality for patients with early oral tongue cancers. Early studies performed in the 1970s compared various techniques of radiation in patients with such lesions and demonstrated a local control superiority of external-beam irradiation plus IB when compared with external beam alone, as well as of brachytherapy versus external-beam irradiation alone.[100,101] In addition, Pernot and colleagues compared external-beam techniques followed by IB with IB alone with or without a neck dissection and found somewhat better local control rates for T2 lesions treated with IB alone as well as better outcomes with shorter intervals between the external-beam radiation and the brachy boost.[102] More recently, investigators from Japan analyzed over 200 cases of stage I and II squamous cell carcinoma of the oral tongue treated either with IB alone or with external-beam radiation followed by IB. They also found excellent results with 5-year local control rates of 92.9%, 81.9%, and 71.8% for T1, T2a (2 to 3 cm), and T2b (3–4 cm) lesions.[97] Based on these and other studies, most radiation oncologists believe that interstitial implantation is an integral part of radiation therapy for carcinoma of the oral tongue. Both high-dose-rate radiation and low-dose-rate radiation appear to be equally efficacious in oral tongue cancer, as demonstrated in a small randomized trial by Inoue and colleagues.[103]

Similarly positive results have been demonstrated with brachytherapy in early lesions of the floor of mouth. French investigators reported recently on their experience with 160 patients treated with low-dose-rate brachytherapy alone, observing local control rates of 93% in T1 and 88% in T2 tumors (Gnd649-120). In addition, excellent results with brachytherapy had been published earlier by other French investigators as well.[98] The American data for brachytherapy in floor of mouth cancer are more limited and date back to the early work of Gilbert Fletcher at MDACC. In that study, local control rates of 97% and 100% were obtained for T1 lesions with IB and external-beam radiation with IB, respectively; the corresponding rates for T2 lesions were 91% and 95%.[100] Nowadays, however, most radiation oncologists in the United States prefer external-beam approaches, preferably after surgical debulking.

In conclusion, brachytherapy is a proven modality of radiation delivery in selected early lesions of the oropharynx and the oral cavity and can be used as a primary treatment or as a boost to complement the external-beam portion of the radiation course. However, its usefulness is somewhat limited by the invasiveness of the procedure as well as the inherent risk for potentially serious complications. In addition, the continued refinements in surgical and external-beam delivery techniques over the coming years, as well as the continued divergence of the surgical and oncologic specialties, are almost certainly going to further diminish the role of this technically challenging procedure in radiation oncology.

Radiation-Related Side Effects

The side effects from radiation for early lesions of the head and neck depend on the dose, fraction size, and radiation volumes and can for all practical purposes be divided into acute and late effects. Because the amount of normal tissue in the treatment port for early T1 or T2 glottic carcinoma is rather small, radiation therapy for these lesions is most commonly associated with only mild and transient side effects. Acutely, patients may experience worsening hoarseness, fatigue, and sore throat, especially toward the end of the radiation. These complications usually subside within 6 to 8 weeks of completion of radiation therapy and can be managed conservatively during radiation with topical anesthetics, opioids, oral rinse solutions, and anti-inflammatory agents. Late effects in these patients are rare and mostly related to voice and swallowing quality due to mild fibrosis of the laryngeal structures. However, more severe complications, such as soft tissue/cartilage necrosis and laryngeal edema, webbing, or stenosis have also been reported. For example, investigators at the MDACC analyzed over 100 patients with T2 glottic tumors treated with radiation and reported a 4.6% actuarial incidence of these complications at 5 years.[38] It is important to note here that continued laryngeal edema for more than 3 months after therapy must be biopsied, since it could be a sign of persistent or recurrent tumor.

In contrast to treatment of early laryngeal cancer, treatment of early oropharyngeal and most oral cavity lesions requires the treatment of nodal drainage basins and hence of a larger total volume. In addition, because the target lesions at these sites receive the largest doses of radiation and because they are located in close proximity to critical structures, such as the mandible and the parotid glands, there is a higher cumulative dose to which these normal tissues are exposed, which translates into a higher incidence of complications. For example, many studies have shown mucositis and esophagitis to be the most prevalent acute adverse effects, occurring between 10% and 25% of reported cases.[43,104] These adverse effects can be detrimental, since they often compromise patients' nutritional status during therapy, which in turn leads to a vicious cycle of worsening mucositis (from inability to heal) and further malnutrition. It is therefore of the utmost importance to approach these patients in a multidisciplinary fashion from the beginning and to arrange for an assessment by the nutritionist and subsequently by gastroenterology if a feeding tube is deemed necessary. In our experience, the prophylactic placement of a feeding tube has allowed many of our patients to maintain a stable weight throughout treatment and, as a result, to minimize treatment breaks during radiation.

Long-term swallowing dysfunction as a result of chemoradiation has also been described and has recently attracted greater attention. Velopharyngeal dysfunction is now thought to be exacerbated by unnecessary irradiation of the uninvolved larynx, cricopharyngeal inlet, and cervical esophagus, prompting many clinicians and investigators to use various techniques (e.g., IMRT, midline blocks, etc) to minimize the dose to these important structures. Even though clinical data in this area are limited, Eisbruch and colleagues[105] have recently developed IMRT planning guidelines in an attempt to limit irradiation of various structures thought to be associated with long-term swallowing dysfunction and aspiration. Furthermore, other investigators have demonstrated some benefit with therapeutic swallowing interventions and advocate various swallowing exercises during and immediately following chemoradiation to maintain and improve long-term swallowing ability.[106]

As far as other long-term complications are concerned, xerostomia and thyroid dysfunction are perhaps the most important and well recognized. With the use of traditional opposed lateral fields, parotid and submandibular gland sparing is minimal at best, and xerostomia rates can be as high as 80% according to some series.[43] Even though multiple agents such as pilocarpine and amifostine have been used as a means of improving salivary function and preventing xerostomia, the data on their efficacy are ambivalent at best, and many of these drugs have additional side effects. Furthermore, great progress has been made over the last few years in adequately sparing the parotid glands from excess dose through the use of IMRT planning. As a result of the continued refinement and adoption of this technology, the role of currently marketed cytoprotective agents has diminished somewhat at our institution.

Another important late complication of radiation therapy is hypothyroidism. Based on recent evidence, the incidence of hypothyroidism after radiation appears to be much higher than generally reported. For example, Mercado and colleagues[107] demonstrated an incidence of 48% at 5 years with a median time to developing the condition of 1.4 years. A more recent study reported similar results with an overall hypothyroidism incidence after radiation of 37%.[108] Hypothyroidism is a significant complication of treatment, which, if left unaddressed, can result in significant morbidity and mortality, particularly in the elderly and in those with preexisting heart conditions. Therefore, clinicians managing patients with head and neck malignancies should actively incorporate screening for hypothyroidism into their follow-up evaluations.

Other serious complications as a result of radiation include osteoradionecrosis of the mandible and upper airway obstruction from severe laryngeal edema. Fortunately, the incidence of these adverse effects is much lower, even with traditional techniques, and hopefully will be further reduced with careful planning and the use of more sophisticated treatment tools. Osteoradionecrosis of the jaw is a severe complication of head and neck radiation therapy and ranges from small asymptomatic bone exposure to severe necrosis and discomfort. Brachytherapy for oropharyngeal and oral cavity disease as well as hyperfractionation seems to be particularly linked to osteonecrosis. For example, French investigators recently reported an 18% rate of bone necrosis as a result of brachytherapy for early lesions of the floor of mouth and noted that this complication correlated significantly with poor dental status and the lack of dental protection at the time of implantation.[98] Furthermore, other studies have shown significantly higher rates of osteoradionecrosis with hyperfractionated treatments (23% versus 9%).[109] Since dental disease and tooth extraction postirradiation appear to be major risk factors for osteoradionecrosis, a serious and concerted effort should be made to repair or extract all nonsalvageable teeth at least 2 weeks before the start of radiation.

Other debilitating adverse effects from radiation include trismus and poor taste, particularly in patients receiving radiation for cancers of the oral cavity. Trismus results from scarring of the pterygoid muscles that open the mouth along with tissues of the buccal region and around the temporomandibular joints. It manifests as a slowly evolving inability to fully open the mouth, making feeding and mastication more difficult over time. It is particularly common in patients receiving radiation for head and neck cancer, with a reported incidence of 15% to 30%.[110] Unfortunately, there is no easy solution once trismus sets in; however, several measures, from jaw exercises to the use of pharmacologic agents (e.g., pentoxifylline), have been shown to minimize the severity and slow the progression of this complication.[111,112]

In addition, many patients receiving radiation for head and neck cancer report changes in taste that prevent them from enjoying food and that can seriously interfere with their appetite and hence with their ability to gain or to maintain a normal weight. Unfortunately, this is one of the last symptoms to resolve after radiation, and it may take from a few months to a full year for the taste to start coming back. Because these symptoms can be distressing to patients and because they can severely impact their quality of life, it is paramount for clinicians to educate their patients on the incidence of changes in taste and counsel them meticulously on available prevention methods.

Chemotherapy

Chemotherapy shows great promise as an approach to treatment of early lesions or even preneoplasias. Given the generally accepted paradigm that treatment of early lesions results in a higher rate of cure, treatment of these and, even more optimally, preneoplasia, promises to either prevent cancer or cure a high percentage of patients.

With the development of a broad array of biologic therapies that target multiple pathways fundamental to molecular carcinogenesis, the option of further exploration into the treatment of early-stage disease is more available than ever. Of particular interest in HNSCC is the role of the EGFR (epidermal growth factor receptor) in tumor biology and therapy (Figs. 9-11 and 9-12). EGFR is expressed in virtually all preinvasive and invasive HNSCC.[113,114] When combined with radiation therapy, targeting EGFR contributes to the cure of advanced disease.[115] As such, current approaches to treatment of early disease are actively investigating drugs that target this protein.

Preneoplasia of the Head and Neck

A common feature of HNSCC is the concept of field cancerization, by which a common exposure across the mucosal landscape of the aerodigestive tract generates clonal populations of premalignant cells. The development from early genetic changes

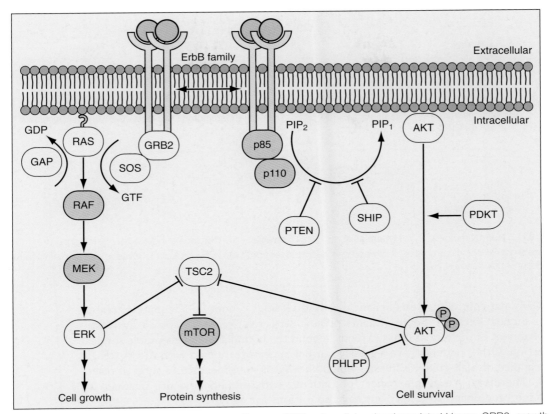

Figure 9-11. Epidermal growth factor receptor pathway. ERK, extracellular signal-regulated kinase; GRB2, growth factor receptor-bound protein 2; mTOR, mammalian target of repamycin; SOS, Son of sevenless. (From Sharma SV, Bell DW, Settleman J, Haber DA: Epidermal growth factor receptor mutations in lung cancer. Nat Rev Cancer 7:169–181, 2007, Fig. 5.)

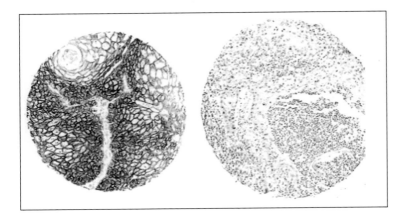

Figure 9-12. Immunohistochemistry of epidermal growth factor in head and neck squamous cell cancer. (From Chen B, van den Brekel MW, Buschers W, et al: Validation of tissue array technology in head and neck squamous cell carcinoma. Head Neck 25(11):922–930, 2003, Fig. 2.)

to invasive cancer progresses through a stepwise series of genetic events that is defined by chromosomal instability, loss of tumor suppressor activity, and gain of function in oncogenes.[116] Concurrent with these genetic events is the development of histologic and visual changes in the mucosal tissue that is described pathologically by categories ranging from low-grade dysplasia to high-grade dysplasia and invasive cancer[117] (Fig. 9-13).

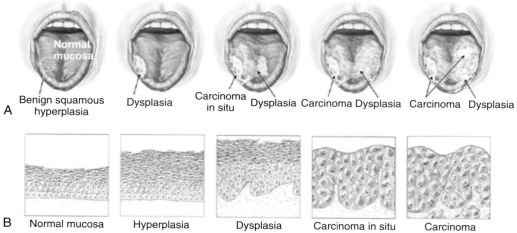

Figure 9-13. Histologic progression of head and neck cancer from benign hyperplasia to invasive carcinoma. (Courtesy of Joseph A. Califano.)

Many patients with premalignant dysplastic lesions cannot be adequately treated with surgical excision. Some patients present with relatively widespread dysplastic involvement of the mucosa that extends beyond the boundaries of acceptable surgical resection. Other patients have a grossly normal-appearing mucosa with the histologic appearance of high-grade dysplasia, which likewise is not amenable to surgical resection. Therefore, a sizeable cohort of patients with preneoplasia are destined to undergo progression to cancer but have no options for early cure.

After progression through the stages of preneoplasia to dysplasia, a subset of patients develop early malignancy, defined here as stage T1 and T2 lesions. The state-of-the-art treatment for such patients is markedly more successful than for those with preneoplasia. As with all approaches to head and neck cancer, treatment aims at both curing the patient and preserving function while minimizing acute and long-term toxicity. A further concern is reserving therapeutic options for use if cancer persists or second lesions develop. The best available treatments in wide use are single-modality approaches with either surgery or radiation. Although the cure rate is high, the aims of function preservation and minimal toxicity are usually not achieved. To better achieve all three aims, again either preventing progression to cancer or developing less toxic but equally effective therapies is paramount.[118]

Premalignancy and Early Malignancy

Primary and Secondary Prevention—Better Options for Cure

Examples of the significant success of primary (preventing development of disease) and secondary prevention (treatment of existing risk factor) are widespread both within and outside traditional medicine. Public health measures constitute the prime example of preventive approaches that save the lives of millions. Perhaps the greatest example is that of sanitation leading to clean water. In medicine, vaccination is the ultimate in primary prevention, whereas treatment of hypertension is an example of secondary prevention. Absence of disease is the best treatment—prevention of disease the next best.

In the setting of cancer, examples of prevention also already exist. Primary prevention of cervical cancer is achieved by avoidance of exposure to the human papillomavirus. Secondary prevention is represented by screening for breast and colorectal cancers. In this case, detection of either preneoplasia (polyp) or early-stage lesions leads to early interventions and high rates of cure. As in these diseases, HNSCC offers another target for prevention. Primary prevention is achieved by avoiding exposure to the carcinogens alcohol and tobacco and viruses (HPV and Epstein-Barr virus). Secondary prevention, however, is less successful. Although this site offers an easily visualizable and accessible region, therapies for early-stage disease, especially preneoplasia, are suboptimal.[119]

Leukoplakia—A Pathway to Squamous Cell Cancer

Head and neck carcinogenesis depends on progression through a stepwise series of genetic events that includes chromosomal instability, loss of tumor suppressor activity, and gain of function in oncogenes[116] as well as epigenetic alterations including hypermethylation of promoter regions of tumor suppressor genes. Concurrent with these genetic and epigenetic events is the development of histologic and visual changes in the mucosal tissue that is described pathologically by categories ranging from low-grade dysplasia to high-grade dysplasia and invasive cancer.[117] In addition to patients with de novo dysplastic lesions, approximately one in three patients with resected early-stage cancers is destined to develop recurrent or second primary cancers. Again, these cancers are likely to arise in areas of mucosal dysplasia. A number of histologic and molecular factors can be used to define a population of patients with dysplasia at particularly high risk for carcinogenic progression. These markers include loss of heterozygosity (LOH) at loci 9p21–22 and 3p, aneuploidy, and toluidine blue staining.[120–122] It has been estimated that the average time between detection of dysplasia and the development of invasive cancer is over 8 years.[123] Some HNSCC appears without detection of visible precursor lesion. This could be due to variability in the timing or detailed pattern of accumulation of genetic alterations or to variability in opportunity for detection based on the availability of screening tools. The detection for such early abnormalities provides a window of opportunity for intervention to prevent malignant progression.

Concurrent with these histologic and cytogenetic events are molecular changes that provide insight into the carcinogenic process as well as targets for therapy. Perhaps the most widely studied target is the retinoic acid receptor (RAR) and its associated pathways. Pioneering work by Lippmann and Hong[124,125] demonstrated, perhaps in reverse order, the fundamental nature of this protein through their experiments with vitamin A replacement for the treatment of preneoplasia as well as the prevention of recurrent lesions of the head and neck. Although this approach ultimately had limited clinical usefulness, it was ground-breaking because it has led to a fundamental understanding of this pathway in molecular carcinogenesis. This understanding of the role of downregulation of the retinoic acid receptor in carcinogenesis led to investigation of additional pathways—specifically cyclooxygenase-2 (COX-2) and EGFR, both of which are overactive in premalignancy and invasive cancer. These two targets provide the basis for current molecular-based therapies for these lesions.[119]

Treatment Options

Available treatments for head and neck preneoplasia range from pharmacotherapy to ablation approaches and surgery. Common to each of these is the fundamental biology of preneoplasia, that of a field effect. Because the field involves all the head and neck mucosa that is exposed to a carcinogen, it follows that any treatment must target the entire exposed field. This explains the failure of ablation or surgery to reduce the development of invasive cancer in these patients.

The experience with retinoic acid, however, shows the beginning of the future for treatment of these lesions. First and foremost, it is a systemic therapy. Unlike surgery and ablation, which are local, this drug is able to reach all potential areas of disease within the field. Second, it has a defined target that is implicated in carcinogenesis. Third, effects on the target can be measured as reversal of target downregulation. What it lacks, however, is long-term benefit and low toxicity. Drugs that target the EGFR and COX-2 may provide an improved second generation of therapy.

Alternative Approaches

Preclinical studies in cell lines and animal models demonstrate cross-talk between the COX-2 and EGFR pathways.[126] This form of cyclooxygenase is upregulated in inflammation, for example, which presents in the head and neck mucosa when exposed to carcinogens. Persistent activation of COX-2 is implicated in carcinogenesis, and inhibition of this molecule results in reduction and prevention of adenomas in colorectal cancer. The EGFR is expressed in nearly 100% of preneoplasia and neoplasia of the head and neck.[113] Given the efficacy of it in treatment of cancers of the lung, colon, and head and neck combined with the overall safety of the drugs that target these cancers, this is the second major target for prevention of HNSCC.[115,127]

Current research efforts are pursuing approaches that target the EGFR, one for recurrent respiratory papillomatosis and the other for leukoplakia with high-risk features. Recurrent respiratory papillomatosis (RRP) is a disease of viral origin that is associated with exophytic lesions of the airway (Fig. 9-14). Although it is a benign

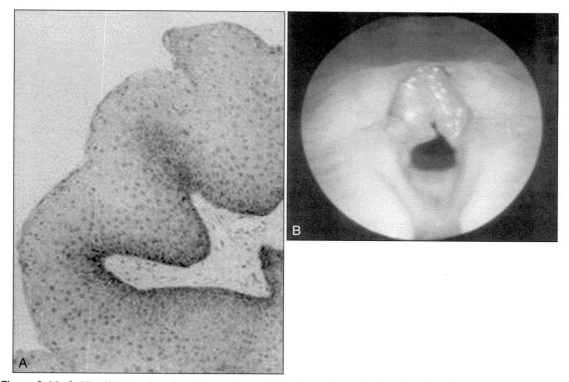

Figure 9-14. A, Histologic section of papilloma, demonstrating finger-like projection of nonkeratinized stratified squamous and vascularized connective tissue stroma. **B,** Sessile papilloma lesions involving the true vocal folds. (From Derkay CS, Darrow DH: Recurrent respiratory papillomatosis of the larynx: current diagnosis and treatment, Otolaryngol Clin North Am 33(5):1127–1141, 2000, Figs. 1 and 2.)

disease, RRP has potentially morbid consequences, due mainly to airway complications in addition to the risk of malignant conversion. The disease is often difficult to treat because of its tendency to recur and spread throughout the respiratory tract. The course of RRP is variable: some patients experience spontaneous remission and others suffer from aggressive papillomatous growth that requires multiple surgical procedures over many years. An estimated 15,000 procedures are performed in the United States each year for adults and children with RRP at a total annual cost of more than $150 million.[128]

Review of the literature reveals a definite relation between expression of EGFR and the occurrence and growth of RRP, and different studies have demonstrated this relation through multiple approaches and methods. Chardonnet and colleagues[129] studied the expression of EGFR in 35 nonregressing cutaneous and mucosal human papillomas, using indirect immunofluorescence on frozen sections. They found that the EGFR mapping was enhanced in mucosal lesions, mainly in laryngeal papillomas.

Because the EGFR is expressed in laryngeal papillomas, Bostrom and colleagues[130] reported a case in which EGFR tyrosine kinase inhibitor (gefitinib) was used in a patient with end-stage RRP in whom other therapies had failed. In addition to surgical debulking, the patient received antiviral medication, photodynamic therapy, interferon, and others, all of which failed. After taking gefitinib, the patient continued to undergo weekly bronchoscopies with papilloma debulking, with minimal to no regrowth of the papillomas, a marked change from the pattern that had occurred before the initiation of gefitinib therapy. In the last 3 months, debulking was performed only three times compared with 15 debulking procedures in the 3 months before the patient began gefitinib therapy.

Based on these preclinical and clinical data, we designed a clinical trial that treats patients with RRP with the anti-EGFR monoclonal antibody, panitumumab. Histologic response will be assessed, with molecular changes evaluated in pre- and post-treatment biopsies. The clinical end point is delay in time to progression of the papillomas.

A second study involves the treatment of high-risk leukoplakia with the anti-EGFR monoclonal antibody, cetuximab. A prospective, multi-arm, randomized, phase II trial of cetuximab versus placebo in patients with high-risk dysplastic upper aerodigestive tract lesions has been initiated. Lesions at particularly high risk for malignant progression include (1) unresectable, diffuse high-grade dysplasia, (2) persistent/recurrent high-grade dysplasia after previously treated HNSCC, and (3) dysplastic lesions with 3p9p loss of heterozygosity. There are no identified interventions that improve outcome in these patients. Patients will receive cetuximab 400 mg/m^2 for week 1, followed by 250 mg/m^2 for weeks 2 through 8, or placebo. The primary outcome is histologic response; the secondary outcome is a clinical assessment by direct visualization of the lesion combined with histologic grade. Exploratory correlatives evaluate EGFR pathway components and molecular alterations in pre- and post-treatment biopsies. Clinical and molecular variables will be correlated with the primary outcome. Safety and feasibility of cetuximab administration in this patient population will also be evaluated.

Finally, the clinical implications of the interaction between COX-2 and the EGFR are under study in a planned phase III trial of celecoxib and the EGFR inhibitor EKB-569. Patients with aneuploid lesions will be recruited in four Nordic countries. The primary endpoint is time to development of cancer.[119]

Conclusion

Both definitive radiation therapy and larynx-preserving surgery offer high cure rates, excellent post-treatment functional results, and acceptable morbidities for patients with early laryngeal cancer. In addition, both modalities can be used for early lesions of the oropharynx and the oral cavity with very similar local control rates. Since both are equally good options for these patients, treatment decisions regarding therapy should be made in a multidisciplinary setting based on a careful evaluation of both disease- and patient-specific parameters. In general, the now standard and preferred approach for early-stage oropharyngeal cancer is definitive conformal radiation, whereas surgery is the preferred initial treatment modality for most early lesions of the oral cavity. Moreover, radiation should be used in the adjuvant setting in the presence of adverse pathologic features as a way of further optimizing locoregional control. Brachytherapy should be considered for selected patients with oropharyngeal and oral cavity lesions, because this method of radiation delivery has a long and well-established record of success in these tumors. Finally, even though the acute and long-term adverse effects of radiation for early cancers of the head and neck can be severe, novel and continuously improving methods of irradiation such as IMRT and altered fractionation hold the potential to ameliorate some of these toxicities while maintaining the effectiveness of radiation as a proven treatment modality for these tumors.

Chemotherapy holds great promise in the long term. Because the precancerous field involves all of the head and neck mucosa that has been exposed to a carcinogen, it follows that any treatment must target the entire exposed field. Radiation and surgery cannot easily address this field effect, whereas systemic therapies such as chemotherapy are able to reach all potential areas of disease within the field. However, current chemotherapeutic candidates have shown mixed results. They have a defined target that is implicated in carcinogenesis. Their effects on the target can be measured as reversal of target downregulation. What they lack, however, is proven long-term benefit and low toxicity.

Newer drugs that target EGFR and COX-2 may provide an improved second generation of chemotherapy. Persistent activation of COX-2 is implicated in carcinogenesis, and inhibition of this molecule results in reduction and prevention of adenomas in colorectal cancer. EGFR is expressed in nearly 100% of preneoplasia and neoplasia of the head and neck.[4] Studies are being put in place to explore the effectiveness of these newer drugs as therapies in the early treatment of HNSCC.

References

1. Jemal A, Murray T, Ward E, et al: Cancer statistics, 2005. CA Cancer J Clin 55:10–30, 2005.
2. Carvalho AL, Nishimoto IN, Califano JA, et al: Trends in incidence and prognosis for head and neck cancer in the United States: a site-specific analysis of the SEER database. Int J Cancer 114:806–816, 2005.
3. Gibson MK, Forastiere AA: Multidisciplinary approaches in the management of advanced head and neck tumors: state of the art. Curr Opin Oncol 16:220–224, 2004.
4. Slaughter DP, Southwick HW, Smejkal W: Field cancerization in oral stratified squamous epithelium: clinical implications of multicentric origin. Cancer 6:963–968, 1953.
5. Califano J, Westra WH, Meininger G, et al: Genetic progression and clonal relationship of recurrent premalignant head and neck lesions. Clin Cancer Res 6:347–352, 2000.
6. Hintz BL, Kagan AR, Nussbaum H, et al: A "watchful waiting" policy for in situ carcinoma of the vocal cords. Arch Otolaryngol 107:746–751, 1981.
7. Pene F, Fletcher GH: Results in irradiation of the in situ carcinomas of the vocal cords. Cancer 37:2586–2590, 1976.
8. Wang CC: Radiation Therapy for Head and Neck Neoplasms, 3rd ed. New York: Wiley-Liss, 1997.
9. Spayne JA, Warde P, O'Sullivan B, et al: Carcinoma-in-situ of the glottic larynx: results of treatment with radiation therapy. Int J Radiat Oncol Biol Phys 49:1235–1238, 2001.
10. Garcia-Serra A, Hinerman RW, Amdur RJ, et al: Radiotherapy for carcinoma in situ of the true vocal cords. Head Neck 24:390–394, 2002.
11. Cellai E, Frata P, Magrini SM, et al: Radical radiotherapy for early glottic cancer: results in a series of 1087 patients from two Italian radiation oncology centers. I. The case of T1N0 disease. Int J Radiat Oncol Biol Phys 63:1378–1386, 2005.
12. Warde P, O'Sullivan B, Bristow RG, et al: T1/T2 glottic cancer managed by external beam radiotherapy: the influence of pretreatment hemoglobin on local control. Int J Radiat Oncol Biol Phys 41:347–353, 1998.
13. Mendenhall WM, Amdur RJ, Morris CG, et al: T1-T2N0 squamous cell carcinoma of the glottic larynx treated with radiation therapy. J Clin Oncol 19:4029–4036, 2001.
14. Frata P, Cellai E, Magrini SM, et al: Radical radiotherapy for early glottic cancer: results in a series of 1087 patients from two Italian radiation oncology centers. II. The case of T2N0 disease. Int J Radiat Oncol Biol Phys 63:1387–1394, 2005.
15. Smitt MC, Goffinet DR: Radiotherapy for carcinoma-in-situ of the glottic larynx. Int J Radiat Oncol Biol Phys 28:251–255, 1994.
16. Mlynarek A, Kost K, Gesser R: Radiotherapy versus surgery for early T1-T2 glottic carcinoma. J Otolaryngol 35:413–419, 2006.

17. Yamazaki H, Nishiyama K, Tanaka E, et al: Radiotherapy for early glottic carcinoma (T1N0M0): results of prospective randomized study of radiation fraction size and overall treatment time. Int J Radiat Oncol Biol Phys 64:77–82, 2006.

18. Ries L: SEER Cancer Statistics Review, 1997–2002. Bethesda, MD: National Cancer Institute, 2005.

19. Greene F: AJCC Cancer Staging Handbook. Chicago: Springer, 2002.

20. Million R: Larynx. In Cassisi NJ, Million R (eds): Management of Head and Neck Cancer: A Multidisciplinary Approach. Philadelphia: JB Lippincott, 1994, pp 315–364.

21. Byers RM, Wolf PF, Ballantyne AJ: Rationale for elective modified neck dissection. Head Neck Surg 10:160–167, 1988.

22. Lindberg R: Distribution of cervical lymph node metastases from squamous cell carcinoma of the upper respiratory and digestive tracts. Cancer 29:1446–1449, 1972.

23. Lee NK, Goepfert H, Wendt CD: Supraglottic laryngectomy for intermediate-stage cancer: U.T. M.D. Anderson Cancer Center experience with combined therapy. Laryngoscope 100:831–836, 1990.

24. Dey P, Arnold D, Wight R, et al: Radiotherapy versus open surgery versus endolaryngeal surgery (with or without laser) for early laryngeal squamous cell cancer. Cochrane Database Syst Rev:CD002027, 2002.

25. Gallo A, de Vincentiis M, Manciocco V, et al: CO2 laser cordectomy for early-stage glottic carcinoma: a long-term follow-up of 156 cases. Laryngoscope 112:370–374, 2002.

26. Marshak G, Brenner B, Shvero J, et al: Prognostic factors for local control of early glottic cancer: the Rabin Medical Center retrospective study on 207 patients. Int J Radiat Oncol Biol Phys 43:1009–1013, 1999.

27. Reddy SP, Mohideen N, Marra S, et al: Effect of tumor bulk on local control and survival of patients with T1 glottic cancer. Radiother Oncol 47:161–166, 1998.

28. McGuirt WF, Blalock D, Koufman JA, et al: Comparative voice results after laser resection or irradiation of T1 vocal cord carcinoma. Arch Otolaryngol Head Neck Surg 120:951–955, 1994.

29. Hirano M, Hirade Y, Kawasaki H: Vocal function following carbon dioxide laser surgery for glottic carcinoma. Ann Otol Rhinol Laryngol 94:232–235, 1985.

30. Epstein BE, Lee DJ, Kashima H, et al: Stage T1 glottic carcinoma: results of radiation therapy or laser excision. Radiology 175:567–570, 1990.

31. Cohen SM, Garrett CG, Dupont WD, et al: Voice-related quality of life in T1 glottic cancer: irradiation versus endoscopic excision. Ann Otol Rhinol Laryngol 115:581–586, 2006.

32. Benninger MS, Gillen J, Thieme P, et al: Factors associated with recurrence and voice quality following radiation therapy for T1 and T2 glottic carcinomas. Laryngoscope 104:294–298, 1994.

33. Stoicheff ML: Voice following radiotherapy. Laryngoscope 85:608–618, 1975.

34. Akimoto T, Nonaka T, Kitamoto Y, et al: Radiation therapy for T2N0 laryngeal cancer: a retrospective analysis for the impact of concurrent chemotherapy on local control. Int J Radiat Oncol Biol Phys 64:995–1001, 2006.

35. Garden AS, Forster K, Wong PF, et al: Results of radiotherapy for T2N0 glottic carcinoma: does the "2" stand for twice-daily treatment? Int J Radiat Oncol Biol Phys 55:322–328, 2003.

36. Howell-Burke D, Peters LJ, Goepfert H, et al: T2 glottic cancer. Recurrence, salvage, and survival after definitive radiotherapy. Arch Otolaryngol Head Neck Surg 116:830–835, 1990.

37. Sessions DG, Ogura JH, Fried MP: The anterior commissure in glottic carcinoma. Laryngoscope 85:1624–1632, 1975.

38. Nomiya T, Nemoto K, Wada H, et al: Advantage of accelerated fractionation regimens in definitive radiotherapy for stage II glottic carcinoma. Ann Otol Rhinol Laryngol 115:727–732, 2006.

39. Schwaibold F, Scariato A, Nunno M, et al: The effect of fraction size on control of early glottic cancer. Int J Radiat Oncol Biol Phys 14:451–454, 1988.

40. Le QT, Fu KK, Kroll S, et al: Influence of fraction size, total dose, and overall time on local control of T1-T2 glottic carcinoma. Int J Radiat Oncol Biol Phys 39:115–126, 1997.

41. Burke LS, Greven KM, McGuirt WT, et al: Definitive radiotherapy for early glottic carcinoma: prognostic factors and implications for treatment. Int J Radiat Oncol Biol Phys 38:1001–1006, 1997.

42. Tateya I, Hirano S, Kojima H, et al: Hyperfractionated radiotherapy for T2 glottic cancer for preservation of the larynx. Eur Arch Otorhinolaryngol 263:144–148, 2006.

43. Fu KK, Pajak TF, Trotti A, et al: A Radiation Therapy Oncology Group (RTOG) phase III randomized study to compare hyperfractionation and two variants of accelerated fractionation to standard fractionation radiotherapy for head and neck squamous cell carcinomas: first report of RTOG 9003. Int J Radiat Oncol Biol Phys 48:7–16, 2000.

44. Dische S, Saunders M, Barrett A, et al: A randomised multicentre trial of CHART versus conventional radiotherapy in head and neck cancer. Radiother Oncol 44:123–136, 1997.

45. Horiot JC, Le Fur R, N'Guyen T, et al: Hyperfractionation versus conventional fractionation in oropharyngeal carcinoma: final analysis of a randomized trial of the EORTC cooperative group of radiotherapy. Radiother Oncol 25:231–241, 1992.

46. Sanchiz F, Milla A, Torner J, et al: Single fraction per day versus two fractions per day versus radiochemotherapy in the treatment of head and neck cancer. Int J Radiat Oncol Biol Phys 19:1347–1350, 1990.

47. Pinto LH, Canary PC, Araujo CM, et al: Prospective randomized trial comparing hyperfractionated versus conventional radiotherapy in stages III and IV oropharyngeal carcinoma. Int J Radiat Oncol Biol Phys 21:557–562, 1991.

48. Garden AS, Morrison WH, Ang K, et al: Larynx and hypopharynx cancer. In Gunderson L, Tepper TJ (eds): Clinical Radiation Oncology. Philadelphia: Elsevier, 2007, pp 727–749.

49. Robbins KT, Davidson W, Peters LJ, et al: Conservation surgery for T2 and T3 carcinomas of the supraglottic larynx. Arch Otolaryngol Head Neck Surg 114:421–426, 1988.

50. Garden AS, Morrison WH, Ang KK, et al: Hyperfractionated radiation in the treatment of squamous cell carcinomas of the head and neck: a comparison of two fractionation schedules. Int J Radiat Oncol Biol Phys 31:493–502, 1995.

51. Pfister DG, Laurie SA, Weinstein GS, et al: American Society of Clinical Oncology clinical practice guideline for the use of larynx-preservation strategies in the treatment of laryngeal cancer. J Clin Oncol 24:3693–3704, 2006.

52. D'Souza G, Kreimer AR, Viscidi R, et al: Case-control study of human papillomavirus and oropharyngeal cancer. N Engl J Med 356:1944–1956, 2007.

53. Harrison LB, Zelefsky MJ, Armstrong JG, et al: Performance status after treatment for squamous cell cancer of the base of tongue—a comparison of primary radiation therapy versus primary surgery. Int J Radiat Oncol Biol Phys 30:953–957, 1994.

54. O'Sullivan B, Warde P, Grice B, et al: The benefits and pitfalls of ipsilateral radiotherapy in carcinoma of the tonsillar region. Int J Radiat Oncol Biol Phys 51:332–343, 2001.

55. Li Y, Taylor JM, Ten Haken RK, et al: The impact of dose on parotid salivary recovery in head and neck cancer patients treated with radiation therapy. Int J Radiat Oncol Biol Phys 67:660–669, 2007.

56. Jabbari S, Kim HM, Feng M, et al: Matched case-control study of quality of life and xerostomia after intensity-modulated radiotherapy or standard radiotherapy for head-and-neck cancer: initial report. Int J Radiat Oncol Biol Phys 63:725–731, 2005.

57. Garden AS, Morrison WH, Wong PF, et al: Disease-control rates following intensity-modulated radiation therapy for small primary oropharyngeal carcinoma. Int J Radiat Oncol Biol Phys 67:438–444, 2007.

58. Wong CS, Ang KK, Fletcher GH, et al: Definitive radiotherapy for squamous cell carcinoma of the tonsillar fossa. Int J Radiat Oncol Biol Phys 16:657–662, 1989.

59. Bataini JP, Asselain B, Jaulerry C, et al: A multivariate primary tumour control analysis in 465 patients treated by radical radiotherapy for cancer of the tonsillar region: clinical and treatment parameters as prognostic factors. Radiother Oncol 14:265–277, 1989.

60. Mendenhall WM, Amdur RJ, Stringer SP, et al: Radiation therapy for squamous cell carcinoma of the tonsillar region: a preferred alternative to surgery? J Clin Oncol 18:2219–2225, 2000.

61. Foote RL, Schild SE, Thompson WM, et al: Tonsil cancer. Patterns of failure after surgery alone and surgery combined with postoperative radiation therapy. Cancer 73:2638–2647, 1994.

62. Candela FC, Kothari K, Shah JP: Patterns of cervical node metastases from squamous carcinoma of the oropharynx and hypopharynx. Head Neck 12:197–203, 1990.
63. Pillsbury HC, III, Clark M: A rationale for therapy of the N0 neck. Laryngoscope 107:1294–1315, 1997.
64. Spanos WJ, Jr, Shukovsky LJ, Fletcher GH: Time, dose, and tumor volume relationships in irradiation of squamous cell carcinomas of the base of the tongue. Cancer 37:2591–2599, 1976.
65. Mak AC, Morrison WH, Garden AS, et al: Base-of-tongue carcinoma: treatment results using concomitant boost radiotherapy. Int J Radiat Oncol Biol Phys 33:289–296, 1995.
66. Mendenhall WM, Stringer SP, Amdur RJ, et al: Is radiation therapy a preferred alternative to surgery for squamous cell carcinoma of the base of tongue? J Clin Oncol 18:35–42, 2000.
67. Baredes S, Leeman DJ, Chen TS, et al: Significance of tumor thickness in soft palate carcinoma. Laryngoscope 103:389–393, 1993.
68. Strong E: Sites of treatment failure in head and neck cancer. Cancer Treat Symp 2:5–20, 1987.
69. Lindberg RD, Fletcher GH: The role of irradiation in the management of head and neck cancer: analysis of results and causes of failure. Tumori 64:313–325, 1978.
70. Keus RB, Pontvert D, Brunin F, et al: Results of irradiation in squamous cell carcinoma of the soft palate and uvula. Radiother Oncol 11:311–317, 1988.
71. Erkal HS, Serin M, Amdur RJ, et al: Squamous cell carcinomas of the soft palate treated with radiation therapy alone or followed by planned neck dissection. Int J Radiat Oncol Biol Phys 50:359–366, 2001.
72. Mackay EN, Sellers AH: A statistical review of carcinoma of the lip. Can Med Assoc J 90:670–672, 1964.
73. de Visscher JG, van den Elsaker K, Grond AJ, et al: Surgical treatment of squamous cell carcinoma of the lower lip: evaluation of long-term results and prognostic factors—a retrospective analysis of 184 patients. J Oral Maxillofac Surg 56:814–820; discussion 820–821, 1998.
74. Mohs FE, Snow SN: Microscopically controlled surgical treatment for squamous cell carcinoma of the lower lip. Surg Gynecol Obstet 160:37–41, 1985.
75. Stranc MF, Fogel M, Dische S: Comparison of lip function: surgery vs radiotherapy. Br J Plast Surg 40:598–604, 1987.
76. de Visscher JG, Grond AJ, Botke G, et al: Results of radiotherapy for squamous cell carcinoma of the vermilion border of the lower lip. A retrospective analysis of 108 patients. Radiother Oncol 39:9–14, 1996.
77. Babington S, Veness MJ, Cakir B, et al: Squamous cell carcinoma of the lip: is there a role for adjuvant radiotherapy in improving local control following incomplete or inadequate excision? ANZ J Surg 73:621–625, 2003.
78. Spiro RH, Huvos AG, Wong GY, et al: Predictive value of tumor thickness in squamous carcinoma confined to the tongue and floor of the mouth. Am J Surg 152:345–350, 1986.
79. O-Charoenrat P, Pillai G, Patel S, et al: Tumour thickness predicts cervical nodal metastases and survival in early oral tongue cancer. Oral Oncol 39:386–390, 2003.
80. Byers RM, Weber RS, Andrews T, et al: Frequency and therapeutic implications of "skip metastases" in the neck from squamous carcinoma of the oral tongue. Head Neck 19:14–19, 1997.
81. Hicks WL, Jr, North JH, Jr, Loree TR, et al: Surgery as a single modality therapy for squamous cell carcinoma of the oral tongue. Am J Otolaryngol 19:24–28, 1998.
82. Fein DA, Mendenhall WM, Parsons JT, et al: Carcinoma of the oral tongue: a comparison of results and complications of treatment with radiotherapy and/or surgery. Head Neck 16:358–365, 1994.
83. Sessions DG, Spector GJ, Lenox J, et al: Analysis of treatment results for oral tongue cancer. Laryngoscope 112:616–625, 2002.
84. Mohit-Tabatabai MA, Sobel HJ, Rush BF, et al: Relation of thickness of floor of mouth stage I and II cancers to regional metastasis. Am J Surg 152:351–353, 1986.
85. Rodgers LW, Jr, Stringer SP, Mendenhall WM, et al: Management of squamous cell carcinoma of the floor of mouth. Head Neck 15:16–19, 1993.
86. Byers RM, Newman R, Russell N, et al: Results of treatment for squamous carcinoma of the lower gum. Cancer 47:2236–2238, 1981.
87. Byers RM, Anderson B, Schwarz EA, et al: Treatment of squamous carcinoma of the retromolar trigone. Am J Clin Oncol 7:647–652, 1984.
88. Lo K, Fletcher GH, Byers RM, et al: Results of irradiation in the squamous cell carcinomas of the anterior faucial pillar-retromolar trigone. Int J Radiat Oncol Biol Phys 13:969–974, 1987.
89. Nair MK, Sankaranarayanan R, Padmanabhan TK: Evaluation of the role of radiotherapy in the management of carcinoma of the buccal mucosa. Cancer 61:1326–1331, 1988.
90. Yorozu A, Sykes AJ, Slevin NJ: Carcinoma of the hard palate treated with radiotherapy: a retrospective review of 31 cases. Oral Oncol 37:493–497, 2001.
91. Hinerman R: Oral cavity cancer. In Gunderson L, Tepper JE (eds): Clinical Radiation Oncology. Philadelphia: Elsevier, 2007, p 662.
92. Jorgensen K, Elbrond O, Andersen AP: Carcinoma of the lip. A series of 869 patients. Acta Otolaryngol 75:312–313, 1973.
93. Esche BA, Haie CM, Gerbaulet AP, et al: Interstitial and external radiotherapy in carcinoma of the soft palate and uvula. Int J Radiat Oncol Biol Phys 15:619–625, 1988.
94. Mazeron JJ, Belkacemi Y, Simon JM, et al: Place of iridium 192 implantation in irradiation of T1-T2 squamous cell carcinoma of the velopharyngeal arch. Bull Cancer Radiother 83:47–53, 1996.
95. Harrison LB, Lee HJ, Pfister DG, et al: Long term results of primary radiotherapy with/without neck dissection for squamous cell cancer of the base of tongue. Head Neck 20:668–673, 1998.
96. Tombolini V, Bonanni A, Valeriani M, et al: Brachytherapy for squamous cell carcinoma of the lip. The experience of the Institute of Radiology of the University of Rome "La Sapienza." Tumori 84:478–482, 1998.
97. Fujita M, Hirokawa Y, Kashiwado K, et al: Interstitial brachytherapy for stage I and II squamous cell carcinoma of the oral tongue: factors influencing local control and soft tissue complications. Int J Radiat Oncol Biol Phys 44:767–775, 1999.
98. Marsiglia H, Haie-Meder C, Sasso G, et al: Brachytherapy for T1-T2 floor-of-the-mouth cancers: the Gustave-Roussy Institute experience. Int J Radiat Oncol Biol Phys 52:1257–1263, 2002.
99. Gerbaulet A: Lip cancer. In Gerbaulet A, Potter R, Mazeron JJ, Meertens H, Van Limbergen E (eds): The GEC-ESTRO handbook of brachytherapy. Leuven, Belgium: ESTRO, 2002, pp 227–236.
100. Chu A, Fletcher GH: Incidence and causes of failures to control by irradiation the primary lesions in squamous cell carcinomas of the anterior two-thirds of the tongue and floor of mouth. Am J Roentgenol Radium Ther Nucl Med 117:502–508, 1973.
101. Lees AW: The treatment of carcinoma of the anterior two-thirds of the tongue by radiotherapy. Int J Radiat Oncol Biol Phys 1:849–858, 1976.
102. Pernot M, Malissard L, Hoffstetter S, et al: Influence of tumoral, radiobiological, and general factors on local control and survival of a series of 361 tumors of the velotonsillar area treated by exclusive irradiation (external beam irradiation+brachytherapy or brachytherapy alone). Int J Radiat Oncol Biol Phys 30:1051–1057, 1994.
103. Inoue T, Inoue T, Yoshida K, et al: Phase III trial of high- vs. low-dose-rate interstitial radiotherapy for early mobile tongue cancer. Int J Radiat Oncol Biol Phys 51:171–175, 2001.
104. Lee DJ, Cosmatos D, Marcial VA, et al: Results of an RTOG phase III trial (RTOG 85-27) comparing radiotherapy plus etanidazole with radiotherapy alone for locally advanced head and neck carcinomas. Int J Radiat Oncol Biol Phys 32:567–576, 1995.
105. Eisbruch A, Schwartz M, Rasch C, et al: Dysphagia and aspiration after chemoradiotherapy for head-and-neck cancer: which anatomic structures are affected and can they be spared by IMRT? Int J Radiat Oncol Biol Phys 60:1425–1439, 2004.
106. Rosenthal DI, Lewin JS, Eisbruch A: Prevention and treatment of dysphagia and aspiration after chemoradiation for head and neck cancer. J Clin Oncol 24:2636–2643, 2006.
107. Mercado G, Adelstein DJ, Saxton JP, et al: Hypothyroidism: a frequent event after radiotherapy and after radiotherapy with

chemotherapy for patients with head and neck carcinoma. Cancer 92:2892–2897, 2001.

108. Ozawa H, Saitou H, Mizutari K, et al: Hypothyroidism after radiotherapy for patients with head and neck cancer. Am J Otolaryngol 28:46–49, 2007.

109. Niewald M, Barbie O, Schnabel K, et al: Risk factors and dose-effect relationship for osteoradionecrosis after hyperfractionated and conventionally fractionated radiotherapy for oral cancer. Br J Radiol 69:847–851, 1996.

110. Stewart FA: Re-treatment after full-course radiotherapy: is it a viable option? Acta Oncol 38:855–862, 1999.

111. Brunello DL, Mandikos MN: The use of a dynamic opening device in the treatment of radiation induced trismus. Aust Prosthodont J 9:45–48, 1995.

112. Dijkstra PU, Kalk WW, Roodenburg JL: Trismus in head and neck oncology: a systematic review. Oral Oncol 40:879–889, 2004.

113. Rubin Grandis J, Melhem MF, Barnes EL, et al: Quantitative immunohistochemical analysis of transforming growth factor-alpha and epidermal growth factor receptor in patients with squamous cell carcinoma of the head and neck. Cancer 78:1284–1292, 1996.

114. Rubin Grandis J, Melhem MF, Gooding WE, et al: Levels of TGF-alpha and EGFR protein in head and neck squamous cell carcinoma and patient survival. J Natl Cancer Inst 90:824–832, 1998.

115. Bonner JA, Harari PM, Giralt J, et al: Radiotherapy plus cetuximab for squamous-cell carcinoma of the head and neck. N Engl J Med 354:567–578, 2006.

116. Kim MM, Califano JA: Molecular pathology of head-and-neck cancer. Int J Cancer 112:545–553, 2004.

117. Forastiere A, Koch W, Trotti A, et al: Head and neck cancer. N Engl J Med 345:1890–1900, 2001.

118. Kelloff GJ, Lippman SM, Dannenberg AJ, et al: Progress in chemoprevention drug development: the promise of molecular biomarkers for prevention of intraepithelial neoplasia and cancer—a plan to move forward. Clin Cancer Res 12:3661–3697, 2006.

119. Lippman SM, Sudbo J, Hong WK: Oral cancer prevention and the evolution of molecular-targeted drug development. J Clin Oncol 23:346–356, 2005.

120. Rosin MP, Lam WL, Poh C, et al: 3p14 and 9p21 loss is a simple tool for predicting second oral malignancy at previously treated oral cancer sites. Cancer Res 62:6447–6450, 2002.

121. Ai H, Barrera JE, Meyers AD, et al: Chromosomal aneuploidy precedes morphological changes and supports multifocality in head and neck lesions. Laryngoscope 111:1853–1858, 2001.

122. Zhang L, Williams M, Poh CF, et al: Toluidine blue staining identifies high-risk primary oral premalignant lesions with poor outcome. Cancer Res 65:8017–8021, 2005.

123. Silverman S, Jr, Gorsky M, Lozada F: Oral leukoplakia and malignant transformation. A follow-up study of 257 patients. Cancer 53:563–568, 1984.

124. Lippman SM, Batsakis JG, Toth BB, et al: Comparison of low-dose isotretinoin with beta carotene to prevent oral carcinogenesis. N Engl J Med 328:15–20, 1993.

125. Hong WK, Endicott J, Itri LM, et al: 13-cis-retinoic acid in the treatment of oral leukoplakia. N Engl J Med 315:1501–1505, 1986.

126. Zhang X, Chen ZG, Choe MS, et al: Tumor growth inhibition by simultaneously blocking epidermal growth factor receptor and cyclooxygenase-2 in a xenograft model. Clin Cancer Res 11:6261–6269, 2005.

127. Cohen EE, Rosen F, Stadler WM, et al: Phase II trial of ZD1839 in recurrent or metastatic squamous cell carcinoma of the head and neck. J Clin Oncol 21:1980–1987, 2003.

128. Lee JH, Smith RJ: Recurrent respiratory papillomatosis: pathogenesis to treatment. Curr Opin Otolaryngol Head Neck Surg 13:354–359, 2005.

129. Chardonnet Y, Viac J, Leval J, et al: Laryngeal papillomas: local cellular immune response, keratinization and viral antigen. Virchows Arch B Cell Pathol Incl Mol Pathol 51:421–428, 1986.

130. Bostrom B, Sidman J, Marker S, et al: Gefitinib therapy for life-threatening laryngeal papillomatosis. Arch Otolaryngol Head Neck Surg 131:64–67, 2005.

10 Head and Neck Cancer Prevention

Oleg Militsakh, Angela Chi, Anthony Alberg, Gabrielle Cannick, Marvella Ford, Matthew Carpenter, Peter Miller, Natalie Sutkowski, and Terry Day

---

KEY POINTS

- Visual, radiographic, and novel technologies including salivary molecular markers offer opportunities for routine screening of at-risk populations for oral and pharyngeal cancers.
- Smoking is one of the two major causes of cancer of the oral cavity and pharynx. Heavy alcohol use by smokers increases the risk even more.
- Heavy alcohol use increases the risk of oral and pharyngeal cancer by up to nine times, and patients should be routinely screened for and counseled about alcohol use by physicians and dentists.
- Increasing evidence suggests that human papillomaviruses may be causative agents in oropharyngeal cancer, resulting in opportunities for prophylactic vaccination and modification of sexual behavior to help prevent HPV infection and viral carcinogenesis.
- Since oral, head, and neck cancers have such high morbidity and mortality rates, comprehensive disease prevention and detection curricula for health professional schools should include training in head and neck cancer prevention and early detection.
- Research is needed to disentangle the effects of biologic and socioeconomic factors on racial and ethnic disparities in survival outcomes due to squamous cell carcinoma of the head and neck (HNSCC). Interventions targeting these factors and their effects could then be developed to reduce the disparities.
- Molecular markers currently exhibiting the most promise as targets for prevention of HNSCC include EGFR and *p53*; additional insights into the molecular pathogenesis of HNSCC may lead to the development of novel chemoprevention strategies in the future.

Introduction

Head and neck cancer prevention opportunities are well known because of the association and relationship of risk factors that include tobacco, alcohol, viruses, and diet. Despite these opportunities, a variety of political, social, and financial obstacles make comprehensive *primary prevention* unlikely in the near future. Primary prevention has historically been addressed through public health efforts and initiatives on the local and national levels. Geopolitical boundaries and variations, therefore, have a significant influence on primary prevention for squamous cell carcinoma of the head and neck. Thus, secondary prevention, which includes early detection, has been a focus of basic and translational research. Tertiary prevention primarily involves reductions in morbidity and mortality related to the disease, making prospective and retrospective clinical trials the major focus of efforts to improve quality of care.

Table 10-1. Types of Cancer Prevention	
Type of Prevention	**Definition**
Primary	Prevention of the onset of a disease
Secondary	Prevention of progression of disease by early detection
Tertiary	Prevention of complications, morbidity, and/or mortality related to a disease that is already present

Table 10-2. Common Head and Neck Cancer Sites and Histologies	
Sites	**Histologies**
Oral cavity	Squamous cell carcinoma
Pharynx (oropharynx, hypopharynx)	Squamous cell carcinoma
Larynx	Squamous cell carcinoma
Nasopharynx	Squamous cell, lymphoepithelioma, undifferentiated
Skin	Squamous cell carcinoma, basal cell carcinoma, melanoma
Thyroid	Papillary, follicular, medullary, anaplastic
Salivary gland	Adenocarcinoma, adenoid cystic carcinoma
Soft tissues	Sarcoma, lymphoma

It is important to understand that "prevention" of head and neck cancer refers to the three major types of prevention (i.e., primary, secondary, and tertiary) (Table 10-1). Primary prevention is prevention of the onset of disease. It can include prevention or cessation of risk factor exposure such as tobacco, education of the public on risk factors, vaccinations, and education of clinicians to counsel patients about risk factors. Secondary prevention includes the early identification of a cancerous or precancerous condition or predisposition thereof that could reverse the progression or could allow treatment before spread occurs. Examples are oral cancer screening, identification of markers/laboratory tests, and radiographic studies. Tertiary prevention involves the reduction of complications, prevention of further dysfunction, and the reduction of long-term sequelae of disease, including speech, dental, and swallowing problems. It can also refer to the reduction in death rates of a preexisting condition.

When defining studies and goals of prevention for head and neck cancer, it is important to clarify *which* head and neck cancer is being discussed. Head and neck cancer may refer to a variety of sites, histologies, and stages, and prevention efforts may be greatly discordant among cancers (Table 10-2).

Epidemiology

Epidemiologic approaches are used to describe the patterns of disease occurrence, to characterize natural history, and to identify determinants of disease. Epidemiologic evidence provides a basis for developing primary and secondary disease prevention strategies. The benefits of intervention programs, whether based on lifestyle modification interventions or early detection, can be assessed using epidemiologic approaches.

Epidemiologic findings are also relevant to patient care, since clinicians can weigh the risk factor profiles of patients as they consider alternative diagnoses.

As mentioned, "head and neck cancer" refers to a diverse array of anatomic sites. This section emphasizes the most common form—cancers of the oral cavity and pharynx combined. Brief descriptions of other malignancies that fall within the rubric of head and neck cancer, such as nasopharyngeal cancer, thyroid cancer, sinonasal cancer, and salivary gland cancer, are provided here to offer a glimpse of unique aspects of their epidemiologic profile. Nasopharyngeal carcinoma, relatively rare in Western nations, poses a major public health burden in certain regions of Southeast Asia. Its etiology is linked to the Epstein-Barr virus in combination with environmental triggers such as fish that is salted and preserved in specific ways that are common in high-risk areas.

Thyroid cancer is a relatively rare cancer with an excellent prognosis, but time trends in the United States indicate that incidence rates have increased during the past two decades.[1] The endocrine function of the thyroid gland along with the higher incidence rates observed in males compared with females suggests a potential etiologic role for the hormonal milieu, but the most clearly established risk factor is radiation exposure.[1] Sinonasal cancers are also rare, with approximately 2000 new cases diagnosed each year in the United States. These cancers are strongly associated with specific occupational exposures, such as nickel and wood dusts.[2] Salivary gland cancers are very rare. Ionizing radiation is an established risk factor, but unlike oral and pharyngeal cancer, salivary gland cancers are not linked to tobacco use or alcohol drinking.[3]

Occurrence of Oral Cavity and Pharynx Cancer

Cancer of the oral cavity and pharynx is a global health problem, accounting for approximately 390,000 new diagnoses and 207,000 deaths in 2000.[4] Unlike many forms of cancer, oral cancer poses a substantial problem in both developing and developed nations.[5] In the United States in 2008, estimates indicate that more than 35,000 new cases of oral cavity and pharynx cancer will be diagnosed and that over 7590 people will die of the disease.[6] From 1975 through 2003, there has been a gradual decline of 23% in age-adjusted incidence (from 13.2 to 10.2 per 100,000) and a 40% decline in mortality rates (from 4.3 to 2.6 per 100,000).[7]

Age is a strong determinant of oral and pharyngeal cancer rates. This cancer is extremely rare in those younger than 35 years, but incidence increases steeply thereafter, with rates peaking among 75- to 79-year-olds.[7] Notable gender and racial differences are present in the population burden of oral and pharyngeal cancer in the United States. From 2000 to 2003, age-adjusted incidence rates for males were 156% greater than for females, and mortality rates were 173% greater than for females. Among males, African Americans suffer a disproportionate share of the burden from oral and pharyngeal cancer, with age-adjusted incidence being 15% greater than for white American males. Moreover, there is an even greater gap (79%) in mortality rates. The similar age-adjusted incidence and mortality rates among African-American and white American women gives rise to optimism that the large racial disparity among men can eventually be eliminated.

The 5-year relative survival rate in the United States (1996 to 2002) was 59%.[7] Survival varies considerably by stage at diagnosis, with 5-year relative survival rates using SEER staging of 81%, 52%, and 26% for local, regional, and distant disease, respectively.[7] The overall survival rate thus reflects the fact that the majority of cases (52%) are diagnosed with disease with regional spread, whereas 33% of cases are diagnosed with localized disease, and 10% with disease with distant spread.[7]

Etiology of Oral Cavity and Pharynx Cancer

Case-control and cohort studies, the epidemiologic study designs used to evaluate exposure disease associations, have provided evidence that cigarette smoking and alcohol drinking are the major causes of cancers of the oral cavity and pharynx. Both cigarette smoking alone and alcohol drinking alone are independent risk factors for head and neck cancer.[8] Taken together, they act synergistically to increase the risk of oral and pharyngeal cancer.[3] Combined, cigarette smoking and alcohol drinking are estimated to account for 75% of oral and pharyngeal cancer deaths in the United States. Forms of tobacco use other than cigarette smoking, such as pipe and cigar smoking and smokeless tobacco use, are also linked to oral cancer risk.[3]

The fact that most oral and pharyngeal cancer deaths are attributable to cigarette smoking and alcohol drinking and that these are potentially modifiable risk factors opens up primary prevention strategies. For example, any step to prevent cigarette smoking initiation or to promote cessation among dependent smokers is a step toward prevention of oral and pharyngeal cancer. This includes tobacco control activities to impact policy, such as cigarette taxes and smoke-free workplace legislation, as well as interventions at the individual level to prevent the onset or continuation of smoking.

An active area of research with relevance to prevention is the observation that infection with oncogenic strains of human papillomavirus (HPV)—particularly HPV-16—are a risk factor, particularly for cancers of the oropharynx.[9] Solid epidemiologic evidence now indicates that HPV is a causal factor in up to 70% of cancers of the oropharyngeal lymphoepithelium (tonsil). HPV vaccines may prevent not only cervical cancer but also certain forms of oropharyngeal cancer. The potential role of dietary factors in relation to the risk of oropharyngeal cancer is another area that could pave pathways for preventive interventions. For example, evidence supporting a protection association between fruit and vegetable intake and risk of oral cancer has been observed.[10]

Background of Head and Neck Cancer Prevention

As with other cancers, the prevention of head and neck cancer can be divided into primary, secondary, and tertiary prevention (Table 10-3) Primary prevention works by decreasing the exposure or effects of extrinsic and intrinsic risk factors implicated in head and neck cancer (Table 10-4). It also encompasses the efforts of educating clinicians and the general public. Secondary prevention is prevention directed at early detection and treatment of cancerous and precancerous lesions. Tertiary prevention

Table 10-3. Prevention of Head and Neck Cancer		
Primary Prevention	**Secondary Prevention**	**Tertiary Prevention**
Decreasing exposure to risk factors	Early detection	Speech and swallow therapy (before, during, and after cancer therapy)
Public education and awareness	Screening (also may act as a primary prevention, because it raises public awareness)	Dental care, fluoride trays and other measures aimed at preventing postradiation dental complications
Clinicians, education	Treatment of precancerous lesions	Measures aimed at preserving postradiation salivary flow (IMRT, amifostine, salivary gland transfer)
Political and social policies and trends		Physical and occupational therapy

IMRT, intensity-modulated radiation therapy.

Table 10-4. Extrinsic and Intrinsic Factors in Head and Neck Cancer

Extrinsic Factors	Intrinsic Factors
Tobacco	Genetic
Alcohol	Iron-deficiency anemia
Dietary intake	Immunodeficiency
Viruses: HPV, HIV	GERD*
GERD*	

*Affected by both intrinsic and extrinsic factors.
GERD, gastroesophageal reflux disease; HPV, human papillomavirus.

aims at decreasing the complications of disease, prevention of further dysfunction, and reduction of long-term sequelae of disease, including speech, dental, and swallowing problems.

Head and Neck Squamous Cell Carcinoma

It is important to understand the various types, histologies, and stages of head and neck cancer (see Table 10-2). In general, the term "head and neck cancer" refers to mucosally derived squamous cell carcinoma that involves the oral cavity, oropharynx, hypopharynx, and laryngeal subsites. Cancers of the thyroid gland, salivary glands, nasopharynx, skin, and melanoma are typically classified under separate categories according to the American Joint Committee on Cancer and the International Union Against Cancer. Thus, for the remainder of the discussion, HNSCC will be used to refer to squamous cell carcinoma of the head and neck (oral, oropharyngeal, hypopharyngeal, and laryngeal). Many reports have combined some or all of these terms into a single category. However, it is important to separate them to avoid confusion and misinterpretation of the data. For example, "oral" cancer (tongue anterior to circumvallate papilla, floor of mouth, buccal, and so on) should not be confused with "oropharyngeal" cancer (base of tongue, soft palate, and tonsil) because often different examinations, instrumentations, and accessibility are required to visualize, diagnose, and biopsy these lesions. In addition, there is emerging evidence of a difference in etiopathogenesis with tobacco and alcohol associated with oral cancers, whereas human papillomavirus is associated with these agents or is an independent risk factor in oropharyngeal cancers.

Prevention of HNSCC is covered in great detail in the sections that follow, whereas other sites of the head and neck region are covered briefly in this section.

Thyroid Cancer

In the United States, papillary thyroid cancer is the most common histologic type (83%) of thyroid cancers, followed by follicular, Hürthle cell, medullary thyroid cancer, and anaplastic carcinoma[11] (Table 10-5).

Radiation is a well-known risk factor for thyroid cancer. In particular, exposure doses of 200 to 500 cGy are associated with cancer development at a rate of 0.5% per year.[12] This risk is higher for those exposed during childhood than for those exposed during adulthood. Indeed after the Chernobyl nuclear accident, the highest rate of thyroid cancer was seen in those who were less than 1 year of age at the time of exposure, and the rate progressively declined from 1 through 12 years of age.[13] With nuclear fallouts, although sheltering and evacuation are mainstays of preventing additional exposure, iodine tablets must be taken within hours of exposure and may

Table 10-5. Thyroid Malignancies	
Histologic Type	**Percent of Thyroid Cancer**
Papillary	83.2
Follicular	6.5
Hürthle cell	3.2
Medullary thyroid cancer	1.7
Anaplastic	1.0

From Davies L, Welch HG: Epidemiology of head and neck cancer in the United States. Otolaryngol Head Neck Surg 135(3):451–457, 2006.

reduce the risk incurred from exposure by a factor of 3. Potassium iodide tablets were not available to the exposed population of affected areas of Ukraine, Belarus, or Russia after the Chernobyl accident. Select few used iodine antiseptic drops mixed with table salt to create an equivalent of iodide tablets. Stable iodine such as potassium iodide saturates the gland and prevents uptake of the radioactive isotope.[14,15]

Medullary Thyroid Cancer

Various RET oncogene mutations are responsible for forms of hereditary medullary thyroid cancer (MTC), including MEN2A (MTC, parathyroid adenoma, pheochromocytoma), MEN2B (MTC, pheochromocytoma, mucosal neuromas, and musculoskeletal abnormalities), and familial MTC. RET mutations effect a number of different codons and thus are responsible for various manifestations of the clinical aggressiveness. In more aggressive forms, such as MEN2B (codon 918), the malignant transformation may occur as early as 8 to 9 months of age, whereas mutations with less aggressive behavior (codons 768, 791) may not manifest until adulthood.[16,17] As a result, genetic testing is recommended for all patients with familial forms of MTC.

Preventive treatment consists of prophylactic total thyroidectomy and perhaps a neck dissection. For patients with MEN2B, current consensus recommends total thyroidectomy before the age of 6 months or as soon as diagnosis is made. MEN2A patients should undergo prophylactic surgical treatment before age 5 years. The risk of nodal metastasis increases with the age of diagnosis, and the patient should be considered for neck dissection if diagnosed at age 10 or older.[18–20] Thus, early diagnosis with molecular typing and prophylactic surgical treatment is crucial for the prevention and treatment of hereditary MTC.

Salivary Gland Cancer

For the most part, the etiology of primary salivary gland malignancies is poorly understood, and thus recommendations for prevention of such neoplasms are limited. The major risk factors that have been identified are radiation exposure, occupational exposures, and viruses.[21]

Radiation exposure is one of the most well-established risk factors for salivary gland cancer.[22] Radiation typically induces salivary neoplasia after a latency period of several years, and both benign and malignant tumors may develop. Several investigators have reported a markedly increased incidence of salivary gland tumors among survivors of the atomic bombs in Hiroshima and Nagasaki, with an estimated relative risk of 3.5 to 11.[21,23–25] In particular, a strong radiation dose response for mucoepidermoid carcinoma and the benign Warthin's tumor has been reported among this cohort.[24,25] Therapeutic radiation also has been linked to salivary neoplasia. Patients receiving radiation therapy for either head and neck malignancies (e.g., carcinomas,

Hodgkin's disease) or benign conditions (e.g., tinea capitis, enlarged tonsils and adenoids, and acne) are at risk.[26–28] In addition, in their study of childhood cancer survivors who went on to develop salivary gland tumors, Whatley and associates[26] suggested that chemoradiation may pose a greater risk than radiation alone. Therefore, limiting therapeutic radiation exposures, particularly for younger patients, appears to be prudent. For benign conditions of the head and neck, radiation therapy generally has fallen out of favor.

In the treatment of head and neck malignancies, intensity-modulated radiation therapy (IMRT) may be used to limit the field of exposure outside the target area. In addition, a small but statistically significant increase in benign and malignant salivary neoplasms, including pleomorphic adenoma, mucoepidermoid carcinoma, and non-Hodgkin's lymphoma, has been described in patients treated with ^{131}I for thyroid malignancies or hyperthyroidism.[29–31] The salivary glands concentrate iodide selectively, and thus radioactive iodine makes them susceptible in the short term to sialadenitis and in the long term to neoplasia.[29] Furthermore, it has been suggested that excessive use of medical or dental diagnostic radiographs increases the risk for salivary tumors. However, the risk seems to be greatest for patients who had radiographs in the remote past, when radiation dosages were higher, and it is uncertain whether the low doses currently used are associated with appreciable risk.[32,33]

Limiting certain occupational exposures may help reduce the risk of salivary cancer development. Associations with various occupations have been suggested, including asbestos mining, rubber manufacturing, plumbing, certain types of woodworking, agriculture, cosmetology, fertilizer production, and automobile manufacturing.[21,22,34,35] Exposures to nickel, chromium, silica, and cement dusts have been implicated as well.[21,36,37] However, in many instances the strength of these associations is limited by the small number of cases examined and by the variability in results reported across studies.[34,38]

Several viruses have been implicated in the etiopathogenesis of salivary gland cancers. For example, Epstein-Barr virus (EBV) is associated with salivary lympho-epithelial carcinoma in Asian patients.[21,39] Additional viruses with potential roles in salivary cancer development include polyomavirus, cytomegalovirus, and human papillomavirus types 16 and 18.[21] However, other than optimizing the host immune system, potential prevention strategies aimed against these viral influences seem limited. Whether the recently developed HPV vaccine will have any effect on preventing salivary neoplasia is purely conjecture at this time.

In contrast to most other head and neck cancers, tobacco use and excessive alcohol consumption have not been consistently associated with malignant salivary gland tumors.[36,38] However, several studies have shown a close association of the benign salivary neoplasm Warthin's tumor with smoking.[40]

A few investigators have proposed a potential role of dietary factors, including antioxidant vitamin deficiencies and dietary lipids, in the development of salivary gland cancers.[36,37,41] However, no definitive role of diet in salivary carcinogenesis or cancer prevention has been established to date.

Nasopharyngeal Cancer

Nasopharyngeal carcinoma comprises a subset of head and neck cancers with distinct etiology. They can be divided into keratinizing or well-differentiated squamous tumors (defined as WHO type I) and nonkeratinizing tumors, which are further divided into poorly differentiated (WHO type II) and undifferentiated (WHO type III) subsets.[42] Undifferentiated tumors are the most common subtype, accounting for approximately 75% of tumors in the West and more than 95% of tumors in China and parts of Southeast Asia, where the overall risk of developing nasopharyngeal carcinoma ranges from 20 to 100 times higher than in the West.[43,44] Although the keratinizing tumors tend to remain localized, patients diagnosed with these cancers often have a poor prognosis.[45–48] Patients with undifferentiated tumors, despite their greater tendency to metastasize, generally have a better prognosis, and such tumors are often characterized histologically by a prominent lymphoid stroma.[49–52] Poorly differentiated nasopharyngeal carcinomas are the least common subtype and have a variable outcome.[45–48]

Worldwide, approximately 80,000 cases of nasopharyngeal carcinoma are diagnosed annually; and each year some 60,000 to 70,000 people die from the disease.[53] The geographic distribution of cases suggests that there are both genetic and environmental predisposing factors.[43–48] Southeast Asians and Cantonese have some of the highest rates of disease, with the peak incidence occurring in these populations in 40- to 50-year-olds. Tunisians and North Africans have a bimodal prevalence, with a small peak in the 10- to 25-year-old population and a much larger incidence in the over-50 population. There are also increased rates in Arctic and Greenland natives, as well as in Pacific Islanders compared with Western countries including the United States, where incidence rates are low (approximately 1/100,000). In the United States, the lowest rates are among Caucasians, with slightly higher rates for African Americans and the highest rates for Asians.[45–48] The prognosis tends to be better for Asian Americans, who predominantly have undifferentiated nasopharyngeal carcinoma, than for Caucasians, who have a comparatively higher incidence of keratinizing disease. The prognosis is worst for African Americans, who have a bimodal prevalence that reflects incidence rates in continental Africa.[47]

Nasopharyngeal carcinogenesis occurs in a stepwise fashion, with environmental carcinogens and genetic predisposition leading to dysplastic changes in the epithelium.[54–56] Genetic analyses of dysplastic tissue have identified frequent losses of heterozygosity in chromosomes 3p, 9p, 11q, 13q, and 14q. Infection of dysplastic tissue with the common herpesvirus, EBV, is an obligatory step in the development of nonkeratinizing carcinomas, whereas there is an inconsistent association with EBV infection for keratinizing tumors. Viral oncogene expression precedes development of intraepithelial neoplasia. Additional chromosomal mutations lead to high-grade neoplasias, with late-stage changes associated with metastasis.[57–60]

Environmental carcinogens with a defined role in nasopharyngeal carcinoma include cured salted fish and other preserved foods, which contain volatile nitrosamines.[61,62] The etiologic importance of nitrosamines is underscored by the finding that genetic polymorphisms have been identified in susceptible populations in CYP2E1, which converts nitrosamines into reactive DNA damaging intermediates.[63–65] Possible occupational hazards with a suspected carcinogenic role include wood dust and formaldehyde,[66] which may contribute to disease in EBV-seropositive patients. Alcohol use and cigarette smoking are risk factors for keratinizing nasopharyngeal carcinoma,[67,68] and betel nut chewing may be associated with increased risk in those with a family history of disease.[69] Other genetic predispositions are suggested by linkages with particular HLA chromosomal sites and the prevalence of specific HLA types, including HLA-A2, Bw46, and B17.[70–73] In addition, genetic polymorphisms in DNA repair proteins have been implicated in disease.[74–76]

There is a 100% association of EBV with nonkeratinizing tumors.[51,54,59,60,64,77–79] The virus is present in all tumor cells but not in surrounding dysplastic tissue, and monoclonal viral genomes have been identified in the tumor cells. This suggests a transforming role.[80] Viral gene expression is characterized by latency program II, consisting of *EBNA1* and *LMP2* oncogene expression, and *BART* and *EBER* transcripts.[57] The *LMP1* oncogene is also detected in about 50% of cases, and this correlates with expression of metastatic and anti-apoptotic genes. EBV appears to contribute to tumor cell immunoevasion, primarily by downregulating *MHC I* molecules and thus endogenous antigen presentation.[81,82] In addition, the virus might be responsible for perpetuation of the lymphoid stroma, which in turn produces cytokines, chemokines, matrix metalloproteases, and angiogenic factors that promote tumor growth and metastasis.[49-52]

Preventive measures against nasopharyngeal carcinoma include early detection through diagnostic screening, dietary modification, reduction of occupational hazards, and EBV vaccination strategies. Late detection of the cancer is a major factor contributing to poor disease prognosis, and unfortunately diagnostic difficulties are common. The early stages of disease are often asymptomatic, and the nasopharynx tends to be inaccessible, with tumors often growing submucosally. Serum IgA antibodies against late EBV proteins are increased in most patients preceding disease diagnosis and can be considered a risk factor for but not diagnostic of nasopharyngeal carcinoma, because they are also increased in a proportion of healthy adults.[83-86] In contrast, quantification of EBV DNA load performed on brush biopsies is diagnostic for nonkeratinizing disease. This screening test has been performed successfully in high-risk Asian populations.

Avoidance of salted fish and preserved foods containing nitrosamines is the most effective known preventive measure against nasopharyngeal carcinoma. (In parts of China, interrupting the traditional practice of weaning babies with cured fish has reduced disease incidence in recent years.[87]) Conversely, consumption of fresh fruits and vegetables correlates with decreased risk.[88] Avoidance of alcohol, smoking, and betel nut chewing are also suggested preventive practices. In addition, minimizing occupational exposure to wood dust and formaldehyde might have some benefit, particularly in individuals with chronic respiratory conditions, who have increased disease incidence.[66]

Prevention of EBV infection is an obvious protective strategy; however, there are no effective prophylactic vaccines against this ubiquitous herpesvirus.[89] More than 90% of adults worldwide have lifelong latent EBV infection; thus, prophylactic vaccines, even if extant, would likely not be useful unless given to young children. Experimental therapeutic vaccines directed against EBV are currently in early clinical testing. These include a chimeric EBV antigen vaccinia virus vaccine against a recombinant EBNA1-LMP2 fusion[90] and an immunotherapy vaccine comprising ex vivo expansion of cytotoxic T cells specific for EBV-LMP2, followed by reinjection into the patient.[91-93] Future therapeutic considerations include antivirals—in particular, cidofovir—in combination with ribonucleotide reductase inhibitors or phosphonated nucleoside analogs.[94,95] Lastly, recent reports implicate nasopharyngeal cancer stem cells in disease progression,[96] possibly generating new opportunities for therapeutic intervention (Fig. 10-1).

Paranasal Sinus Cancer

A variety of occupational risk factors have been described in association with paranasal sinus (i.e., sinonasal carcinomas). These include woodworking and in particular exposure to wood dust, as well as exposure to paint, oil fumes, and chromium-containing materials.[97-101] In contrast to oral, laryngeal, and pharyngeal carcinomas, with sinonasal malignancies tobacco use has not proved to be a consistent risk factor.[102] Woodworking, however, has been linked to sinonasal adenocarcinoma, particularly in the ethmoid region, with a notable male predominance (75% to 90%).[102] It is interesting that the deficiency of the immunoglobulin A and mucosal metaplasia has been demonstrated in workers with over 10 years of exposure to wood and wood dusts.[98] Even more interesting is that sinonasal squamous cell carcinomas have been associated with exposure to nickel, softwood dust, and mustard gas,

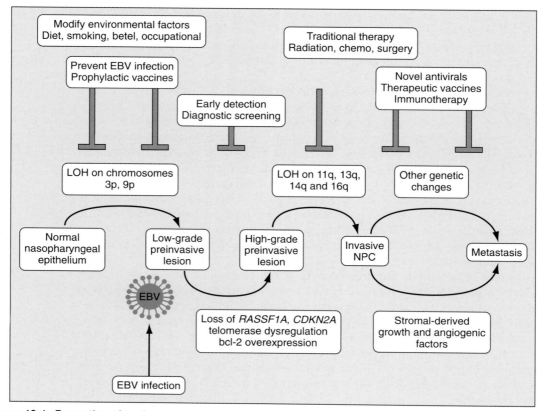

Figure 10-1. Prevention of nonkeratinizing nasopharyngeal carcinoma. The multistep nasopharyngeal carcinogenesis process offers many opportunities for therapeutic intervention. Modification of environmental factors could prevent the loss of heterozygosity[287] of putative tumor suppressors on chromosomes 3p and 9p, which are associated with development of preinvasive lesions. Prophylaxis against the oncogenic Epstein-Barr virus (EBV) would prevent the subsequent genetic events associated with infection, halting progression to high-grade invasive lesions. Early detection at this stage through screening would maximize the response to traditional therapeutic options, preventing late-stage disease and obviating the need for novel experimental therapeutics. LOH, loss of heterozygosity; NPC, nasopharyngeal carcinoma.

whereas sinonasal adenocarcinomas have been related to exposure to hardwood, chrome pigment, and leather dust.[103]

Sarcomas of sinonasal cavities may develop several years after radiation exposure and should be considered in the differential diagnosis for patients with prior exposure.[104]

Skin Cancer (Squamous Cell and Basal Cell) and Melanoma Cancer

Ultraviolet light exposure is a known risk factor for cutaneous malignancies, including basal cell carcinoma, squamous cell carcinoma, and melanoma. Because of the potential for sun exposure, the head and neck area is a common site for skin cancer development. In particular, squamous cell carcinoma of the lip vermilion is strongly associated with a history of chronic sun exposure, although other factors may play a role.[105–108]

Several risk factors have been described to have an association with skin melanoma formation. Besides sun exposure, genetics and history of melanoma or dysplastic nevi have been implicated in the development of melanomas.[109] People who are classified as Fitzpatrick type I have the highest risk of skin cancer[110–114] (Table 10-6). When patients are stratified by skin type, sun exposure appears to be the strongest and

Table 10-6. Fitzpatrick Classification of Skin Types

Skin Type	Skin Color	Characteristics
I	White; very fair; red or blond hair; blue eyes; freckles	Always burns, never tans
II	White; fair; red or blond hair; blue, hazel, or green eyes	Usually burns, tans with difficulty
III	White; fair with any eye or hair color; very common	Sometimes mild burn, gradually tans
IV	Brown; typical Mediterranean Caucasian skin	Rarely burns, tans with ease
V	Dark brown; middle Eastern skin types	Very rarely burns, tans very easily
VI	Black	Never burns, tans very easily

most consistent risk factor. Note that intermittent intense sun exposure may have more deleterious effects than continuous sun exposure. This could explain the increased distribution of melanomas that occur on the back and trunk.[109,115]

Prior dysplastic nevi can be found in one third of patients diagnosed with melanoma. Moreover, patients with a previous diagnosis of melanoma are 30 times more likely to develop subsequent skin melanomas.[116]

Familial syndromes and genetic mutations have been described in association with cutaneous melanomas. Familial multiple mole melanoma syndrome is probably the most common hereditary syndrome. Several recently discovered genes (such as CMM1(1p36), CDKN2A(9p21), CDK4(12q14), and CMM4(9p21)) have been linked to the development of cutaneous melanomas.[117]

Continued investigations are directed at revealing molecular markers and targets for diagnosis, staging, prognosis, and treatment of skin cancer.[118]

Prevention of Head and Neck Squamous Cell Carcinoma

Prevention Related to Tobacco Use

Prevention of tobacco use, or cessation among current users, remains the primary objective by which to prevent head and neck cancer. Most smokers start smoking before the age of 18, and almost all smokers have initiated smoking by age 25.[119] Primary prevention efforts targeted toward adolescents and young adults will yield significant cancer prevention benefits to the extent that they offer an enduring preventive impact. Many school-based prevention programs are effective over the short term,[120] but the long-term effectiveness of these programs remains modest.[121] Recent data from the Monitoring the Future project suggest that recent declines in adolescent smoking may be ending.[122] This calls attention to the need for comprehensive tobacco prevention strategies that include media and countermarketing methods.[123]

Among current smokers, cessation is a top priority, and indeed quitting smoking has direct benefits to cancer prevention and reversal of the premalignant changes (Figs. 10-2 and 10-3). Unfortunately, the quit ratio (percentage of ever smokers who have quit) has remained largely unchanged in recent years (Fig. 10-4). Moreover, the quit ratio remains significantly lower among nonwhite smokers, highlighting the growing health disparity that smoking incurs. The U.S. Public Health Service (USPHS) guidelines for smoking cessation recommend pharmacotherapy as a first-line strategy to assist in quitting.[124] Nicotine replacement therapies (NRT), along with bupropion and varenicline, have all been shown to be effective for smoking cessation.[125–127] However, use of proven cessation aids remains disappointingly low. One population-based study noted that 78% of smokers have never used pharmacotherapy,[128] a finding replicated elsewhere.[129,130] Wider dissemination of these effective cessation tools could likely increase the rate of successful quitting. However, given that the incidence of quit attempts (percentage of smokers making a 24-hour quit attempt in a given year) has also not substantively changed in the past decade

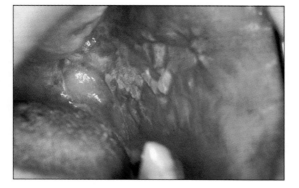

Figure 10-2. Oral leukoplakia in the pipe smoker.

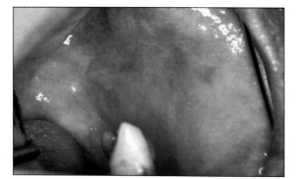

Figure 10-3. The same patient as in Figure 10-2 with oral leukoplakia resolved 2 months after cessation of tobacco use.

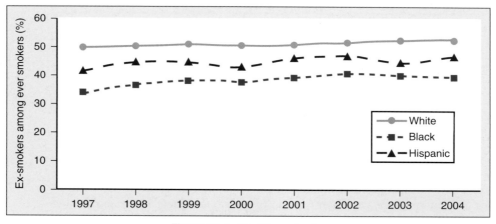

Figure 10-4. Smoking quit ratio.

(Fig. 10-5), clinicians and researchers need to examine novel interventions to increase interest in quitting among smokers who are unmotivated to quit. Physician advice to quit smoking is a strong tool to assist large numbers of smokers to quit,[124] but delivery of effective cessation interventions within the healthcare system remains inconsistent.[131,132] One potential novel strategy to induce quitting is the harm reduction approach of reduced smoking, which often motivates recalcitrant smokers to quit.[133,134]

Comprehensive tobacco control includes important policy level initiatives as well. Among these, taxation and environmental restrictions (e.g., smoke-free laws) are effective strategies to lower the prevalence of smoking.[135–137] The Master Settlement

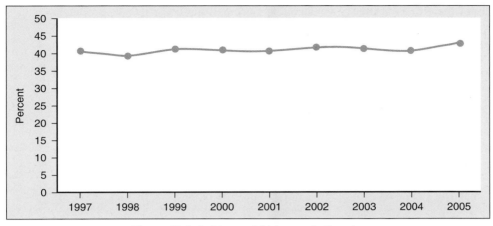

Figure 10-5. Incidence of 24-hour quit attempts.

Agreement significantly strengthened the infrastructure for tobacco control,[138] although the fact that tobacco is still unregulated by the FDA remains a significant impediment to policy change.[139]

In all, prevention and control of tobacco use require a comprehensive approach that prevents adolescents and young adults from initiating tobacco use and that motivates and assists existing smokers to successfully quit—all within a framework of aggressive policy efforts that collectively support long-term reduced exposure to the leading risk factor for head and neck cancer.

Prevention Related to Alcohol Use

There is strong and consistent evidence that heavy alcohol consumption increases the risk of cancer of the oral cavity and pharynx (OPC).[140] The National Institute on Alcohol Abuse and Alcoholism (NIAAA) estimates that nearly 50% of OPC is associated with heavy drinking.[141] Although the combined use of alcohol and tobacco poses the greatest risk, the major risk factor for those who have never smoked is alcohol consumption, with an odds ratio threefold higher in drinkers than in non-drinkers.[142] In addition, the risk of second primary tumors (SPTs) is 50% higher in OPC patients who continue to drink heavily after treatment, even after adjusting for smoking status.

In a meta-analysis of over 200 studies investigating the effects of alcohol on the risk of developing cancer, Bagnardi and colleagues[142] concluded that alcohol consumption of 50 g (i.e., four standard drinks) or more per day significantly increased the risk of developing OPC. Significant increases in risk existed even at 25 g or two standard drinks per day. Relative risk increased with increasing alcohol consumption. Relative risk was 1.73, 2.77, and 5.75 for alcohol intakes of 25, 50, and 100 g of alcohol a day, respectively. Other studies have shown even higher relative risks of up to nine times greater for moderate to heavy drinkers and up to 35 times greater risk when alcohol consumption exceeds 100 g of alcohol per day.[105] An important conclusion from these findings is that research has yet to identify a threshold level of alcohol consumption below which no increased risk is evident.

Although no studies on OPC have investigated binge versus daily drinking, such patterns have been shown to be important with other alcohol-sensitive medical conditions, with binge drinkers showing greater variations in blood pressure than heavy daily drinkers.[143] Merletti and colleagues[144] suggest that risk of oral cancer may also be related to consumption patterns of drinking either during or between meals.

Studies of the effects of the type of alcoholic beverage on OPC risk have produced equivocal results. Some studies have shown that more potent beverages such as hard liquor pose more of a risk than either beer or wine, whereas others have not shown this relationship. Still other investigations contradict these results by finding that wine consumption has the greatest risk. Because studies of this nature have been conducted in various countries around the world, some feel that the divergent findings simply reflect the fact that the most frequently consumed beverage in each region or country tends to be the beverage associated with the highest relative risk.[142]

Alcohol and tobacco smoking are closely linked in that people who drink are more likely to smoke and vice versa. Smoking rates in alcohol-dependent individuals are as high as 90%.[145] In addition, smokers who are nicotine-dependent have a 2.7 times greater chance of becoming alcohol-dependent than do nonsmokers.[146] Some studies indicate that the prevalence of alcohol dependence in patients with OPC exceeds 50%.[147]

The combination of moderate to heavy alcohol use and tobacco smoking dramatically increases the risk of OPC. In a case-control study, Andre and colleagues[148] found that the odds ratio for OPC in those smoking a pack or more of cigarettes per day increased dramatically with increased drinking. Smokers who drank two drinks or less per day had an odds ratio for OPC of 4.5, whereas the odds ratio for smokers who drank three drinks per day almost tripled to 12.8. Smokers consuming over 80 g of alcohol per day (six or more drinks) were at extremely high risk, with an odds ratio of 36.2. Even light smokers (smoking less than a pack a day) had an odds ratio six times higher if they drank three or more drinks per day compared with drinking two drinks or less.

The combined risk is especially dramatic in very heavy drinkers (five or more standard drinks per day) who also smoke heavily (two or more packs per day), with studies showing these individuals to have up to 100 times greater risk for developing a malignancy.[148]

Alcohol Screening

Based on the strong relationship between heavy alcohol use and the development of OPC, screening to identify patients at risk for OPC because of heavy alcohol use should be conducted routinely. In fact, brief screening procedures designed for medical and dental settings have been developed and validated. According to NIAAA guidelines, all adult patients should initially be asked (via health questionnaires or orally) "Do you sometimes drink beer, wine, or other alcoholic beverages?" This initial question is designed to screen out the approximate 40% of patients who are nondrinkers or who drink very rarely. Drinkers would then be asked a single heavy-drinking-day screening question: "How many times in the past year have you had five or more drinks in a day [for men] or four or more drinks in a day [for women]." A standard drink would be defined for the patient as 12 ounces of beer, 5 ounces of wine, or 1½ ounces of spirits. This heavy-drinking-day screening question is a sensitive, specific, and time-efficient screening instrument that has a sensitivity of 0.86 for detecting alcohol use disorders. A positive screen would be one or more heavy drinking days. Although it is possible for someone to have had a once- or twice-only heavy drinking day in the past year (e.g., New Year's Eve) and therefore not be a routine heavy drinker, 98% of heavy daily drinkers answer the heavy-drinking-day question in the affirmative.

If the health professional is unsure of the validity of the patient's response, he or she can ask about the quantity and frequency of the patient's alcohol consumption. Heavy or at-risk drinking is defined as more than 14 drinks a week for men and more than 7 drinks a week for women and for men over the age of 65 years. However, a positive response to the heavy-drinking-day question is considered a positive screen and should trigger a general discussion of the patient's drinking along with advice and counseling to reduce consumption.

If time allows, health professionals can also screen using the Alcohol Use Disorders Identification Test (AUDIT), a ten-item alcohol screening questionnaire developed by the World Health Organization (WHO) for use in primary health care. A shorter three-question version known as the AUDIT-C is also available. However, in most busy medical, dental, or surgical practices, the single heavy-drinking-days question is the most practical and efficient way to screen all patients.

Some clinicians may wish to add alcohol biomarker blood tests such as gamma-glutamyltransferase (GGT) or carbohydrate-deficient transferrin (%CDT) as additional screening aids. Biochemical tests are useful when the clinician feels a need for more concrete evidence of heavy drinking or when he or she questions the veracity or memory of the patient. The %CDT test is especially useful in detecting heavy alcohol consumption (five or more drinks per day) over the past 2 weeks. The combined use of these biomarkers with alcohol screening questions can lead to rates of detection of alcohol use disorders of more than 90%.

Brief Intervention

Brief counseling and advice for patients who screen positively can be effective in reducing a patient's alcohol use and alcohol-related morbidity. If screening indicates the need for brief alcohol intervention, clinicians should state their conclusions and recommendations clearly: "You are drinking more than is medically safe and alcohol is putting you at risk for mouth and throat cancer. I strongly recommend that you cut down on drinking to no more than one beer a day or quit altogether." This should be followed by a discussion of the relationship between heavy alcohol use and OPC.

In addition, clinicians should attempt to gauge the patient's motivational readiness to change (i.e., "Are you willing to consider changes in your drinking?"). If the patient is willing to change, the clinician should help set a drinking goal, agree on a plan of action, and provide educational materials on oral cancer risk factors as well as ways to reduce alcohol intake (available from the NIAAA website). If the patient is not willing to change, the clinician should restate his or her concern about OPC risk and encourage the patient to think about what has been discussed and the pros and cons of continued heavy drinking. At-risk but nondependent drinkers can benefit from such counseling.

Patients with more severe alcohol use disorders require referral to an alcoholism counseling specialist or to Alcoholics Anonymous. Unfortunately, there are often not enough affordable resources in the community, or the patient does not follow through on the referral. This should not deter the clinician from advising and monitoring patients about their alcohol use, because such intervention is significantly effective with many patients.

Prevention Related to Dietary Intake Factors

Increased risk of oral cancers has been described in people with dietary deficiencies, often from inadequate intake of fruits and vegetables.[149,150] Moreover, a recent prospective EPIC study demonstrated a 9% (12% for men and 4% for women) reduced risk of squamous cell carcinoma of the upper aerodigestive tract with an 80-g daily intake of fruits and vegetables.[151]

Several recent studies have focused on particular vegetable groups (e.g., lycopene-containing vegetables and allium vegetables) and have been able to establish a link between a reduced risk of upper aerodigestive tract squamous cell carcinoma and vegetable intake.[152,153]

Deficiency states of iron, zinc, and beta carotene seem to be especially important in increasing risk for head and neck cancers.[154–156] A recent prospective study, however, showed that while dietary vitamin C had protective effects for oral premalignant lesions, supplemental vitamin C did not offer a reduced risk. Furthermore, supplementation of vitamin E and beta carotene had an increased risk of oral premalignant lesions in smokers.[157]

In India and Southeast Asia, the chronic placement of betel quid, or *paan*, in the mouth has been strongly associated with an increased risk of oral cancer.[158] The quid is made from a betel leaf that is wrapped around a combination of areca nut and slaked lime and often includes tobacco, sweeteners, and condiments. Notably, betel quid users have been reported to have a nearly 8% lifetime risk of developing oral cancer.[159]

Prevention Related to Viral Etiologies

In recent years, the human papillomavirus has been increasingly identified as a predisposing factor in the development of oropharyngeal carcinoma.[160] The virus is found in approximately 50% of oropharyngeal cancers, with high-risk HPV type 16 accounting for about 90% of the cases and other high-risk types, including HPV 18, 31, 33, 35, accounting for the remainder.[161] Most of the HPV-associated oropharyngeal tumors are located in the tonsils and in the base of the tongue region.[162–165] Histologically, the tumor cells are typically nonkeratinizing and are poorly differentiated, with a basaloid appearance. They exhibit diffuse nuclear and cytoplasmic staining for p16, a biomarker that is commonly found on normal epithelial cells of the tonsillar crypt and that is not associated with keratinizing HPV-negative tumors.[164,166] As reviewed by Syrjanen,[160] there is a lesser association of HPV with cancers of the oral cavity and with laryngeal carcinomas, and rates of detection in these cancers vary significantly in a number of different studies from less than 5% to 30%. This variance is likely due to the different methods of detection used and to different study designs.

Some cases catalogued as supraglottic in origin may actually arise from neighboring lingual tonsils, and lingual and palatine tonsil cancer may encroach on oral tongue, resulting in mistaken assignment of site. In addition, the virus has been detected in several precancerous conditions and benign squamous cell proliferations, including oral leukoplakia, in which approximately 25% of cases reportedly contain HPV; oral verrucous carcinomas, with a 50% to 60% association; and laryngeal papillomas or recurrent respiratory papillomatosis, in which HPV is detected in about 80% of cases (mainly low-risk types HPV 6 and 11). It is not yet known whether these benign conditions lead to further development of carcinoma. HPV seropositivity and oral HPV prevalence in particular are risk factors for subsequent development of disease. Depending on the population studied, the rate of oral HPV prevalence ranges from 2% to 10% of healthy volunteers and is found in about 2% of pediatric tonsillectomy samples in the United States.[167] It has been reported that HPV-associated cancers often occur in patients with a younger median age (less than 55 years old), whereas HPV-negative tumors occur more frequently in the over-55 population.[168]

For oropharyngeal carcinomas in general, recent evidence suggests that four independent risk factors collectively account for 90% of HPV-positive and -negative cases.[9] These factors include poor oral hygiene, comprising poor dentition and infrequent tooth-brushing; a family history of head and neck squamous cell carcinoma; a heavy smoking history, which is strongly correlated with HPV-negative disease; and HPV 16 seropositivity for the L1 major virus capsid protein. HPV 16 L1 seropositivity alone accounted for 55% of cases. A history of heavy alcohol use synergized with smoking history for HPV-negative disease, whereas these factors were underrepresented in patients with HPV-associated disease, suggesting that smoking and drinking were not important factors in viral transformation. Instead, the prevailing view currently emerging is that there are two main carcinogenic pathways, with one resulting from heavy tobacco and alcohol exposure and the other from HPV infection.[9,169] Although poor diet (a lack of particular micronutrients) is known to play a role in the former, it is unclear whether diet is a risk factor for HPV-associated disease.

Sexual transmission appears to be a primary mode of oral HPV infection. Sexual history correlates with HPV-associated oropharyngeal carcinoma, with a higher number of lifetime vaginal and oral sex partners conferring increased risk.[9,168] In addition, self-reported practice of oral-anal and oral-genital sex, engagement in casual sex, infrequent condom use, and early age at first intercourse are disease risk factors, as is having a partner with cervical cancer or with genital warts.[9,168] Furthermore, women over age 50 with in situ and invasive cervical carcinoma have an increased risk. Oral infections are more common in women with cervical infections, although not necessarily the same virus types are found at both sites. This indicates that some women may have increased susceptibility, possibly resulting from immune deficits.[170-172] Immunodeficiency resulting from HIV, or from the use of antirejection medication following organ transplantation, increases oral HPV prevalence.[171,173,174] Also, patients with Fanconi's anemia have an increased genetic susceptibility to HPV infection and thus an increased risk for cancer.[175-177] Finally, infection with the common herpesvirus HSV-1 has been proposed as a possible cofactor in HPV tumorigenesis.[178]

During sexual contact, HPV may be transmitted through microabrasions in mucous membranes, infecting basal cells, which then divide as the viral genome replicates (although this does not explain the high rate of tonsillar cancer in heterosexual men). As the infected cells differentiate, they move into the sub-basal layer, where the virus completes the replication process and is eventually released from terminally differentiated squamous cells. The viral genome encodes six nonstructural proteins, including the E6 and E7 oncoproteins, and two capsid proteins, L1 and L2. Viral integration correlates with carcinogenesis and is not found in normal tonsil but is limited to dysplasias and invasive cancers.[179-182] Viral integration deregulates expression of the E6 and E7 oncoproteins, which act to disrupt the cell cycle and DNA repair pathways, causing genomic instability. E6 targets p53 for degradation, while E7 inactivates pRb, leading to accumulation of p16, E2F activation, and DNA replication. Ordinarily, this would signal p53 to activate the apoptotic pathway, but with E6 inactivation of p53, the cell undergoes unregulated growth. HPV-associated oropharyngeal carcinomas overexpress p16, and HIF-1α; c-*myc* is amplified after integration; and there is a decreased finding of epidermal growth factor receptor (EGFR) amplification.[179] E6 and E7 inactivation of the p53 and pRb pathways parallel the mutagenic effects of alcohol and smoking on these tumor suppressor genes in HPV-negative disease.

HPV-associated oropharyngeal carcinomas reportedly have a better prognosis than do HPV-negative tumors. Moreover, in tonsillar cancer, high viral load correlates with better prognosis.[162,163,183-185] The reasons for this are uncertain, with theories including a better response to radiation, increased immunosurveillance due to presentation of viral antigens, and absence of field cancerization effects. Also, E6-mediated degradation of p53 may be incomplete in HPV tumors, compared with the effects of p53 mutations in HPV-negative tumors. Hence, in HPV tumors, residual p53 may still be functional, allowing for apoptosis induction after radiation or chemotherapy.[183] In addition, the HPV-associated tumors rarely amplify EGFR, and tumors with low EGFR expression are known to have better prognosis.[183]

Modification of risky sexual behavior—for example, by increasing condom use, abstaining from casual sex, and limiting the number of sexual partners—would reduce viral transmission.[9,168] Other measures that may contribute to prevention of HPV-associated oropharyngeal cancer are early diagnosis through screening for oral HPV 16 in saliva or brush biopsies or through screening for HPV 16 seropositivity (an early risk factor),[9] and prophylactic vaccination. Screening is particularly important in immunosuppressed patients who are more susceptible to HPV infection, such as HIV and transplant patients. Also, maintaining good oral hygiene decreases risk, since poor dentition correlates with carcinoma development.[9] Tooth loss is generally caused by chronic bacterial infection and is associated with inflammation, which is known to promote carcinogenesis.[186-190]

Prophylactic HPV vaccines currently undergoing clinical trials in the United States for prevention of cervical cancer are reportedly very effective in preventing cervical infection[191-194] and may likewise prevent oral infection and subsequent oropharyngeal cancer, although the data for this are not yet available. The current vaccines are based on the ability of the virus capsid protein L1 by itself or with L2 to create virus-like particles (VLP) when expressed in eukaryotic cells.[193,194] The L1 major capsid protein induces strong type-specific immunity, whereas inclusion of the L2 minor capsid protein induces cross-reactive immunity to multiple HPV types. There is a quadri-valent VLP vaccine that protects against both low- and high-risk HPV types 6, 11, 16, and 18 and a bivalent vaccine that protects against high-risk HPV 16 and 18.[194] The vaccines are reportedly most effective in young individuals who have never been infected with HPV, because they mount the highest antiviral titers.[195] Vaccination of HPV-seropositive women was not harmful; however, it was not sufficient to protect this population from developing cervical neoplasias.

The prophylactic VLP vaccines are not therapeutic because the viral capsid pro-teins L1 and L2, which form the VLP, are generally not expressed in the tumor cells. After integration, viral replication no longer occurs; instead, only the E6 and E7 oncoproteins are consistently expressed in the tumors. Therefore, efforts to create therapeutic vaccines have concentrated on increasing immunity to HPV 16 E6 and E7.[192,196-199] Experimental vaccines in early-stage clinical trials include E7 subunit and DNA vaccines, peptides and proteins in adjuvant, recombinant virus vector vaccines, and immunotherapy vaccines in which the patients' dendritic cells are pulsed with E7 peptides and infused back into the patients. The difficulties involved in making an effective therapeutic vaccine involve overcoming the local immunosuppressive effects caused by IL (interleukin)-18, TGFβ (transforming growth factor β). T-regulatory cells, and other factors in the tumor microenvironment.[191,192,200] Thus, targeting the appropriate dendritic cell population for the most effective antigen presentation is a therapeutic vaccine goal. Finally, a promising chimeric prophylac-tic/therapeutic VLP vaccine containing E6 and E7 is currently under investigation[201] (Fig. 10-6).

Prevention Related Gastroesophageal Reflux Disease and Laryngopharyngeal Reflux

The association of gastroesophageal reflux disease with laryngeal cancer was first described in the 1980s, and more evidence has emerged that supports GERD as an independent risk factor. Over the last two decades, otolaryngic manifestations of GERD and laryngopharyngeal reflux with or without gastroesophageal reflux has been brought into the spotlight, including the model for developing laryngeal injury as the result of gastric acid and pepsin exposure to laryngeal mucosa.[202] Although there are no prospective studies to date that identify an increased incidence of laryngeal cancer in patients with GERD, there are several retrospective studies, including a recent

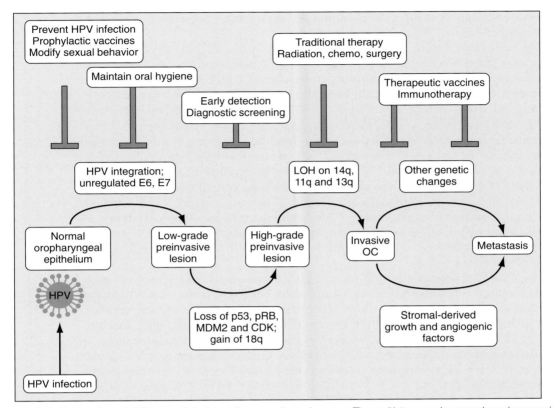

Figure 10-6. Prevention of HPV-associated oropharyngeal carcinoma.   The multistep oropharyngeal carcinogenesis process offers multiple opportunities for therapeutic intervention. Inhibiting oral human papillomavirus (HPV) infection and integration, through vaccines or behavior modification, would prevent viral oncogenes from targeting the p53 and pRb pathways, which create genomic instability in preinvasive lesions. This would prevent the subsequent chromosomal changes that result in the loss of heterozygosity[99] on particular chromosomes carrying putative tumor suppressor genes, halting progression to high-grade preinvasive lesions and ultimately to invasive carcinoma. Maintenance of proper oral hygiene would prevent the tumor-promoting chronic inflammation associated with bacterial tooth decay. Early detection through screening would maximize the response to traditional therapeutic options, preventing late-stage disease and obviating the need for novel experimental therapeutics. OC, oropharyngeal carcinoma.

matched case-control study that identified GERD as an independent risk factor for laryngeal cancer development.[203-205] Furthermore, acid suppression therapy after treatment of laryngeal cancer may have a protective effect on the rate of local recurrences.[206]

Prevention Related to Genetic Factors

Although head and neck cancers represent a heterogeneous group of tumor types with complex molecular and genetic aberrations, there are four major categories of molecular markers of pathogenetic significance in these tumors: (1) markers of tumor growth, proliferation, and apoptosis (e.g., EGFR, cyclin D1, the apoptotic mediator Fas and its ligand FasL, the antiapoptotic protein bcl-2); (2) markers of tumor suppression (e.g., p53, p27, p16); (3) markers of angiogenesis (e.g., the vascular endothelial growth factor family); and (4) markers of tumor invasion and metastatic potential (e.g., matrix metalloproteinases, E-cadherin).[207] Insights into the molecular pathogenesis of head and neck cancers may lead to the development of targeted therapies in the future, including novel chemoprevention strategies. Those markers that currently appear to offer the most promise as targets for prevention of HNSCC are described below.

The epidermal growth factor receptor maps to 7p13-q22 and encodes a transmembrane protein with tyrosine kinase activity. When bound by its ligands epidermal growth factor and transforming growth factor α (TGFα), EGFR mediates a complex cascade of signaling pathways influencing cellular proliferation, differentiation, and strong mitogenic activity.[207,208] Overexpression of proteins within the EGFR family (including EGFR, Her-2/neu, and c-erB 3 and 4) has been identified in premalignant and malignant lesions of the head and neck and is associated with poor outcome in patients with squamous cell carcinoma of the oral cavity, larynx, and other head and neck sites.[208-212] Strategies being developed for blocking EGFR activity in HNSCC include monoclonal antibodies (e.g., cetuximab), tyrosine kinase inhibitors (e.g., gefitinib [Iressa] and erlotinib [Tarceva]), ligand-linked immunotoxins, and antisense approaches.[213,214] In addition, tyrosine kinase inhibitors in combination with COX-2 inhibitors are in the early stages of clinical testing for prevention of squamous cell carcinoma in patients with oral or other head and neck premalignant lesions.[213]

The tumor suppressor gene *p53* located on chromosome 17p13 serves as a gatekeeper against carcinogenesis.[215] In normal cells, stresses such as DNA damage, hypoxia, oncogene activation, and viral replication stimulate *p53* activation, which in turn leads to cycle arrest or apoptosis, thereby maintaining genomic stability. Inactivation of *p53* or other components within the *p53* network is extremely common in human neoplasia, and approximately 50% of HNSCC possess mutant *p53*.[215,216] Mutations in *p53* appear to represent an early event in carcinogenesis, for they can be detected in dysplastic mucosa.[217] In addition, in a subset of HNSCC cases—particularly those arising in the oropharynx—HPV is present. The virally encoded E6 protein can promote degradation of the *p53* gene product and thus contribute to carcinogenesis.[218]

Therapeutic strategies aimed at restoring wild-type *p53* function or exploiting the *p53* null phenotype in cancer cells are being developed.[219] One strategy is to use adenoviral vectors to carry the wild-type gene into cancer cells. Upon restoration of *p53* function, the cells are sensitized to DNA damaging anticancer agents and undergo apoptosis. Initial clinical testing in patients with HNSCC demonstrated the safety of intratumoral injection of this *p53*-carrying adenoviral vector and induced regression or stabilization of disease in a few patients.[220] Results of clinical trials of this therapy in combination with chemotherapeutic agents such as docetaxel are awaited.[219,221]

Another strategy is to use adenoviral vectors to exploit the *p53* null phenotype of cancer cells. Efficient replication of adenovirus requires p53 degradation by association of the virally encoded E1B 55K protein with the N-terminus of p53. The engineered ONYX-015 adenovirus lacks the E1B 55K protein, and thus the rationale is that it can only replicate in and destroy cells that lack p53, such as tumor cells. However, it subsequently has been shown that an mRNA export function of E1B 55K—rather than mediation of p53 destruction—gives ONYX-015 its oncolytic activity.[222] In terms of chemoprevention, a phase I trial of ONYX-015 mouthwash for patients with oral premalignant lesions showed this therapy to be feasible with demonstrable activity.[223] As for HNSCC therapy, phases I and II clinical trials of intratumoral ONYX-015 alone or in combination with cisplatin and 5-fluorouracil have been conducted, and combination therapy has produced substantial and durable objective responses in patients with recurrent HNSCC.[224] Development of ONYX-015 has been halted in the United States for nonmedical reasons, although subsequent trials using this modified adenovirus (renamed H101) in China have been conducted for treatment of head and neck and esophageal carcinoma.[225]

Prevention Related to Environmental Factors

Practically speaking, the environment encompasses all conditions surrounding an individual's way of life. Major environmental factors relevant to head and neck cancer development, including tobacco, alcohol, diet, and infectious agents, have been discussed previously. Additional environmental factors to be considered are occupational, radiation, and ultraviolet light exposures. It is often difficult to obtain conclusive evidence of the etiologic role of specific environmental factors in cancer development because (1) the time between carcinogenic exposure and cancer diagnosis may be years or decades; (2) it is typically difficult to quantify accurately the amount of carcinogen exposure in retrospect; and (3) most carcinogens induce cancer development in only a small proportion of exposed persons.[226]

Various occupational exposures have been suggested as contributing to head and neck cancer development. For instance, strong evidence exists that intense exposure to wood dusts leads to an increased risk of sinonasal and nasopharyngeal carcinomas.[227,228] In particular, the incidence of intestinal-type sinonasal adenocarcinomas among woodworkers exposed to fine hardwood dusts is nearly 1000 times that of the general public.[228] Other suspected carcinogen associations include asbestos and laryngeal cancer as well as formaldehyde and coal dust and hypopharyngeal cancer.[229,230] In addition, the polycyclic aromatic hydrocarbons (PAHs) are well-known carcinogens. Although HNSCC is most often associated with PAH exposure from tobacco smoke, high levels of PAH exposure also can be found in industrial settings (e.g., among steel, foundry, and gas workers).[229]

Guidelines for limiting such occupational exposures are essential for prevention. Such guidelines may include personal protective equipment, process modification, ventilation, and filtration measures. An optimal approach to occupational health and safety should address employee education and behavior as well as engineering and administrative improvements.[231]

Radiation exposure is another potential environmental factor. In particular, radiation is a well-known risk factor for thyroid cancer, as discussed previously in the thyroid cancer section of this chapter. Studies also have shown an association between radiation exposure and salivary neoplasia. Therapeutic irradiation for primary lesions of the head and neck rarely may be complicated by the development of secondary sarcomas. Therapeutic radiation exposure should be minimized when possible by judicious treatment planning and use of field-limiting techniques such as intensity-modulated radiation therapy.

Ultraviolet light exposure is a known risk factor for cutaneous malignancies. A primary prevention program should include measures to reduce ultraviolet light exposure, such as wearing protective clothing, applying sunscreens, minimizing outdoor activities during peak sun exposure hours, and avoiding sunlamps and tanning beds.

Public Education and Awareness as Prevention Modalities

Several studies have demonstrated a lack of knowledge by the American public about HNSCC and inadequate media coverage of the disease.[232-240] It is interesting that a recent survey conducted by Harris revealed that only 42% of Americans interviewed were aware that tobacco is a risk factor for HNSCC, and only 26% could recall ever being examined for head and neck cancers.[234] Furthermore, only 12% of the American public realized that red or white sores in the mouth could represent an early sign of oral cancer (Fig. 10-7). Similarly, less than 2% of the nonsmoking population and 1% of smokers realized that hoarseness could be an early sign of laryngeal cancer.[234] Several organizations have aimed at educating medical and dental professionals on the risk factors, treatment, and rehabilitation related to HNSCC.[241-244] However, we

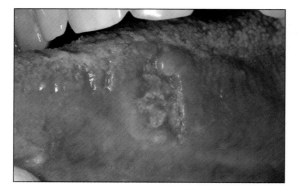

Figure 10-7. T1 squamous cell carcinoma of the oral cavity. Early detection reduces the extent of required therapy and improves post-treatment outcomes.

have found only one organization dedicated to public education on laryngeal cancer.[241] Several organizations have provided materials that enhance public and professional education, support, awareness, and prevention for HNSCC. The National Institute of Dental and Craniofacial Research (NIDCR) provides an oral health information clearinghouse that includes oral cancer educational materials free to interested individuals (www.nidcr.nih.gov/OralHealth/Topics/CancerTreatment). The International Agency for Research on Cancer (www.iarc.fr) has a printable screening exam poster (screening.iarc.fr/doc/schartoral.pdf) that allows individuals to visualize the appearance of suspicious lesions of the oral cavity. The Oral Cancer Foundation (www.oralcancerfoundation.org) provides a detailed website with links and updates related to oral cancer and has teamed with the American Dental Association and others to enhance screening efforts. Support for People with Oral, Head and Neck Cancer Foundation (SPOHNC; www.spohnc.org) provides a newsletter, local support groups, and information for survivors, the public, and health professionals. Since 1998 the International Oral and Head and Neck Cancer Awareness Week (OHANCAW), sponsored by the Yul Brynner Head and Neck Cancer Foundation (www.headandneck.org), has brought this issue to communities and the public through media campaigns, an annual awareness week, and free cancer screenings.[243]

Prevention through education of the public aims at changing behaviors and enhancing early detection. It is important to extend the education efforts to low-income populations as well, since individuals with lower economic status have a higher prevalence of tobacco use and therefore have a greater risk of developing HNSCC.[155,245-248]

Health Professional Education

Training Providers in Oral, Head, and Neck Cancer Prevention and Early Detection

Competency in the prevention and early detection of disease begins during predoctoral education. Competency in oral, head, and neck cancer prevention and detection is important because increased early and accurate detection may improve the percentage of cancers diagnosed before metastasis to the lymphatic system or other organs in the body.[249] As a component of continuing education for practicing dentists, the American Dental Association launched a $1.2 million campaign sponsored by the National Cancer Institute to train dentists in oral cancer prevention and tobacco cessation practices.[250-251] New York State has passed legislation requiring practicing dentists to have at least 2 hours of continuing education in oral cancer prevention and early detection.[252] However, this training also needs to be enforced during predoctoral education. Although most dental students are taught how to conduct an oral cancer examination, state dental boards do not currently require competency in this practice for licensure.[249]

Health professional schools have not uniformly incorporated prevention and detection content into their curricula.[253] This situation has been addressed in Developmental Objective 1–7 of Healthy People 2010, which aims to increase the number of health professional schools that include core competencies in health promotion and disease prevention.[254] Subsequently, the Healthy People Curriculum Task Force developed a Clinical Prevention and Population Health Framework calling for health professional students to be trained in screening and counseling skills.[253]

Because oral, head, and neck cancers have such high morbidity and mortality rates, comprehensive disease prevention and detection curricula for health professional schools should include training in head and neck cancer prevention and early detection. The National Strategic Planning Conference for the Prevention and Control of Oral and Pharyngeal Cancer has recommended that predoctoral dental and medical curricula be developed to "require competency in prevention, diagnosis, and multidisciplinary management of oral and pharyngeal cancer."[251] However, surveys of dental and medical schools found that this area is not being adequately addressed in all schools. In 1998 only 64% (30 of 47) of U.S. dental schools included direct patient contact in their predoctoral instruction on identifying precancerous lesions.[255] Similarly, at the turn of the century only 15% (21 of 136) of medical schools taught all intraoral components of a head and neck cancer examination to students.[256]

When dental and medical students are asked about their training in oral, head, and neck cancer examination, they report feeling inadequately prepared to conduct such examinations with patients.[256-261] However, studies suggest that expanding the predoctoral curriculum to include focused instruction on oral, head, and neck cancer prevention and detection may improve students' confidence and competency pertaining to examination skills.[256,257,260] This is supported by findings that medical students' general cancer prevention and detection skills improved after targeted education in cancer prevention and detection and smoking cessation counseling.[262-266]

Training Resources for Providers

Available multimedia resources for instructing health care providers in oral, head, and neck cancer prevention and early detection include training videos available from the University of Michigan (Voices of Detroit Initiative) and The Oral Cancer Center at the University of Pittsburgh.[267,268] The University of Michigan video, *Oral Health and Tobacco Cessation in a Primary Care Setting*, features specific training in oral cancer screening as well as tobacco cessation counseling.[268] From the Oral Cancer Center at the University of Pittsburgh, the video *Oral Cancer Screening: A Brief Review* provides step-by-step instruction in conducting an oral cancer examination.[267] Both resources are downloadable via the Internet and could be included in a head and neck cancer prevention and early detection program for both health professional students and current healthcare providers.

Another available resource is an interactive tobacco cessation CD-ROM educational program. This program, entitled *Helping Your Patients Quit Tobacco*, was developed specifically to teach tobacco cessation interventions to dental and dental hygiene students.[269] The program content of the CD-ROM includes a detailed section on a five-step tobacco cessation counseling process,[124] a resource library about the health effects of tobacco use, and a self-test on information contained in the program. A three-phase evaluation of the CD-ROM showed that dental and dental hygiene students responded positively to the usefulness of this type of educational program.[270]

Health professional schools have a responsibility to train competent and confident future providers. By assessing the oral, head, and neck cancer prevention and early detection training of health professionals, educators can understand the factors related to current and future healthcare providers' examination and counseling skills.

Racial Disparities in Head and Neck Cancer

Racial disparities in head and neck carcinoma incidence and survival have been previously documented in this chapter. The cause of these disparities requires further examination. This section briefly addresses reasons for the noted disparities and offers suggestions for future research.

Risk factors related to incidence of HNSCC include alcohol and tobacco use. Higher levels of smoking and drinking have independent effects on the risk of developing oral and pharyngeal cancer.[271] In an earlier study, Day and associates[272] found that a large proportion of racial differences in incidence of oral and pharyngeal cancer are due to racial differences in alcohol intake, particularly among current smokers.

However, no study exists that has identified a specific biologic factor or mechanism related to differences in survival between African Americans and Caucasians related to tobacco and alcohol use. Gourin and Podolsky[273] conducted a study examining racial disparities in patients with HNSCC. These investigators found that the lower survival rates among African Americans in the study were related to several factors. For example, African Americans were less likely than other patients to have health insurance ($P < .001$), which limited their access to health care and early detection of disease. In addition, African Americans were more likely than other patients to have nonoperative treatment performed because of the greater incidence of stage IV disease and extracapsular spread ($P < .0001$). The study sample consisted of 478 African Americans and 650 Caucasians identified by tumor registry data from patients treated at a single institution in the South. These findings are important because they highlight the fact that racial differences in survival outcomes related to HNSCC are strongly related to differences in access to health care.

Similarly, Al-Othman and associates[274] examined the impact of race on outcome after definitive radiation therapy for HNSCC. Their sample consisted of 686 patients who completed definitive, twice-daily radiation therapy alone or combined with a planned neck dissection between the years 1983 and 1997. Patients were followed up for a minimum of 2 years after treatment, with a median follow-up period of 7 years. Fifty-five (8%) of the 686 patients were African Americans; the remainder were Caucasian. Results show that despite similar 5-year local-regional control rates (70% versus 76% [$P = .275$]), the risk for distant recurrence was twice as high for the African-American patients as for the Caucasian patients (27% versus 13% [$P < .012$]). In addition, African-American patients had lower 5-year cause-specific and absolute survival rates (52% versus 74% [$P < .001$] and 29% versus 52% [$P < .001$], respectively). Al-Othman and associates[274] attribute the decreased survival of African-American patients in their study to an increased risk of distant metastases, the cause of which remains unknown. Other investigators suggest that racial differences in survival of oral and pharyngeal malignancies may be due in large part to lower socioeconomic status, more advanced stage at diagnosis, differences in treatment, patient comorbidities, access to health care, and quality of care received among racial and ethnic minorities.[271,274-277]

It is unclear whether the mechanisms related to survival differences in outcomes between African Americans and Caucasians with squamous cell carcinoma of the head and neck are biologic, socioeconomic, or both.[274] Future research is needed to disentangle the effects of these factors on survival outcomes. When the mechanisms have been clearly identified, interventions can be developed to reduce these survival differences.

Secondary Prevention

Secondary prevention of HNSCC implies that a person has developed genetic, molecular, and/or histologic evidence of the disease and that the disease can be diagnosed as early as possible in the cascade of events. Thus, early detection or secondary prevention can include a serum, salivary, or tissue-based molecular test that reveals the disease. Further detection techniques can include population screening, routine physical examination, radiographic studies, and biopsy.

Early detection by screening is discussed in detail in Chapters 3 through 5 with techniques including molecular studies, markers, public health approaches, clinical examinations, and radiographic studies.

Molecular relationships to the onset and diagnosis of HNSCC are described in the aforementioned section on molecular genetics. Screening for HPV has also been described as a potential primary and secondary prevention technique.

The oral cancer examination has been advocated by many groups as an opportunity for dentists and physicians to identify the disease early (see Fig. 10-7). A recent study in India is the first prospective study to provide confirmation of survival improvement in a large population of at-risk individuals.[278]

New visualization-enhancing technologies are being developed and used. A chemoluminescent light (ViziLite, Zila Pharmaceuticals, Inc, Phoenix, AZ) can improve visualization of the premalignant and malignant oral lesions. Unfortunately, the early reports using this technology do not provide enough support for its use as a general screening device for oral lesions.[279,280] The Velscope (LED Dental, Inc, White Rock, BC, Canada) is an instrument that has been marketed as an aid in the diagnosis of early oral cancer and precancerous lesions without published prospective or controlled trials to date. It is hoped that future studies with both trained and untrained clinicians will further elucidate the usefulness and indications for these techniques.

Other studies have assessed the role of autofluorescence and fluorescence visualization in the clinical setting and the operating room to assess for premalignant and malignant areas of the oral cavity. Although interest in these technologies is increasing, the exact role and indications for their use are yet to be defined.[281,282]

Studies also support the use of a brush biopsy technique to assess the level of risk or suspicion of lesions of the oral cavity and to promote early detection.[283] OralCDx (OralCDx Laboratories, Inc, Suffern, NY) is a commercially available brush for performing these types of biopsies. Further studies are necessary to identify which patients and lesions should be assessed with this technique. The role of staining methods has also been promoted to assess patients at risk for the development of oral cancer and/or to determine the most appropriate location for biopsy using a toluidine blue rinse. Oratest (Zila Pharmaceuticals, Inc, Phoenix, AZ) is a commercially available mixture that has been studied and is currently used in some centers for these indications.

Radiographic techniques including CT scans, MRI, and CT/PET scans continue to play a role in assessing primary, regional, and distant disease in HNSCC while also providing information related to staging.[284] Many of these techniques for secondary prevention are covered in greater detail in Chapters 1–5 and 12 (Box 10-1).

Tertiary Prevention

Tertiary prevention typically refers to a reduction in morbidity, complications, or mortality related to an acute or chronic disease that has recently been diagnosed and partially or entirely treated (Figs. 10-8). For HNSCC, this commonly includes reducing recurrence, second primary, metastasis, speech and swallowing dysfunction, dental and chewing problems, xerostomia and mucositis, cosmetic deformity, and

Box 10-1. Examples of Secondary Prevention in HNSCC

Molecular Test
Serum marker
Salivary marker
Tissue marker

Physical Examination
Unaided clinical examination
Enhanced visualization technologies
    Fluorescence
    Enhanced lighting—Vizilite, Velscope
    Toluidine blue—Oratest

Radiographic Study—CT, MRI, CT/PET

Biopsy
Needle
Brush
Incisional
Excisional

HNSCC, squamous cell cancer of the head and neck.

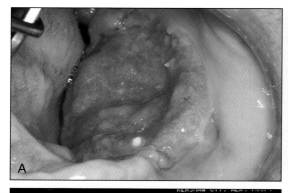

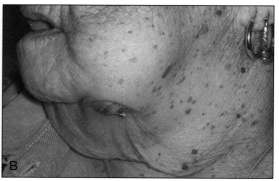

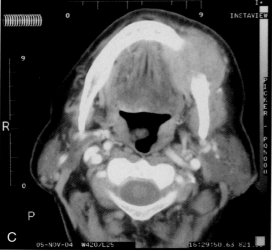

Figures 10-8. Clinical photographs (A and B) and CT scan (C) of the patient with T4 squamous cell carcinoma of the oral cavity.   Treatment of this advanced lesion requires multimodality therapy. Post-treatment functional outcomes can be improved significantly with tertiary prevention.

Table 10-7. Tertiary Prevention in HNSCC

Problem	Example of Intervention
Recurrence	Smoking cessation
Second primary	Screening
Metastasis	CT/PET scan
Dysphagia	Swallowing therapy, dilation
Malnutrition	Gastrostomy tube
Airway obstruction	Tracheotomy
Cosmetic deformity	Free tissue transfer reconstruction
Trismus	Jaw exercises
Osteoradionecrosis	Fluoride carriers
Xerostomia	Medical prophylaxis
Dysarthria	Speech therapy
Depression	Psychotherapy, medical therapy
Shoulder dysfunction	Physical therapy
Death	Adjuvant therapy, second-line treatment

other problems common in head and neck cancer patients (Table 10-7). Studies assessing the many problems along with disease-specific and overall quality of life are important to understand during and after treatment for head and neck cancer.[285,286]

Summary

Head and neck squamous cell carcinoma of both the skin and mucosal sites is clearly associated with lifestyle-related risk factors. Primary prevention efforts have largely failed in the United States and most countries worldwide, although reducing tobacco exposure is an obvious opportunity. Education of children with an emphasis on avoidance of risk factors may have potential for a reduction in incidence and mortality for the next generation. Vaccinations for viral-related cancers may also result in similar improvements. Secondary prevention efforts may have more of an impact with novel technologies, education, and screening efforts. Recent efforts in early detection with new technologies and molecular studies should provide earlier diagnosis in the coming decade. Although screening for head and neck cancers cannot yet be universally recommended for the entire population, close evaluation of those at high risk may improve survival statistics. The first prospective prevention trial in India has already shown a 34% reduction in oral cancer mortality, with future potential to prevent 37,000 oral cancer deaths worldwide.[278] Further studies are necessary for the non-squamous carcinomas of the head and neck region to further analyze risk factors, genetic predisposition, and molecular markers of disease.

References

1. Ron E, Schneider A: Thyroid cancer. In Schottenfeld D, Fraumeni JF (eds.): Cancer Epidemiology and Prevention. New York: Oxford University Press, 2006.
2. Littman AJ, Vaughan TL: Cancers of the nasal cavity and paranasal sinuses. In Schottenfeld D, Fraumeni JF (eds.): Cancer Epidemiology and Prevention. New York: Oxford University Press, 2006.
3. Mayne ST, Winn DM: Cancers of the oral cavity and pharynx. In Schottenfeld D, Fraumeni JF (eds.): Cancer Epidemiology and Prevention. New York: Oxford University Press, 2006.
4. Parkin DM, Bray FI, Devesa SS: Cancer burden in the year 2000: the global picture. Eur J Cancer 37(Suppl 8):S4–S66, 2001.
5. Mucci L, Adami H-O: Oral and pharyngeal cancer. In Adami H-O, Hunter D, Trichopoulos D (eds.): Textbook of Cancer Epidemiology. New York: Oxford University Press, 2002.
6. National Cancer Institute. Surveillance Epidemiology and End Results (SEER). Available at: http://seer.cancer.gov/statfacts/html/oralcav.html.
7. Ries LAG, Krapcho M, Mariotto A, et al: SEER Cancer Statistics Review, 1975–2004. Available at: http://seer.cancer.gov/csr/1975_2004/.
8. Hashibe M, Brennan P, Benhamou S, et al: Alcohol drinking in never users of tobacco, cigarette smoking in never drinkers, and the risk of head and neck cancer: pooled analysis in the Inter-

national Head and Neck Cancer Epidemiology Consortium. J Natl Cancer Inst 99(10):777–789, 2007.

9. D'Souza G, Kreimer AR, Viscidi R, et al: Case-control study of human papillomavirus and oropharyngeal cancer. N Engl J Med 356(19):1944–1956, 2007.

10. World Cancer Research Fund: Food, Nutrition and the Prevention of Cancer: A Global Perspective. Washington, DC: American Institute for Cancer Research, 1997.

11. Davies L, Welch HG: Epidemiology of head and neck cancer in the United States. Otolaryngol Head Neck Surg 135(3):451–457, 2006.

12. Schneider AB: Radiation-induced thyroid tumors. Endocrinol Metab Clin North Am 19:495–508, 1990.

13. Becker DV, Robbins J, Beebe GW, et al: Childhood thyroid cancer following the Chernobyl accident: a status report. Endocrinol Metab Clin North Am 25:197–211, 1996.

14. Jaworska A: [Iodine prophylaxis following nuclear accidents.] Tidsskr Nor Laegeforen 127(1):28–30, 2007.

15. Moysich KB, Menezes RJ, Michalek AM: Chernobyl-related ionising radiation exposure and cancer risk: an epidemiological review. Lancet Oncol 3(5):269–279, 2000.

16. Machens A, Holzhausen HJ, Thanh PN, et al: Malignant progression from C-cell hyperplasia to medullary thyroid carcinoma in 167 carriers of RET germline mutations. Surgery 134(3):425–431, 2003.

17. Machens A, Niccoli-Sire P, Hoegel J, et al: Early malignant progression of hereditary medullary thyroid cancer. N Engl J Med 349(16):1517–1525, 2003.

18. Brandi ML, Gaziel RF, Angeli A, et al: Guidelines for diagnosis and therapy of MEN type 1 and type 2. J Clin Endocrinol Metab 86(12):5658–5671, 2001.

19. Weber TT, Schilling T, Buchler MW: Thyroid carcinoma. Curr Opin Oncol 18(1):30–35, 2006.

20. National Comprehensive Cancer Network (NCCN): Thyroid carcinoma. In NCCN Clinical Practice Guidelines in Oncology, 2007. Available at: www.nccn.org.

21. Ellis GL, Auclair PL: Salivary gland tumors: general considerations. In Tumors of the Salivary Glands. Washington, DC: Armed Forces Institute of Pathology, 1996, pp 31–38.

22. Sun EC, Curtis R, Melbye M, et al: Salivary gland cancer in the United States. Cancer Epidemiol Biomarkers Prev 8:1095–1100, 1999.

23. Belsky JL, Takeichi N, Yamamoto T, et al: Salivary gland neoplasms following atomic radiation: additional cases and reanalysis of combined data in a fixed population. Cancer 35:555–559, 1975.

24. Saku T, Hayashi Y, Takahara O, et al: Salivary gland tumors among atomic bomb survivors, 1950–1987. Cancer 79:1465–1475, 1997.

25. Land CE, Saku T, Hayashi Y, et al: Incidence of salivary gland tumors among atomic bomb survivors, 1950–1987: evaluation of radiation-related risk. Radiat Res 146:28–36, 1996.

26. Whatley WS, Thompson JW, Rao B: Salivary gland tumors in survivors of childhood cancer. Otolaryngol Head Neck Surg 134:385–388, 2006.

27. Beal KP, Singh B, Kraus D, et al: Radiation-induced salivary gland tumors: a report of 18 cases and a review of the literature. Cancer J 9:467–471, 2003.

28. Modan B, Chetrit A, Alfandary E, et al: Increased risk of salivary gland tumors after low-dose radiation. Laryngoscope 108:1095–1097, 1998.

29. Mandel SJ, Mandel L: Radioactive iodine and the salivary glands. Thyroid 13:265–271, 2003.

30. Holm LE, Hall P, Wiklund K, et al: Cancer risk after iodine-131 therapy for hyperthyroidism. J Natl Cancer Inst 83:1072–1077, 1991.

31. Hall P, Holm LE, Lundell G, et al: Cancer risks in thyroid cancer patients. Br J Cancer 64:159–163, 1991.

32. Preston-Martin S, Thomas DC, White SC, et al: Prior exposure to medical and dental x-rays related to tumors of the parotid gland. J Natl Cancer Inst 80:943–949, 1988.

33. Preston-Martin S, White SC: Brain and salivary gland tumors related to prior dental radiography: implications for current practice. J Am Dent Assoc 120:151–158, 1990.

34. Wilson RT, Moore LE, Dosemeci M: Occupational exposures and salivary gland cancer mortality among African American and white workers in the United States. J Occup Environ Med 46:287–297, 2004.

35. Swanson GM, Burns PB: Cancers of the salivary gland: workplace risks among women and men. Ann Epidemiol 7:369–374, 1997.

36. Horn-Ross PL, Ljung BM, Morrow M: Environmental factors and the risk of salivary gland cancer. Epidemiology 8:414–419, 1997.

37. Zheng W, Shu BT, Gao YT, et al: Diet and other risk factors for cancer of the salivary glands: a population-based case-control study. Int J Cancer 67:194–198, 1996.

38. Muscat JE, Wynder EL: A case/control study of risk factors for major salivary gland cancer. Otolaryngol Head Neck Surg 118:195–198, 1998.

39. Tsai CC, Chen CL, Hsu HC: Expression of Epstein-Barr virus in carcinomas of major salivary glands. Hum Pathol 27:258–262, 1996.

40. Pinston JA, Cole P: Cigarette smoking and Warthin's tumor. Am J Epidemiol 144:183–187, 1996.

41. Actis A, Eynard AR: Influence of environmental and nutritional factors on salivary gland tumorigenesis with a special reference to dietary lipids. Eur J Clin Nutr 54:805–810, 2000.

42. Shanmugaratnam K, Sobin LH: The World Health Organization histological classification of tumours of the upper respiratory tract and ear: a commentary on the second edition. Cancer 71(8):2689–2697, 1993.

43. Yu MC, Yuan JM: Epidemiology of nasopharyngeal carcinoma. Semin Cancer Biol 12(6):421–429, 2002.

44. Chang ET, Adami HO: The enigmatic epidemiology of nasopharyngeal carcinoma. Cancer Epidemiol Biomarkers Prev 15(10):1765–1777, 2006.

45. Sun LM, Li CI, Huang EY, et al: Survival differences by race in nasopharyngeal carcinoma. Am J Epidemiol 165(3):271–278, 2007.

46. Ou SH, Zell JA, Ziogas A, et al: Epidemiology of nasopharyngeal carcinoma in the United States: improved survival of Chinese patients within the keratinizing squamous cell carcinoma histology. Ann Oncol 18(1):29–35, 2007.

47. Richey LM, Olshan AF, George J, et al: Incidence and survival rates for young blacks with nasopharyngeal carcinoma in the United States. Arch Otolaryngol Head Neck Surg 132(10):1035–1040, 2006.

48. Lee JT, Ko CY: Has survival improved for nasopharyngeal carcinoma in the United States? Otolaryngol Head Neck Surg 132(2):303–308, 2005.

49. Agathanggelou A, Niedobitek G, Chen R, et al: Expression of immune regulatory molecules in Epstein-Barr virus–associated nasopharyngeal carcinomas with prominent lymphoid stroma: evidence for a functional interaction between epithelial tumor cells and infiltrating lymphoid cells. Am J Pathol 147(4):1152–1160, 1995.

50. Niedobitek GA, Agathanggelou A, Nicholls JM: Epstein-Barr virus infection and the pathogenesis of nasopharyngeal carcinoma: viral gene expression, tumour cell phenotype, and the role of the lymphoid stroma. Semin Cancer Biol 7(4):165–174, 1996.

51. Niedobitek G: Epstein-Barr virus infection in the pathogenesis of nasopharyngeal carcinoma. Mol Pathol 53(5):248–254, 2000.

52. Beck A, Pazolt D, Grabenbauer GG, et al: Expression of cytokine and chemokine genes in Epstein-Barr virus–associated nasopharyngeal carcinoma: comparison with Hodgkin's disease. J Pathol 194(2):145–151, 2001.

53. Parkin DM, Bray F, Ferlay J, et al: Global cancer statistics, 2002. CA Cancer J Clin 55(2):74–108, 2005.

54. Lo KW, To KF, Huang DP: Focus on nasopharyngeal carcinoma. Cancer Cell 5(5):423–428, 2004.

55. Young LS, Rickinson AB: Epstein-Barr virus: 40 years on. Nat Rev Cancer 4(10):757–768, 2004.

56. Chan AT, Teo PM, Huang DP: Pathogenesis and treatment of nasopharyngeal carcinoma. Semin Oncol 31(6):794–801, 2004.

57. Cho WC: Nasopharyngeal carcinoma: molecular biomarker discovery and progress. Mol Cancer 6:1, 2007.

58. Jeyakumar A, Brickman TM, Jeyakumar A, et al: Review of nasopharyngeal carcinoma. Ear Nose Throat J 85(3):168–170, 172–173, 184, 2006.

59. Liu JP, Cassar L, Pinto A, et al: Mechanisms of cell immortalization mediated by EB viral activation of telomerase in nasopharyngeal carcinoma. Cell Res 16(10):809–817, 2006.

60. Wei WI, Sham JS: Nasopharyngeal carcinoma. Lancet 365(9476):2041–2054, 2005.

61. Yu MC, Mo CC, Chong WX, et al: Preserved foods and naso-pharyngeal carcinoma: a case-control study in Guangxi, China. Cancer Res 48(7):1954–1959, 1988.

62. Shao YM, Poirier S, Ohshima H, et al: Occurrence of volatile nitrosamines in food samples collected in three high-risk areas for nasopharyngeal carcinoma. IARC Sci Publ 84:415–419, 1987.

63. Tiwawech D, Srivatanakul P, Karalak A, et al: Cytochrome P450 2A6 polymorphism in nasopharyngeal carcinoma. Cancer Lett 241(1):135–141, 2006.

64. Tiwawech D, Ishida T: Glutathione S-transferase M1 gene polymorphism in Thai nasopharyngeal carcinoma. Asian Pac J Cancer Prev 6(3):270–275, 2005.

65. Tiwawech D, Srivatanakul P, Karalak A, et al: The p53 codon 72 polymorphism in Thai nasopharyngeal carcinoma. Cancer Lett 198(1):69–75, 2003.

66. Hildesheim A, Dosemici M, Chan CC, et al: Occupational exposure to wood, formaldehyde, and solvents and risk of nasopharyngeal carcinoma. Cancer Epidemiol Biomarkers Prev 10(11):1145–1153, 2001.

67. Chow WH, McLaughlin JK, Hrubec Z, et al: Tobacco use and nasopharyngeal carcinoma in a cohort of U.S. veterans. Int J Cancer 55(4):538–540, 1993.

68. Nam JM, McLaughlin JK, Blot WJ: Cigarette smoking, alcohol, and nasopharyngeal carcinoma: a case-control study among U.S. whites. J Natl Cancer Inst 84(8):619–622, 1992.

69. Yang XR, Diehl S, Pfeiffer R, et al: Evaluation of risk factors for nasopharyngeal carcinoma in high-risk nasopharyngeal carcinoma families in Taiwan. Cancer Epidemiol Biomarkers Prev 14(4):900–905, 2005.

70. Lu CC, Chen JC, Jin YT, et al: Genetic susceptibility to naso-pharyngeal carcinoma within the HLA-A locus in Taiwanese. Int J Cancer 103(6):745–751, 2003.

71. Goldsmith DB, West TM, Morton R: HLA associations with nasopharyngeal carcinoma in Southern Chinese: a meta-analysis. Clin Otolaryngol Allied Sci 27(1):61–67, 2002.

72. Burt RD, Vaughan TL, Nisperos B, et al: A protective association between the HLA-A2 antigen and nasopharyngeal carcinoma in U.S. caucasians. Int J Cancer 56(4):465–467, 1994.

73. Lu SJ, Day NE, Degos L, et al: Linkage of a nasopharyngeal carcinoma susceptibility locus to the HLA region. Nature 346(6283):470–471, 1990.

74. Dodd LE, Sengupta S, Chen IH, et al: Genes involved in DNA repair and nitrosamine metabolism and those located on chromosome 14q32 are dysregulated in nasopharyngeal carci-noma. Cancer Epidemiol Biomarkers Prev 15(11):2216–2225, 2006.

75. Kuo ML, Hwang HS, Sosnay PR, et al: Overexpression of the R2 subunit of ribonucleotide reductase in human nasopharyn-geal cancer cells reduces radiosensitivity. Cancer J 9(4):277–285, 2003.

76. Cho EY, Hildesheim A, Chen CJ, et al: Nasopharyngeal carci-noma and genetic polymorphisms of DNA repair enzymes XRCC1 and hOGG1. Cancer Epidemiol Biomarkers Prev 12(10):1100–1104, 2003.

77. Burgos JS: Involvement of the Epstein-Barr virus in the naso-pharyngeal carcinoma pathogenesis. Med Oncol 22(2):113–121, 2005.

78. Pagano JS, Blaser M, Buendia MA, et al: Infectious agents and cancer: criteria for a causal relation. Semin Cancer Biol 14(6):453–471, 2004.

79. Raab-Traub N: Epstein-Barr virus in the pathogenesis of NPC. Semin Cancer Biol 12(6):431–441, 2002.

80. Jiang X, Yao KT: The clonal progression in the neoplastic process of nasopharyngeal carcinoma. Biochem Biophys Res Commun 221(1):122–128, 1996.

81. Sengupta S, den Boon JA, Chen IH, et al: Genome-wide expression profiling reveals EBV-associated inhibition of MHC class I expression in nasopharyngeal carcinoma. Cancer Res 66(16):7999–8006, 2006.

82. Ogino T, Moriai S, Ishida Y, et al: Association of immunoescape mechanisms with Epstein-Barr virus infection in nasopharyn-geal carcinoma. Int J Cancer 120(11):2401–2010, 2007.

83. Fachiroh J, Paramita DK, Hariwiyanto B, et al: Single-assay combination of Epstein-Barr virus (EBV) EBNA1– and viral capsid antigen-p18–derived synthetic peptides for measuring anti-EBV immunoglobulin G (IgG) and IgA anti-

84. Karray H, Ayadi W, Fki L, et al: Comparison of three different serological techniques for primary diagnosis and monitoring of nasopharyngeal carcinoma in two age groups from Tunisia. J Med Virol 75(4):593–602, 2005.

85. Stevens SJ, Verkuijlen SA, Hariwiyanto B, et al: Diagnostic value of measuring Epstein-Barr virus (EBV) DNA load and carcinoma-specific viral mRNA in relation to anti-EBV immu-noglobulin A (IgA) and IgG antibody levels in blood of naso-pharyngeal carcinoma patients from Indonesia. J Clin Microbiol 43(7):3066–3073, 2005.

86. Stevens SJ, Verkuijlen SA, Hariwiyanto B, et al: Noninvasive diagnosis of nasopharyngeal carcinoma: nasopharyngeal brush-ings reveal high Epstein-Barr virus DNA load and carcinoma-specific viral BARF1 mRNA. Int J Cancer 119(3):608–614, 2006.

87. Lee AW, Foo W, Mang O, et al: Changing epidemiology of nasopharyngeal carcinoma in Hong Kong over a 20-year period (1980–1999): an encouraging reduction in both incidence and mortality. Int J Cancer 103(5):680–685, 2003.

88. Gallicchio L, Matanoski G, Tao XG, et al: Adulthood con-sumption of preserved and nonpreserved vegetables and the risk of nasopharyngeal carcinoma: a systematic review. Int J Cancer 119(5):1125–1135, 2006.

89. Bharadwaj M, Moss DJ: Epstein-Barr virus vaccine: a cytotoxic T-cell–based approach. Expert Rev Vaccines 1(4):467–476, 2002.

90. Taylor GS, Haigh YA, Gudgeon NH, et al: Dual stimulation of Epstein-Barr virus (EBV)–specific CD4+- and CD8+-T-cell responses by a chimeric antigen construct: potential therapeu-tic vaccine for EBV-positive nasopharyngeal carcinoma. J Virol 78(2):768–778, 2004.

91. Lin CL, Lo WF, Lu TH, et al: Immunization with Epstein-Barr virus (EBV) peptide-pulsed dendritic cells induces functional CD8+ T-cell immunity and may lead to tumor regression in patients with EBV-positive nasopharyngeal carcinoma. Cancer Res 62(23):6952–6958, 2002.

92. Ma BB, Chan AT: Systemic treatment strategies and therapeu-tic monitoring for advanced nasopharyngeal carcinoma. Expert Rev Anticancer Ther 6(3):383–394, 2006.

93. Masmoudi A, Toumi N, Khanfir A, et al: Epstein-Barr virus–tar-geted immunotherapy for nasopharyngeal carcinoma. Cancer Treat Rev 33(6):499–595, 2007.

94. Murono SN, Raab-Traub N, Pagano JS: Prevention and inhibi-tion of nasopharyngeal carcinoma growth by antiviral phospho-nated nucleoside analogs. Cancer Res 61(21):7875–7877, 2001.

95. Wakisaka N, Yoshizaki T, Raab-Traub N, et al: Ribonucleotide reductase inhibitors enhance cidofovir-induced apoptosis in EBV-positive nasopharyngeal carcinoma xenografts. Int J Cancer 116(4):640–645, 2005.

96. Wang J, Guo LP, Chen LZ, et al: Identification of cancer stem cell–like side population cells in human nasopharyngeal carci-noma cell line. Cancer Res 67(8):3716–3724, 2007.

97. Leclerc A, Martinez Cortes M, Gerin M, et al: Sinonasal cancer and wood dust exposure: results from a case-control study. Am J Epidemiol 140(4):340–349, 1994.

98. Bussi M, Gervasio CF, Riontino E, et al: Study of ethmoidal mucosa in a population at occupational high risk of sinonasal adenocarcinoma. Acta Otolaryngol 122(2):197–201, 2002.

99. Gordon I, Boffetta P, Demers PA: A case study comparing a meta-analysis and a pooled analysis of studies of sinonasal cancer among wood workers. Epidemiology 9(5):518–524, 1998.

100. Luce D, Leclerc A, Begin D, et al: Sinonasal cancer and occu-pational exposures: a pooled analysis of 12 case-control studies. Cancer Causes Control 13(2):147–157, 2002.

101. Van den Oever R: Occupational exposure to dust and sinonasal cancer: an analysis of 386 cases reported to the N.C.C.S.F. Cancer Registry. Acta Otorhinolaryngol Belg 50(1):19–24, 1996.

102. Mannetje A, Kogevinas M, Luce D, et al: Sinonasal cancer, occupation, and tobacco smoking in European women and men. Am J Ind Med 36(1):101–107, 1999.

103. Slootweg PJ, Richardson MR: Squamous cell carcinoma of the upper aerodigestive system. In Gnepp DR (ed.): Diagnostic Surgical Pathology of the Head and Neck. Philadelphia: W.B. Saunders, 2001, p 20.

104. Sale KA, Wallace DI, Girod DA, et al: Radiation-induced malignancy of the head and neck. Otolaryngol Head Neck Surg 131(5):643–645, 2004.

105. Mashberg A, Boffetta P, Winkelman R, et al: Tobacco smoking, alcohol drinking, and cancer of the oral cavity and oropharynx among U.S. veterans. Cancer 72(4):1369–1375, 1993.

106. Thornhill MH: The sun, the ozone layer and the skin: the role of ultraviolet light in lip and skin cancer. Dent Update 20(6):236–240, 1993.

107. Moore S, Johnston N, Pierce A, et al: The epidemiology of lip cancer: a review of global incidence and aetiology. Oral Dis 5(3):185–195, 1999.

108. Neville BW, Day TA: Oral cancer and precancerous lesions. CA Cancer J Clin 52(4):195–215, 2002.

109. Bulliard JL: Site-specific risk of cutaneous malignant melanoma and pattern of sun exposure in New Zealand. Int J Cancer 85(5):627–632, 2000.

110. Naldi L, Lorenzo Imberti G, Parazzini F, et al: Pigmentary traits, modalities of sun reaction, history of sunburns, and melanocytic nevi as risk factors for cutaneous malignant melanoma in the Italian population: results of a collaborative case-control study. Cancer 88(12):2703–2710, 2000.

111. Rafnsson V, Hrafnkelsson J, Tulinius H, et al: Risk factors for malignant melanoma in an Icelandic population sample. Prev Med 39(2):247–252, 2004.

112. Bakos L, Wagner M, Bakos RM, et al: Sunburn, sunscreens, and phenotypes: some risk factors for cutaneous melanoma in southern Brazil. Int J Dermatol 41(9):557–562, 2002.

113. Fargnoli MC, Piccolo D, Altobelli E, et al: Constitutional and environmental risk factors for cutaneous melanoma in an Italian population: a case-control study. Melanoma Res 14(2):151–157, 2004.

114. Youl P, Aitken J, Hayward N, et al: Melanoma in adolescents: a case-control study of risk factors in Queensland, Australia. Int J Cancer 98(1):92–98, 2002.

115. Bulliard JL, Cox B, Semenciw R: Trends by anatomic site in the incidence of cutaneous malignant melanoma in Canada, 1969–1993. Cancer Causes Control 10(5):407–416, 1999.

116. Nashan D, Kocer B, Schiller M, et al: Significant risk of a second melanoma in patients with a history of melanoma but no further predisposing factors. Dermatology 206(2):76–77, 2003.

117. Gillgren P, Brattstrom G, Frisell J, et al: Body site of cutaneous malignant melanoma: a study on patients with hereditary and multiple sporadic tumours. Melanoma Res 13(3):279–286, 2003.

118. McMasters KM, Noyes RD, Reintgen DS, et al: Lessons learned from the Sunbelt Melanoma Trial. J Surg Oncol 86(4):212–223, 2004.

119. U.S. Department of Human Services: The Health Consequences of Involuntary Exposure to Tobacco Smoke: A Report of the Surgeon General. Washington, DC: U.S. Government Printing Office, 1994.

120. Backinger CL, Fagan P, Matthews E, et al: Adolescent and young adult tobacco prevention and cessation: current status and future directions. Tob Control 12(Suppl 4):IV46–IV53, 2003.

121. Institute of Medicine: Growing Up Tobacco Free: Preventing Nicotine Addiction in Children and Youth. Washington, DC: National Academy Press, 2004.

122. Johnston L, O'Malley PM, Bachman JG, et al: Monitoring the Future: National Results on Adolescent Drug Use: Overview of Key Findings, 2005. Bethesda, MD: National Institute on Drug Abuse, 2006.

123. Farrelly MC, Niederdeppe J, Yarsevich J: Youth tobacco prevention mass media campaigns: past, present, and future directions. Tob Control 12(Suppl 1):i35–i47, 2003.

124. Fiore M, Jaen C, Baker T, et al: Treating Tobacco Use and Dependence: 2008 Update. Clinical Practice Guideline. Rockville, MD: Public Health Service, 2008.

125. Gonzales D, Rennard SI, Nides M, et al: Varenicline, an alpha-4beta2 nicotinic acetylcholine receptor partial agonist versus sustained-release bupropion and placebo for smoking cessation: a randomized controlled trial. JAMA 296(1):47–55, 2006.

126. Hughes JR, Stead LF, Lancaster T: Antidepressants for smoking cessation. Cochrane Database Syst Rev 1:CD000031, 2007.

127. Silagy C, Lancaster T, Stead L, et al: Nicotine replacement therapy for smoking cessation. Cochrane Database Syst Rev 3: CD000146, 2004.

128. Cokkinides VE, Ward E, Jemal A, et al: Under-use of smoking-cessation treatments: results from the National Health Interview Survey, 2000. Am J Prev Med 28(1):119–122, 2005.

129. Fu SS, Sherman SE, Yano EM, et al: Ethnic disparities in the use of nicotine replacement therapy for smoking cessation in an equal access health care system. Am J Health Promot 20(2):108–116, 2005.

130. Zhu S, Mercer T, Sun J, et al: Smoking cessation with and without assistance: a population-based analysis. Am J Prev Med 18(4):305–311, 2000.

131. Doescher MP, Saver BG, Franks P, et al: Racial and ethnic disparities in perceptions of physician style and trust. Arch Fam Med 9(10):1156–1163, 2000.

132. Pbert L, Adams A, Quirk M, et al: The patient exit interview as an assessment of physician-delivered smoking intervention: a validation study. Health Psychol 18(2):183–188, 1999.

133. Carpenter MJ, Hughes JR, Solomon LJ, et al: Both smoking reduction with nicotine replacement therapy and motivational advice increase future cessation among smokers unmotivated to quit. J Consult Clin Psychol 72(3):371–381, 2004.

134. Hughes JR, Carpenter MJ: Does smoking reduction increase future cessation and decrease disease risk? A qualitative review. Nicotine Tob Res 8(6):739–749, 2006.

135. Chaloupka FJ, Cummings KM, Morley CP, et al: Tax, price and cigarette smoking: evidence from the tobacco documents and implications for tobacco company marketing strategies. Tob Control 11(Suppl 1):I62–I72, 2002.

136. Farkas AJ, Gilpin EA, Distefan M, et al: The effects of household and workplace smoking restrictions on quitting behaviours. Tob Control 8(3):261–265, 1999.

137. Sung HY, Hu TW, Ong M, et al: A major state tobacco tax increase, the master settlement agreement, and cigarette consumption: the California experience. Am J Public Health 95(6):1030–1035, 2005.

138. Schroeder SA: Tobacco control in the wake of the 1998 master settlement agreement. N Engl J Med 350(3):293–301, 2004.

139. Givel M, Glantz SA: The "global settlement" with the tobacco industry: 6 years later. Am J Public Health 94(2):218–224, 2004.

140. Miller PM, Day TA, Ravenel MC: Clinical implications of continued alcohol consumption after diagnosis of upper aerodigestive tract cancer. Alcohol and Alcoholism 41:140–142, 2005.

141. National Institute on Alcohol Abuse and Alcoholism (NIAAA): Alcohol and Cancer. No. 21 PH 345, July, 1993. Bethesda, MD: NIAAA, 1993.

142. Bagnardi V, Blangiardo M, La Vecchia C, et al: Alcohol consumption and the risk of cancer: a meta-analysis. Alcohol Res Health 25(4):263–270, 2001.

143. Marmot MG, Elliott P, Shipley M, et al: Alcohol and blood pressure: the INTERSALT study. Br Med J 308:1263–1267, 1994.

144. Merletti F, Boffetta P, Ciccione G, et al: Role of tobacco and alcoholic beverages in the etiology of cancer of the oral cavity/oropharynx in Torino, Italy. Cancer Res 49(17):4919–4924, 1989.

145. Patten CA, Martin JE, Owen N: Can psychiatric and chemical dependency treatment units be smoke free? J Subst Abuse Treat 13(2):107–118, 1996.

146. Breslau N: Psychiatric comorbidity of smoking and nicotine dependence. Behav Genet 25(2):95–101, 1995.

147. Seitz HK, Simanowski UA: Ethanol and carcinogenesis of the alimentary tract. Alcohol Clin Exp Res 10(6 Suppl):33S–40S, 1986.

148. Andre K, Schraub S, Mercier M, et al: Role of alcohol and tobacco in the aetiology of head and neck cancer: a case-control study in the Doubs region of France. Eur J Cancer B Oral Oncol 31B(5):301–309, 1995.

149. Winn DM: Diet and nutrition in the etiology of oral cancer. Am J Clin Nutr 61(2):437S–445S, 1995.

150. Llewellyn CD, Lanklater K, Bell J, et al: An analysis of risk factors for oral cancer in young people: a case-control study. Oral Oncol 40(3):304–313, 2004.

151. Boeing H, Dietrich T, Hoffmann K, et al: Intake of fruits and vegetables and risk of cancer of the upper aero-digestive tract: the prospective EPIC-study. Cancer Causes Control 17(7):957–969, 2006.

152. Galeone C, Pelucchi C, Levi F, et al: Onion and garlic use and human cancer. Am J Clin Nutr 84(5):1027–1032, 2006.

153. De Stefani E, Oreggia F, Boffetta P, et al: Tomatoes, tomato-rich foods, lycopene and cancer of the upper aerodigestive tract: a case-control study in Uruguay. Oral Oncol 36(1):47–53, 2000.

154. Gupta PC, Hebert JR, Bhonsie RB, et al: Influence of dietary factors on oral precancerous lesions in a population-based case-control study in Kerala, India. Cancer 85(9):1885–1893, 1999.

155. Gupta PC, Hebert JR, Bhonsie RB, et al: Dietary factors in oral leukoplakia and submucous fibrosis in a population-based case control study in Gujarat, India. Oral Dis 4(3):200–206, 1998.

156. Hebert JR, Gupta PC, Bhonsie RB, et al: Dietary exposures and oral precancerous lesions in Srikakulam District, Andhra Pradesh, India. Public Health Nutr 5(2):303–312, 2002.

157. Maserejian NN, Giovannucci E, Rosner B, et al: Prospective study of vitamins C, E, and A and carotenoids and risk of oral premalignant lesions in men. Int J Cancer 120(5):970–977, 2007.

158. Shiu MN, Chen TH: Impact of betel quid, tobacco and alcohol on three-stage disease natural history of oral leukoplakia and cancer: implications for prevention of oral cancer. Eur J Cancer Prev 13(1):39–45, 2004.

159. Murti PR, Bhonsie RB, Pindborg JJ, et al: Malignant transformation rate in oral submucous fibrosis over a 17-year period. Community Dent Oral Epidemiol 13(6):340–341, 1985.

160. Syrjanen S: Human papillomavirus (HPV) in head and neck cancer. J Clin Virol 32(Suppl 1):S59–S66, 2005.

161. Kreimer AR, Clifford GM, Boyle P, et al: Human papillomavirus types in head and neck squamous cell carcinomas worldwide: a systematic review. Cancer Epidemiol Biomarkers Prev 14(2):467–475, 2005.

162. Badaracco G, Rizzo C, Mafera B, et al: Molecular analyses and prognostic relevance of HPV in head and neck tumours. Oncol Rep 17(4):931–939, 2007.

163. Dahlgren L, Dahlstrand HM, Lindquist D, et al: Human papillomavirus is more common in base of tongue than in mobile tongue cancer and is a favorable prognostic factor in base of tongue cancer patients. Int J Cancer 112(6):1015–1019, 2004.

164. El-Mofty SK, Patil S: Human papillomavirus (HPV)–related oropharyngeal nonkeratinizing squamous cell carcinoma: characterization of a distinct phenotype. Oral Surg Oral Med Oral Pathol Oral Radiol Endod 101(3):339–345, 2006.

165. Pintos J, Black MJ, Sadeghi N, et al: Human papillomavirus infection and oral cancer: a case-control study in Montreal, Canada. Oral Oncol April 26, 2007. Epub ahead of print. Available at: www.ncbi.nlm.nih.gov.

166. El-Mofty SK, Lu DW: Prevalence of high-risk human papillomavirus DNA in nonkeratinizing (cylindrical cell) carcinoma of the sinonasal tract: a distinct clinicopathologic and molecular disease entity. Am J Surg Pathol 29(10):1367–1372, 2005.

167. Sisk J, Schweinfurth JM, Wang XT, et al: Presence of human papillomavirus DNA in tonsillectomy specimens. Laryngoscope 116(8):1372–1374, 2006.

168. Smith EM, Ritchie JM, Summersgill KF, et al: Age, sexual behavior and human papillomavirus infection in oral cavity and oropharyngeal cancers. Int J Cancer 108(5):766–772, 2004.

169. Dahlstrom KR, Adler-Storthz K, Etzel CJ, et al: Human papillomavirus type 16 infection and squamous cell carcinoma of the head and neck in never-smokers: a matched pair analysis. Clin Cancer Res 9(7):2620–2626, 2003.

170. D'Souza G, Fakhry C, Sugar EA, et al: Six-month natural history of oral versus cervical human papillomavirus infection. Int J Cancer 121(1):143–150, 2007.

171. Fakhry C, D'Souza G, Sugar EA, et al: Relationship between prevalent oral and cervical human papillomavirus infections in human immunodeficiency virus–positive and –negative women. J Clin Microbiol 44(12):4479–4485, 2006.

172. Smith EM, Ritchie JM, Yankowitz J, et al: HPV prevalence and concordance in the cervix and oral cavity of pregnant women. Infect Dis Obstet Gynecol 12(2):45–56, 2004.

173. Baccaglini L, Atkinson JC, Patton LL, et al: Management of oral lesions in HIV-positive patients. Oral Surg Oral Med Oral Pathol Oral Radiol Endod 103(Suppl): S50.e1–23, 2007.

174. Palefsky J: Biology of HPV in HIV infection. Adv Dent Res 19(1):99–105, 2006.

175. Kutler DI, Wreesmann VB, Goberdhan A, et al: Human papillomavirus DNA and p53 polymorphisms in squamous cell carcinomas from Fanconi anemia patients. J Natl Cancer Inst 95(22):1718–1721, 2003.

176. Carvalho JP, Dias ML, Carvalho FM, et al: Squamous cell vulvar carcinoma associated with Fanconi's anemia: a case report. Int J Gynecol Cancer 12(2):220–222, 2002.

177. Socie G, Scieux C, Gluckman E, et al: Squamous cell carcinomas after allogeneic bone marrow transplantation for aplastic anemia: further evidence of a multistep process. Transplantation 66(5):667–670, 1998.

178. Starr JR, Daling JR, Fitzgibbons ED, et al: Serologic evidence of herpes simplex virus 1 infection and oropharyngeal cancer risk. Cancer Res 61(23):8459–8464, 2001.

179. Kim SH, Koo BS, Kang S, et al: HPV integration begins in the tonsillar crypt and leads to the alteration of p16, EGFR and c-myc during tumor formation. Int J Cancer 120(7):1418–1425, 2007.

180. Begum S, Cao D, Gillison M, et al: Tissue distribution of human papillomavirus 16 DNA integration in patients with tonsillar carcinoma. Clin Cancer Res 11(16):5694–5699, 2005.

181. Wentzensen N, Vinokurova S, von Knebel Doeberitz M: Systematic review of genomic integration sites of human papillomavirus genomes in epithelial dysplasia and invasive cancer of the female lower genital tract. Cancer Res 64(11):3878–3884, 2004.

182. Hafkamp HC, Speel EJ, Haesevoets A, et al: A subset of head and neck squamous cell carcinomas exhibits integration of HPV 16/18 DNA and overexpression of p16INK4A and p53 in the absence of mutations in p53 exons 5–8. Int J Cancer 107(3):394–400, 2003.

183. Reimers N, Kasper HU, Weissenborn SJ, et al: Combined analysis of HPV-DNA, p16 and EGFR expression to predict prognosis in oropharyngeal cancer. Int J Cancer 120(8):1731–1738, 2007.

184. Weinberger PM, Yu Z, Haffty BG, et al: Molecular classification identifies a subset of human papillomavirus–associated oropharyngeal cancers with favorable prognosis. J Clin Oncol 24(5):736–747, 2006.

185. Ritchie JM, Smith EM, Summersgill KF, et al: Human papillomavirus infection as a prognostic factor in carcinomas of the oral cavity and oropharynx. Int J Cancer 104(3):336–344, 2003.

186. Tan TT, Coussens LM: Humoral immunity, inflammation and cancer. Curr Opin Immunol 19(2):209–216, 2007.

187. Affara NI, Coussens LM: IKKα at the crossroads of inflammation and metastasis. Cell 129(1):25–26, 2007.

188. de Visser KE, Eichten A, Coussens LM: Paradoxical roles of the immune system during cancer development. Nat Rev Cancer 6(1):24–37, 2006.

189. de Visser KE, Korets LV, Coussens LM: De novo carcinogenesis promoted by chronic inflammation is B lymphocyte dependent. Cancer Cell 7(5):411–423, 2005.

190. Coussens LM, Tinkle CL, Hanahan D, et al: MMP-9 supplied by bone marrow–derived cells contributes to skin carcinogenesis. Cell 103(3):481–490, 2000.

191. Leggatt GR, Frazer IH: HPV vaccines: the beginning of the end for cervical cancer. Curr Opin Immunol 19(2):232–238, 2007.

192. Dillner J, Arbyn M, Dillner L: Translational mini-review series on vaccines: monitoring of human papillomavirus vaccination. Clin Exp Immunol 148(2):199–207, 2007.

193. Villa LL: Prophylactic HPV vaccines: reducing the burden of HPV-related diseases. Vaccine 24(Suppl 1):S23–S28, 2006.

194. Washam C: Two HPV vaccines yielding similar success. J Natl Cancer Inst 97(14):1030, 2005.

195. Block SL, Nolan T, Sattler C, et al: Comparison of the immunogenicity and reactogenicity of a prophylactic quadrivalent human papillomavirus (types 6, 11, 16, and 18) L1 virus-like particle vaccine in male and female adolescents and young adult women. Pediatrics 118(5):2135–2145, 2006.

196. Lin YY, Alphs H, Hung CF, et al: Vaccines against human papillomavirus. Front Biosci 12:246–264, 2007.

197. Govan VA: Strategies for human papillomavirus therapeutic vaccines and other therapies based on the E6 and E7 oncogenes. Ann NY Acad Sci 1056:328–343, 2005.

198. Roden R, Wu TC: Preventative and therapeutic vaccines for cervical cancer. Expert Rev Vaccines 2(4):495–516, 2003.

199. Stanley MA: Progress in prophylactic and therapeutic vaccines for human papillomavirus infection. Expert Rev Vaccines 2(3):381–389, 2003.

200. Arbyn M, Dillner J: Review of current knowledge on HPV vaccination: an appendix to the European Guidelines for

Quality Assurance in Cervical Cancer Screening. J Clin Virol 38(3):189–197, 2007.

201. Gambhira R, Gravitt PE, Bossis I, et al: Vaccination of healthy volunteers with human papillomavirus type 16 L2E7E6 fusion protein induces serum antibody that neutralizes across papillomavirus species. Cancer Res 66(23):11120–11124, 2006.

202. Koufman JA: The otolaryngologic manifestations of gastro-esophageal reflux disease (GERD): a clinical investigation of 225 patients using ambulatory 24-hour pH monitoring and an experimental investigation of the role of acid and pepsin in the development of laryngeal injury. Laryngoscope 101(4 Part 2, Suppl 53):1–78, 1991.

203. Copper MP, Smit LD, Stanajcic PP, et al: High incidence of laryngopharyngeal reflux in patients with head and neck cancer. Laryngoscope 110(6):1007–1011, 2000.

204. Vaezi MF, Qadeer MA, Lopez R, et al: Laryngeal cancer and gastroesophageal reflux disease: a case-control study. Am J Med 119(9):768–776, 2006.

205. Ward PH, Hanson DG: Reflux as an etiological factor of carcinoma of the laryngopharynx. Laryngoscope 98(11):1195–1199, 1988.

206. Qadeer MA, Lopez R, Wood BG, et al: Does acid suppressive therapy reduce the risk of laryngeal cancer recurrence? Laryngoscope 115(10):1877–1881, 2005.

207. Lothaire P, de Azambuja E, Dequanter D, et al: Molecular markers of head and neck squamous cell carcinoma: promising signs in need of prospective evaluation. Head Neck 28:256–269, 2006.

208. Ke LD, Adler-Storhz K, Clayman GL, et al: Differential expression of epidermal growth factor receptor in human head and neck cancers. Head Neck 20:320–327, 1998.

209. Xia W, Lau YK, Zhang HZ, et al: Combination of EGFR, HER-2/neu, and HER-3 is a stronger predictor for the outcome of oral squamous cell carcinoma than any individual family members. Clin Cancer Res 5:4164–4174, 1999.

210. Grandis JR, Tweardy DJ, Melhem MF: Asynchronous modulation of transforming growth factor protein expression in progression of premalignant lesion to head and neck squamous cell carcinoma. Clin Cancer Res 4:13–20, 1998.

211. Maurizi M, Almadori G, Ferrandina G, et al: Prognostic significance of epidermal growth factor receptor in laryngeal squamous cell carcinoma. Br J Cancer 74:1253–1257, 1996.

212. Shin DM, Ro JY, Hong WK, et al: Dysregulation of epidermal growth factor receptor expression in premalignant lesion during head and neck tumorigenesis. Cancer Res 54:3153–3159, 1994.

213. Choe MS, Zhang X, Shin HJ, et al: Interaction between epidermal growth factor receptor– and cyclooxygenase 2–mediated pathways and its implication for the chemoprevention of head and neck cancer. Mol Cancer Ther 4:1448–1455, 2005.

214. Choong NW, Cohen EEW: Epidermal growth factor receptor directed therapy in head and neck cancer. Crit Rev Oncol Hematol 57:25–43, 2006.

215. Levine AJ: p53, the cellular gatekeeper for growth and division. Cell 88:323–331, 1997.

216. Field JK: Oncogenes and tumor suppressor genes in squamous cell carcinoma of the head and neck. Eur J Cancer B Oral Oncol 28B:67–76, 1992.

217. Girod SC, Krueger G, Pape HD: p53 and Ki67 expression in preneoplastic and neoplastic lesions of the oral mucosa. Int J Oral Maxillofac Surg 22:285–288, 2003.

218. Campisi G, Panzarella V, Giuliani M, et al: Human papillomavirus: its identity and controversial role in oral carcinogenesis, premalignant and malignant lesions. Int J Oncol 30:813–824, 2007.

219. Gasco M, Crook T: The p53 network in head and neck cancer. Oral Oncol 39:222–231, 2003.

220. Clayman GL, el-Naggar AK, Lippmann SM, et al: Adenovirus-mediated p53 gene transfer in patients with advanced recurrent head and neck squamous cell carcinoma. J Clin Oncol 16:2221–2232, 1998.

221. Yoo GH, Piechocki MP, Oliver J, et al: Enhancement of Ad-p53 therapy with docetaxel in head and neck cancer. Laryngoscope 114:1871–1879, 2004.

222. O'Shea CC, Soria C, Bagus B, et al: Heat shock phenocopies E1B-55K late functions and selectively sensitizes refractory tumor cells to ONYX-015 oncolytic viral therapy. Cancer Cell 8:61–74, 2005.

223. Rudin CM, Cohen EE, Papadimitrakopolou VA, et al: An attenuated adenovirus, ONYX-015, as mouthwash therapy for premalignant oral dysplasia. J Clin Oncol 21:4546–4552, 2003.

224. Khuri FR, Nemunaitis J, Ganly I, et al: A controlled trial of intratumoral ONYX-015, a selectively replicating adenovirus, in combination with cisplatin and 5-fluorouracil in patients with recurrent head and neck cancer. Nature Med 6:879–885, 2000.

225. Xia ZJ, Chang JH, Zhang L, et al: Phase III randomized clinical trial of intratumoral injection of E1B gene–deleted adenovirus (H101) combined with cisplatin-based chemotherapy in treating squamous cell cancer of head and neck or esophagus. Ai Zheng 23:1666–1670, 2004.

226. Neugut AI, Li FP: Cancer epidemiology and prevention: environmental carcinogens, 2002. Available at: www.medscape.com/viewarticle/534484.

227. Yu MC, Yuan JM: Epidemiology of nasopharyngeal carcinoma. Semin Cancer Biol 12:421–429, 2002.

228. Perez-Ordonez B, Huvos A: Intestinal-type sinonasal adenocarcinoma. In Gnepp DR (ed.): Diagnostic Surgical Pathology of the Head and Neck. Philadelphia: W.B. Saunders, 2001, pp 99–100.

229. Gustavsson P, Jakobsson R, Nyberg F, et al: Occupational exposures and squamous cell carcinoma of the oral cavity, pharynx, larynx, and oesophagus: a case-control study in Sweden. Occup Environ Med 55:393–400, 1998.

230. LaForest L, Luce D, Goldberg P, et al: Laryngeal and hypopharyngeal cancers and occupational exposure to formaldehyde and various dusts: a case-control study in France. Occup Environ Med 57:767–773, 2000.

231. Lazovich D, Parker DL, Brosseau M, et al: Effectiveness of a worksite intervention to reduce an occupational exposure: the Minnesota wood dust study. Am J Public Health 92:1498–1505, 2002.

232. Horowitz AM, Canto MT, Child WL: Maryland adults' perspectives on oral cancer prevention and early detection. J Am Dent Assoc 133(8):1058–1063, 2002.

233. Horowitz AM, Moon HS, Goodman HS, et al: Maryland adults' knowledge of oral cancer and having oral cancer examinations. J Public Health Dent 58(4):281–287, 1998.

234. Day TA, Reed SG, Cannick GF, et al: Survey of Oral and Head and Neck Cancer Knowledge Among the American Public. Washington, DC: Sixth International Conference on Head and Neck Cancer, 2004.

235. Shetty KV, Johnson NW: Knowledge, attitudes and beliefs of adult South Asians living in London regarding risk factors and signs for oral cancer. Community Dent Health 16(4):227–231, 1999.

236. Canto MT, Horowitz AM, Goodman HS, et al: Oral health knowledge, practices, and status among outpatient veterans at the VA Maryland Health Care System. Spec Care Dentist 19(4):186–189, 1999.

237. Canto MT, Horowitz AM, Goodman HS, et al: Maryland veterans' knowledge of risk factors for and signs of oral cancers and their use of dental services. Gerodontology 15(2):79–86, 1998.

238. Yellowitz JA, Goodman HS, Farooq NS: Knowledge, opinions, and practices related to oral cancer: results of three elderly racial groups. Spec Care Dentist 17(3):100–104, 1997.

239. Horowitz AM, Nourjah P, Gift HC: U.S. adult knowledge of risk factors and signs of oral cancers: 1990. J Am Dent Assoc 126(1):39–45, 1995.

240. Canto MT, Kawaguchi Y, Horowitz AM: Coverage and quality of oral cancer information in the popular press: 1987–1998. J Public Health Dent 58(3):241–247, 1998.

241. WebWhispers. Available at: www.webwhispers.org.

242. Support for People with Oral, Head and Neck Cancer. Available at: www.spohnc.org.

243. Yul Brynner Head and Neck Cancer Foundation. Available at: www.headandneck.org.

244. Oral Cancer Foundation. Available at: www.oralcancerfoundation.org.

245. Gupta PC, Aghi MB, Bhonsie RB, et al: An intervention study of tobacco chewing and smoking habits for primary prevention of oral cancer among 12,212 Indian villagers. IARC Sci Publ 74:307–318, 1986.

246. Gupta PC, Mehta FS, Pindborg JJ, et al: Intervention study for primary prevention of oral cancer among 36,000 Indian tobacco users. Lancet 1(8492):1235–1239, 1986.

247. Zhu S, Giovino GA, Mowery PD, et al: The relationship between cigarette smoking and education revisited: implications for categorizing persons' educational status. Am J Public Health 86(11):1582–1589, 1996.

248. Balluz L, Aluwalia IB, Murphy W, et al: Surveillance for certain health behaviors among selected local areas: United States: Behavioral Risk Factor Surveillance System, 2002. MMWR Surveill Summ 53(5):1–100, 2004.

249. Horowitz AM, Goodman HS, Yellowitz JA, et al: The need for health promotion in oral cancer prevention and early detection. J Public Health Dent 56(6):319–330, 1996.

250. American Dental Association: ADA News: $1 Million NCI Grant Targets Oral Cancer. Available at: www.ada.org/public/media/releases/0209_release01.asp.

251. American Dental Association, Centers for Disease Control and Prevention, National Institute of Dental Research/National Institutes of Health: National Strategic Planning Conference for the Prevention and Control of Oral and Pharyngeal Cancer. Chicago, 1996.

252. State Requirements for Dental Licensure: Oral Cancer Education Now the Law in NYS. Available at: www.nysdental.org/education.

253. Allan J, Barwick TA, Cashman S, et al: Clinical prevention and population health: curriculum framework for health professions. Am J Prev Med 27(5):471–476, 2004.

254. U.S. Department of Health and Human Services: Healthy People 2010: With Understanding and Improving Health and Objectives for Improving Health, 2nd ed. Washington, DC: U.S. Government Printing Office, 2000.

255. Rankin KV, Burzynski NJ, Silverman S Jr, et al: Cancer curricula in U.S. dental schools. J Cancer Educ 14(1):8–12, 1999.

256. Ahluwalia KP, Yellowitz JA, Goodman HS, et al: An assessment of oral cancer prevention curricula in U.S. medical schools. J Cancer Educ 13(2):90–95, 1998.

257. Burzynski NJ, Rankin KV, Silverman S, Jr, et al: Graduating dental students' perceptions of oral cancer education: results of an exit survey of seven dental schools. J Cancer Educ 17(2):83–84, 2002.

258. Cannick GF, Horowitz AM, Drury TF, et al: Assessing oral cancer knowledge among dental students in South Carolina. J Am Dent Assoc 136(3):373–378, 2005.

259. Cannick GF, Horowitz AM, Reed SG, et al: Opinions of South Carolina dental students toward tobacco use interventions. J Public Health Dent 66(1):44–48, 2006.

260. Rankin KV, Jones DL, McDaniel RK: Oral cancer education in dental schools: survey of Texas dental students. J Cancer Educ 11(2):80–83, 1996.

261. Reed SG, Duffy NG, Walters KC, et al: Oral cancer knowledge and experience: a survey of South Carolina medical students in 2002. J Cancer Educ 20(3):136–142, 2005.

262. Allen SS, Bland CJ, Dawson SJ: A mini-workshop to train medical students to use a patient-centered approach to smoking cessation. Am J Prev Med 6(1):28–33, 1990.

263. Eyler AE, Dicken LL, Fitzgerald JT, et al: Teaching smoking-cessation counseling to medical students using simulated patients. Am J Prev Med 13(3):153–158, 1997.

264. Geller AC, Prout MN, Miller DR, et al: Evaluation of a cancer prevention and detection curriculum for medical students. Prev Med 35(1):78–86, 2002.

265. Roche AM, Eccleston P, Sanson-Fisher R: Teaching smoking cessation skills to senior medical students: a block-randomized controlled trial of four different approaches. Prev Med 25(3):251–258, 1996.

266. Yip JK, Hay JL, Ostroff JS, et al: Dental students' attitudes toward smoking cessation guidelines. J Dent Educ 64(9):641–650, 2000.

267. University of Pittsburgh. Oral Cancer Screening: A Brief Review. January 10, 2004. Available at: www.upci.upmc.edu/news/upci_news/2002/051602_oral_video.html.

268. Ismail A: Oral Health and Tobacco Cessation in a Primary Care Setting. Available at: http://oralhealth.dent.umich.edu/VODI/html/00/about.html.

269. Severson HH, Christiansen GJ, Jacobs T: Helping Your Patients Quit Tobacco. Eugene, OR: Applied Behavior Science Press, 2001.

270. Gordon JS, Severson HH, Seeley JR, et al: Development and evaluation of an interactive tobacco cessation CD-ROM educational program for dental students. J Dent Educ 68(3):361–369, 2004.

271. Morse DE, Kerr AR: Disparities in oral and pharyngeal cancer incidence, mortality and survival among black and white Americans. J Am Dent Assoc 137(2):203–212, 2006.

272. Day GL, Blot WJ, Austin DF, et al: Racial differences in risk of oral and pharyngeal cancer: alcohol, tobacco, and other determinants. J Natl Cancer Inst 85(6):465–473, 1993.

273. Gourin CG, Podolsky RH: Racial disparities in patients with head and neck squamous cell carcinoma. Laryngoscope 116(7):1093–1106, 2006.

274. Al-Othman MO, Morris CG, Logan HL, et al: Impact of race on outcome after definitive radiotherapy for squamous cell carcinoma of the head and neck. Cancer 98(11):2467–2472, 2003.

275. Mandelblatt JS, Yabroff KR, Kerner JF: Suitable access to cancer services: a review of barriers to quality care. Cancer 86(11):2378–2390, 1999.

276. Shavers VL, Brown ML: Racial and ethnic disparities in the receipt of cancer treatment. J Natl Cancer Inst 94(5):334–357, 2002.

277. Wong MD, Shapiro MF, Boscardin WJ, et al: Contribution of major diseases to disparities in mortality. N Engl J Med 347(20):1585–1592, 2002.

278. Sankaranarayanan R, Ramadas K, Thomas G, et al: Effect of screening on oral cancer mortality in Kerala, India: a cluster-randomised controlled trial. Lancet 365(9475):1927–1933, 2005.

279. Oh ES, Laskin DM: Efficacy of the ViziLite system in the identification of oral lesions. J Oral Maxillofac Surg 65(3):424–426, 2007.

280. Epstein JB, Gorsky M, Lonky S, et al: The efficacy of oral lumenoscopy (ViziLite) in visualizing oral mucosal lesions. Spec Care Dentist 26(4):171–174, 2006.

281. De Veld DC, Witjes MJ, Sterenborg HJ, et al: The status of in vivo autofluorescence spectroscopy and imaging for oral oncology. Oral Oncol 41(2):117–131, 2005.

282. Gillenwater A, Jacob R, Ganeshappa R, et al: Noninvasive diagnosis of oral neoplasia based on fluorescence spectroscopy and native tissue autofluorescence. Arch Otolaryngol Head Neck Surg 124(11):1251–1258, 1998.

283. Sciubba JJ: Improving detection of precancerous and cancerous oral lesions. computer-assisted analysis of the oral brush biopsy: U.S. Collaborative OralCDx Study Group. J Am Dent Assoc 130(10):1445–1457, 1999.

284. Rumboldt Z, Day TA, Michel M: Imaging of oral cavity cancer. Oral Oncol 42(9):854–865, 2006.

285. Sciubba JJ, Goldenberg D: Oral complications of radiotherapy. Lancet Oncol 7(2):175–183, 2006.

286. Weymuller EA, Jr, Yueh B, Deleyiannis F, et al: Quality of life in head and neck cancer. Laryngoscope 110(3 Part 3):4–7, 2000.

287. Hoffmann M, Gottschlich S, Gorogh T, et al: Human papillomaviruses in lymph node neck metastases of head and neck cancers. Acta Otolaryngol 125(4):415–421, 2005.

11 Sentinel Lymph Node Biopsy for Oral Cancer

Francisco J. Civantos, Robert Zitsch, and Anthony Bared

KEY POINTS

- The goal of sentinel lymph node biopsy (SLNB) is to achieve more accurate staging of the neck through a less invasive means than selective neck dissection. The procedure is most useful in a population with low risk of lymphatic metastases, with no major comorbidity that precludes staged completion neck dissection, and with particular concern about the potential morbidity of selective neck dissection.

- The sentinel node technique, though more accurate in diagnosis of lymphatic metastases, leaves the at-risk basins untreated unless the completion neck dissection is performed. Selective neck dissection, on the other hand, may treat lymphatic metastases that remain unrecognized, precluding the possibility of closer follow-up or adjuvant therapy. Gamma probe–guided neck dissection combines the benefits of both types of dissection but adds complexity to the standard selective neck dissection.

- For the sentinel node technique to be most effective, proper training and significant experience are necessary. With proper technique and carefully followed procedures, false-negatives and lymphatic recurrences can be reduced.

- Proper, but also rapid, pathologic assessment is integral to the sentinel node procedure. Step sectioning and immunohistochemistry should be completed within a few days to allow early re-exploration in the minority of patients with positive sentinel nodes.

- Training in this technique includes instruction on the proper injection method, use of the gamma probe, and proper pathologic analysis of the sentinel nodes. Subsequently, the surgeon should develop experience through the practice of gamma probe–guided neck dissection. In this procedure, the surgeon simulates SLNB in the context of a planned selective neck dissection.

- Although formal quality-of-life studies have not been carried out, it is clear that the expected and potential morbidities of SLNB are lower than the well-documented morbidities of formal neck dissection.

- The concept that injection of a tracer will mark first echelon lymph nodes, and that the status of these lymph nodes correctly predicts that of the completion neck specimen, has been shown to apply in oral cancer, just as it does for melanoma. As these technologies progress, this procedure will likely move from one that can be applied to a selected group of patients to one suited for all T1 and T2 oral cancers.

Introduction

Sentinel lymph node biopsy (SLNB) is a minimally to moderately invasive technique that allows the surgeon to excise and meticulously examine the primary draining lymph nodes in the clinically N0 neck. Morton and associates[1,2] reintroduced this concept to surgical practice in a landmark publication describing the technique and their early prospective clinical experience with SLNB using blue dye in patients with clinically node-negative cutaneous malignant melanoma. Using injection of blue dye at the primary site, this team identified 259 sentinel nodes in 194 of 237 lymphatic nodal basins and found that the incidence of false-negative sentinel nodes (i.e., the identified sentinel node is found to be disease-free when metastatic disease is present in the regional lymphatic vessels) was less than 1%.[2] Their model of initial SLNB followed by completion lymphadenectomy and detailed pathologic analysis and correlation of findings has been used to validate this technique at multiple anatomic sites in subsequent trials. SLNB has been validated as an accurate means of staging the lymphatics relative to formal lymphadenectomy in cutaneous melanoma.[3]

Alex and Krag and associates[4,5] subsequently developed the use of radionuclides, nuclear imaging, and a hand-held gamma probe to identify sentinel lymph nodes in the clinically N0 neck. Based on their work, SLNB has more recently been performed using peritumoral intradermal injections of unfiltered technetium (^{99m}Tc)-sulfur colloid, or other radiotracer, and intraoperative gamma detection probes. The use of ^{99m}Tc-sulfur colloid and the gamma probe allows placement of the biopsy incision directly over the radiolabeled sentinel node(s), and the probe directs dissection straight to the node without disturbance of surrounding tissues. SLNB in melanoma using the gamma probe resulted in retrieval of sentinel nodes in 82% to 100% of cases, with a very low incidence of false-negative results confirmed by early follow-up.[6-10] In addition, a higher than expected incidence of bilateral drainage, "skip" drainage to a more distant node in a group than might be anticipated from the location of the primary melanoma, drainage to multiple lymph node groups in the neck, and unorthodox ipsilateral patterns of lymphatic drainage have been documented.[9-11]

Management of the N0 neck in patients with early invasive squamous cell carcinoma of the head and neck is controversial. This controversy is particularly well illustrated for early oral cancers that can be excised transorally. Simple close observation of the lymphatic basin has traditionally been used to avoid the morbidity of prophylactic neck dissection or irradiation in the majority of patients in whom neck metastases will truly never develop.[12-15] On the contrary, the weight of opinion in the recent literature argues against a generalized "watchful waiting" approach[16-18] and favors treatment of patients at risk for cervical metastases. Patients at risk have been identified by characteristics of the primary lesion, such as thickness greater than 4 mm, size greater than 2 cm, anatomic location, microinvasion, perineural infiltration, and so on.[19-24]

Computed tomography (CT), magnetic resonance imaging (MRI), and ultrasonography have been used to better identify grossly involved nonpalpable nodes and to increase the safety of the watchful waiting approach. However, significant limitations exist in terms of specificity and sensitivity because imaging modalities are incapable of identifying very small, and even microscopic, subclinical metastases.

The controversy surrounding the management of the N0 neck in mucosal squamous cell carcinoma of the head and neck is analogous to that of elective regional lymphadenectomy in patients with invasive, intermediate-risk, clinical node-negative melanoma. Experience from multiple centers has demonstrated that the presence or absence of occult melanoma metastases to regional nodes can be determined with a high degree of accuracy using the less invasive SLNB technique. Patients with negative sentinel nodes can thereby be spared the expense and morbidity of surgery from which they could realize no benefit, whereas those with positive sentinel nodes proceed to lymphadenectomy for compelling therapeutic indications.

As has occurred in clinically node-negative melanoma, SLNB ultimately offers the exciting possibility of identifying patients with clinically node-negative carcinomas of the other head and neck sites and with histologies that harbor occult metastases in the cervical lymphatics. It is important that a complete understanding of the technique, including an established false-negative rate, is available for each tumor type before incorporating it into routine clinical practice.

Background of Sentinel Lymph Node Biopsy for Head and Neck Squamous Cell Carcinoma

Between 1996 and 2000, multiple sites initiated single-institutional trials studying SLNB for oral cancer, the most accessible mucosal site.[25-32] More than 60 single institution trials, two international conference consensus documents, and a meta-analysis have since been published regarding this topic.[33-35] In particular, the group in Canniesburn, Scotland, has been a major advocate of this technique in Europe, where a considerable number of institutions and groups have published elegant validation series comparing the pathologic results of sentinel node biopsies with those of immediate completion neck dissection. These groups were not only looking at overall results, but assessing such issues as learning curves, proper pathologic analysis, and various details of surgical technique. Ross and associates[33] are the first to publish preliminary results regarding SLNB alone, without completion neck dissection, for oral cavity cancer.

Several smaller series have extended the technique to hypopharyngeal and supraglottic sites, in conjunction with endoscopic resection.[36] There are also series that described the experience with head and neck cutaneous lesions other than melanomas, including selected high-risk squamous cell carcinomas of the skin, Merkel cell carcinomas, and other lesions.[37-40] It has been demonstrated in the literature that predictive values of a negative sentinel lymph node vary between 90% and 100%, that significant upstaging of the lymphatic basins occurs with this technique relative to standard formal lymphadenectomy, and that unexpected patterns of lymphatic drainage can occur, including unanticipated contralateral drainage, which may be missed with standard lymphadenectomies. In addition, fine step sectioning and immunohistochemistry are essential in properly evaluating the sentinel lymph node and significantly improve the negative predictive value.

On the contrary, there has been reluctance to adopt SLNB, and it is not yet widely used for mucosal cancers, particularly in North America. Significant concerns exist regarding the possible need for staged surgery in patients whose sentinel nodes are detected to be positive in a delayed fashion as well as the risk of false-negatives in a highly curable setting. A false-negative SLNB takes on great importance because although a selective neck dissection does not always accurately diagnose metastases, it provides therapy to the lymphatic field, whereas SLNB leaves the highest-risk lymphatic basins untreated. False-negative results can occur for technical reasons, such as incomplete injection, inadequate radiologic imaging, failure to remove all radioactive nodes due to background radioactivity or desire to avoid more complex anatomic areas, and many other factors. However, even when SLNB is technically perfect, there are theoretical limitations in the ability of this technique to pick up every lymphatic metastasis. These limitations include the failure of standard histopathologic techniques to detect minimal disease, the theoretical potential for metastases to lodge in distal nodes while being eliminated in more proximal ones (termed "skip" metastases), and the potential for nonlymphatic gross disease that is below the threshold of imaging. Given the fairly moderate morbidity of selective neck dissection, these concerns are enough to keep many surgeons from offering patients SLNB for mucosal cancers.[41]

Selective neck dissection remains attractive as an accurate, minimally invasive technique for staging the cervical lymphatics in spite of these issues. It is therefore important that statistically significant, quality-controlled data be generated before the less invasive SLNB approach is accepted. Excellent pathologic validation data exist, but trials with long-term follow-up on patients with oral cancer having SLNB alone are limited. On the other hand, patients occasionally present with lesions that clinically appear relatively superficial (i.e., less than 4 mm depth of invasion suspected), and these represent a group for which the watchful waiting approach remains the standard of care. In this group, the SLNB approach might theoretically represent a more aggressive approach for patients who desire an evaluation of the lymphatics beyond what is currently standard.

Gamma Probe–Guided Selective Neck Dissection

The introduction of SLNB for sites such as breast and oral cavity, where there is an established pattern of lymphatic drainage and a generally accepted procedure for selective lymphadenectomy with acceptable morbidity, has led to the concept of "gamma probe–guided selective neck dissection," in which patients who are advised to consider lymphadenectomy are offered concurrent sentinel node mapping and biopsy along with the formal dissection (Fig. 11-1). This procedure allows the performance of validation studies but also is offered to obtain the benefit of more accurate mapping and staging through fine sectioning and immunohistochemistry of the sentinel node. Many patients who would have been staged as N0 are upstaged to N1 on the basis of this technique. This allows for closer follow-up evaluation, consideration of radiologic imaging, and possible adjuvant radiation. In review of the literature for oral cancer, upstaging could be anticipated to occur in 10% to 20% of cases.[27,28,31,42,43]

The gamma probe–guided selective neck dissection technique also allows for the identification of unusual patterns of lymphatic drainage and for better selective neck dissection by ensuring that all lymph nodes at risk are removed (Fig. 11-2). For example, with oral cavity cancer, one might detect contralateral nodes, perifacial nodes, and very posterior nodes in the jugular region bordering on level V, which might have been left out of a selective neck dissection but proved to represent important direct drainage patterns from the primary tumor. Sufficient data on the use of this technique are available, and the potential benefits are sufficiently documented. Therefore, an argument can be made that the use of this approach as an adjunct to formal lymphadenectomy is justifiable, could potentially benefit the patient, and is of low risk. The addition of a preoperative tumoral injection and prolongation of the surgery, by less than 1 hour in most cases, are unlikely to harm the patient and are outweighed by the benefits of more accurate staging and knowledge of drainage patterns as a guide to a better lymphadenectomy. This is generally the approach used to gain experience with sentinel node technology by surgeons experienced in selective neck dissection.

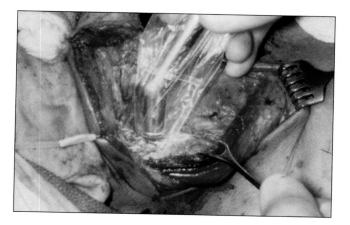

Figure 11-1. Gamma probe-guided neck dissection involves use of the gamma probe to remove sentinel nodes in the context of a planned selective neck dissection.

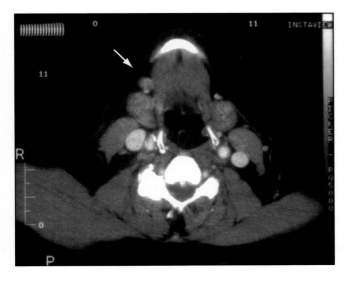

Figure 11-2. Asymmetric lymph node (*arrow*) in the expected drainage area of the primary tumor, seen on CT, would evoke suspicion enough to require biopsy of the imaged node and probable selective neck dissection.

The University of Miami Experience

The University of Miami experience in 106 sentinel lymph node biopsies in the head and neck region has been previously published.[42] The procedure was found to be extremely safe, and re-exploration could be safely accomplished in experienced hands without any untoward events. No shoulder symptoms, lip asymmetry, contour changes, or other unexpected side effects occurred. Precautions at the initial surgery, such as tagging of important nerves, and accelerated pathologic analysis of sentinel nodes combined with early re-exploration, helped make secondary surgeries safer. Among the 43 patients with oral cancer, primary site locations included 28 tongue, 2 floor of mouth, 1 alveolar ridge, 6 buccal mucosa, and 5 retromolar trigone. Stages included 11 T1 lesions, 27 T2 lesions, and 5 T3 lesions. Because the sentinel node evaluation for oral cancer was considered less standard than for melanoma, neck dissection specimens were initially examined in routine fashion, with representative sampling of 20 to 30 randomly selected lymph nodes in the neck, and pathology reports generated.

Frozen section was performed in the initial 18 cases and resulted in the identification of only 6 of 10 positive results. Fine sectioning at 2 mm and immunohistochemistry of the banked sentinel node blocks were performed separately at a later date by protocol. Twenty patients (46.5%) had positive results on final pathology. In nine patients, the sentinel node was the only positive node identified. In seven of these (16% of total), micrometastases not seen on initial hematoxylin and eosin were detected on extended sectioning and/or immunohistochemistry within the sentinel node. These seven patients were upstaged from N0 to N1 as a result of more detailed pathologic analysis of the sentinel node (95% CI: 6.8% to 30.7%).

The procedure was 100% accurate for T1 lesions in our single-institution series, with three true positives, eight true-negatives, and no false-negative results. Two false-negative sentinel node biopsies occurred among the 43 patients with oral cancer, all of whom had pathologic correlation with levels I to IV neck dissection. In patients with negative sentinel nodes, the presence of cancer in any nonradioactive lymph node was considered definitive evidence of disease missed by the sentinel node procedure. Among 43 oral cancers, there were 20 of 43 patients (46.5%) with metastases, 18 of which were identified on SLNB, giving a false-negative rate of 10% (95% CI: 1.2% to 31.7%) and a negative predictive value of 92% (95% CI: 74% to 99%). Both false-negative cases were similar in that they represented grossly abnormal nodes replacing the lymph node architecture and in juxtaposition to the sentinel node.

The strict definition of a sentinel node may produce an overestimate of the risk of missing cancer in such cases, since the gamma probe led the surgeon to the palpable node that was identified on the narrow-exposure sentinel node procedure. In both cases, positive nodes were identified and excised during the sentinel node exploration before initiating the completion of neck dissection. Two additional cases displayed microscopically positive levels III and IV sentinel nodes along with gross disease in level II that was not radioactive. The latter two cases, though not false-negatives, were notable because the sentinel nodes had microscopic disease, whereas grossly involved nodes did not take up radioactivity. Especially interesting is the contrast in patterns of tumor progression in the lymphatics of squamous cell carcinoma versus melanoma. Positive melanoma and Merkel cell carcinoma often involved multiple micrometastases in nodes that maintained their radioactivity and were therefore apparently functional. However, in 4 of 43 oral cancer patients grossly positive non-radioactive nodes were present, whereas sentinel nodes were negative or contained microscopic disease. Sentinel nodes were adjacent to these grossly involved nodes in three patients and located at a more distant distal location in one patient. We postulated that tumor destruction of the lymph node led to lymphatic obstruction and the development of new lymphatic pathways. Two of the four patients in question had T3 lesions, and two had T2 lesions, despite the fact that the group as a whole consisted primarily of T1 and T2 lesions. Our inclusion of a small number of T3 lesions, which naturally are at greater risk for subclinical gross disease, may have made this phenomenon more notable. Our impression is that, particularly for squamous cell carcinoma, efforts must be made via imaging to rule out subclinical gross disease that can lead to false-negatives and redirection of lymphatic flow.

Others have reported similar findings.[44] For oral cancer, it appears that the sentinel node procedure is an excellent test for microscopic disease but is not as good a test for subclinical gross disease that must be sought by radiologic studies and intraoperative palpation.

We also concluded that T3 oral lesions were less well suited for the SLNB procedure because of the higher incidence of gross nodal involvement and because the wider bed of radionuclide results in an impractically high number of sentinel nodes. The procedure was 100% accurate in 11 significantly invasive T1 oral lesions, in which there were three true-positives.

The ACOSOG Pathologic Validation Trial

Early data from the University of Miami series[42] as well as a series from the University of Missouri[32] were presented to the American College of Surgeons Oncology Group (ACOSOG) in 2001 and ultimately led to the development of a multi-institutional validation trial of SLNB for early invasive oral cancer, which recently completed accrual[45] (Fig. 11-3). This trial involved 25 institutions and 34 certified surgeons and included a formal training program. The group consisted of a mix of relatively experienced and inexperienced surgeons. Strict imaging criteria, based on CT or MRI, were used to rule out nonpalpable gross disease. Patients underwent injection of the lesion with unfiltered ^{99m}Tc-sulfur colloid, nuclear imaging, narrow-exposure sentinel lymphadenectomy, subsequent immediate selective neck dissection of levels I through IV, and routine pathologic analysis of the sentinel lymph nodes and nonsentinel lymph nodes. Blue dye was not injected because of concerns regarding the effect of blue coloration of the primary site on the resection of the primary tumor, where margins are generally not as wide as in the skin or breast. It was felt that the ability to visualize the tissue around the primary tumor must not be compromised.

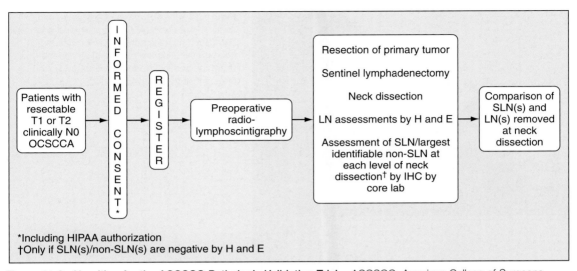

*Including HIPAA authorization
†Only if SLN(s)/non-SLN(s) are negative by H and E

Figure 11-3. Algorithm for the ACOSOG Pathologic Validation Trial. ACOSOG, American College of Surgeons Oncology Group; H&E, hematoxylin & eosin; OCSCCA, oral cavity squamous cell carcinoma; SLN, sentinel lymph node.

Lymphatic tissues, from both sentinel and nonsentinel lymph nodes, were submitted centrally for step sectioning at 2 to 3 mm intervals and immunohistochemistry for cytokeratin. Data were collected for routine pathologic assessment at the sites, comparing the sentinel node with the completion neck dissection specimen. Central tissue acquisition, step sectioning, and immunohistochemistry are still in progress. The major end point for the trial is the negative predictive value (NPV) of SLNB, which is defined as the proportion of patients with negative sentinel nodes who also have no positive nonsentinel nodes on pathologic evaluation of the neck dissection specimen. This end point was assessed by routine pathology, with limited sections through each node and hematoxylin and eosin stain, and will also be assessed via central step sectioning and immunohistochemistry (Fig. 11-4).

The data from the ACOSOG trial are summarized in Tables 11-1 through 11-3. A total of 161 patients enrolled in the study, of whom 140 were evaluated (Box 11-1). The median age was 58. There was one failure to map the lymphatics, representing a 99.3% technical success rate. There were 52 T1 lesions (56.2%) and 88 T2 lesions (42.3%). The median number of sentinel nodes removed per patient was three. There were 26 floor-of-mouth lesions (18.6%) and 95 tongue lesions (67.9%). On final analysis, including macrometastases, micrometastases, and single tumor cells believed to represent viable tumor, there were 41 patients (29%) who had cancer in the cervical nodes. The negative predictive value of a negative sentinel node, based only on routine pathology and hematoxylin and eosin stain, was 93 (95% CI: 0.865, 0.972). With central step sectioning and immunohistochemistry, this percentage improved to 96%. Of note, the negative predictive value was 100 for T1 lesions, with 13 positives of 52 patients. The number of sentinel nodes removed did correlate with stage ($P = .014$). The negative predictive value is the closest equivalent to the clinical situation in a patient with low to moderate risk of harboring cervical metastases and represents true-negatives as a fraction of total negatives. It answers the following question: If the sentinel node is negative, what is the percentage of risk that there is occult cancer in the neck?[45]

Although negative predictive values were similar, false-negative rates (false-negatives as a fraction of total positives) were worse for floor of mouth. The number

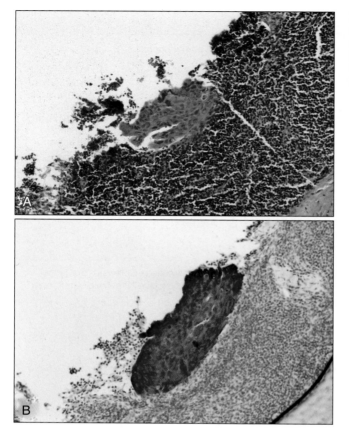

Figure 11-4. A micrometastasis is seen in a sentinel node with (**A**) hematoxylin and eosin stain and (**B**) immunohistochemistry for cytokeratin. Micrometastases are more likely to be found using the sentinel node technique and often go undiagnosed after selective neck dissection.

Table 11-1. Patient Characteristics for ACOSOG Trial: Sentinel Node Biopsy in Early Invasive Oral Cancer (*n* = 140)

Age (years)		
Median	58	
Minimum	24	
Maximum	90	
Gender		
Male	85	60.7%
Female	55	39.3%
Clinical T Stage		
T1	52	37.1%
T2	88	62.9%
Path. T Stage		
T1	77	56.2%
T2	58	42.3%
T3	1	0.7%
T4	1	0.7%

Table 11-1. Patient Characteristics for ACOSOG Trial: Sentinel Node Biopsy in Early Invasive Oral Cancer (n = 140)—cont'd

Path. Tumor Size (cm)		
Median	1.9	
Minimum	0.1	
Maximum	6.0	
No. of Sentinel Nodes Removed (Path.)		
Median	3	
Minimum	1	
Maximum	13	
No. of Sentinel Nodes Removed (Path.)		
1	24	17.1%
2	30	21.4%
3	26	18.6%
4	32	22.9%
5	10	7.1%
6	6	4.3%
7	2	1.4%
8	6	4.3%
9	2	1.4%
11	1	0.7%
13	1	0.7%
Tumor Location		
Tongue	95	67.9%
Floor of mouth	26	18.6%
Alveolar ridge	4	2.9%
Retromolar trigone	8	5.7%
Hard palate	0	0.0%
Buccal mucosa	7	5.0%
Oral vestibule	0	0.0%
H&E Status (NPV = 0.93)		
True-negative	100	71.4%
False-negative	7	5.0%
Positive	33	23.6%
H&E Status Positive Breakdown		
SN only positive	20	60.6%
SN and ON positive	13	39.4%
H&E False-Negatives		
False-negatives	7	17.5%
All other-positives	33	82.5%
Central Path. Status (NPV = 0.96)		
True-negative	99	70.7%
False-negative	4	2.9%
Positive	37	26.4%
Central Path. Status Positive Breakdown		
SN only positive	21	56.8%
SN and ON positive	16	43.2%
Central Path., False-Negatives		
False-negatives	4	9.8%
All other positives	37	90.2%

ACOSOG, American College of Surgeons Oncology Group; H&E, hematoxylin & eosin; NPV, negative predictive value; path., pathologic.
Data provided directly by ACOSOG Head and Neck Working Group.

Table 11-2. ACOSOG Trial, Number of Lymph Nodes Removed during SLNB by Stage

No. of Sentinel Nodes Removed (Path.)	Clinical T Stage		Total
	T1	T2	
1	12 (23.1%)	12 (13.6%)	24
2	12 (23.1%)	18 (20.4%)	30
3	10 (19.2%)	16 (18.2%)	26
4	10 (19.2%)	22 (25.0%)	32
5+	8 (15.4%)	20 (22.7%)	28
Total	52	88	140

Table 11-3. ACOSOG Trial, Number of Lymph Nodes Removed during Surgery by Anatomic Site

No. of Sentinel Nodes Removed (Path.)	Tumor Location					Total
	Tongue	Floor of Mouth	Alveolar Ridge	Retromolar Trigone	Buccal Mucosa	
1	14 (14.7%)	4 (15.4%)	0 (0.0%)	4 (50.0%)	2 (28.6%)	24
2	24 (25.3%)	2 (7.7%)	0 (0.0%)	2 (25.0%)	2 (28.6%)	30
3	19 (20.0%)	4 (15.4%)	2 (50.0%)	1 (12.5%)	0 (0.0%)	26
4	22 (23.2%)	6 (23.1%)	1 (25.0%)	1 (12.5%)	2 (28.6%)	32
5+	16 (16.8%)	10 (38.5%)	1 (25.0%)	0 (0.0%)	1 (14.3%)	28
Total	95	26	4	8	7	140

Box 11-1. Enrollment Summary for ACOSOG Trial

Patients enrolled	161
Ineligible or inevaluable	24
Failed SLNB	2
Aborted SLNB	5
Withdrew before surgery	1
Ineligible	10
Much missing data	3
Eligible and evaluable (enrolled by 32 surgeons at 26 institutions)	140

ACOSOG, American College of Surgeons Oncology Group; SLNB, sentinel lymph node biopsy.
Data provided directly by ACOSOG Head and Neck Working Group.

of positives in this smaller group was small relative to tongue (one false-negative and three false-positives), but the false-negative rate of 25% versus 8.1% for the other oral sites indicates a need for caution in this group. Presumably, this is due to technical issues related to the proximity of the primary site to the lymphatic basin.[45] At this point, we can say that if we presume that a SLNB in the context of a planned completion neck dissection is analogous to an isolated SLNB compared with an isolated neck dissection, then there is only a 4% chance of missing cancer in the lymph nodes based on meticulous pathology including step sections at 2 to 3 mm and immunohistochemistry for cytokeratin. However, very little observational data of SLNB alone in oral cancer are available, and this needs to be generated, preferably in a prospective fashion, before we can consider that the procedure has truly been tested. At this point, further technical progress is needed before we can consider SLNB to be reasonable for lesions of the floor of mouth to manage the issues related to "shine-through" radioactivity from the primary site. It is unclear whether the use of blue dye, or other new techniques, such as long-term staining with carbon dye, single-photon emission computed tomography (SPECT) imaging, ultrasound detectable injectable agents, or other developing techniques, might someday allow us to more accurately identify sentinel nodes in this group of patients.

The standard approach at this point for management of the N0 neck in a patient at significant risk is the selective neck dissection. Given the growing body of data regarding the reasonable predictive value of SLNB, this technique could be offered for those in whom watchful observation of the lymphatic basin would represent a reasonable traditional option. However, it is important that patients fully understand that the moderate morbidity that selective neck dissection entails must be balanced against the small risk of a false-negative result from SLNB. Given the existence of many supportive pathologic validation trials, including the ACOSOG cooperative group trial, which involved rigorous independent oversight, the most appropriate next step would be to acquire rigorous data on the results of SLNB alone—without completion of neck dissection—for this group of patients. The ideal study would involve a randomized comparison between selective neck dissection versus initial SLNB with neck dissection for proven positive results. But appropriately designing such a study would require thousands of patients. Thus, a more practical approach would be the generation of prospective, quality-controlled normative data of the results of the sentinel node technique, including long-term follow-up and quality-of-life assessment. Without such data we cannot be certain that the number of micrometastases picked up by both sentinel node technique and selective neck dissection is actually much less than the true presence of cancer in the neck. In other words, could we be treating many more undetected cancers with our selective neck dissection than we think? While these data are being collected, we should still view this as a cutting edge technique, not fully proven, but appropriate for patients unwilling to accept the moderate morbidity of selective neck dissection.

Controversies Regarding Surgical Technique

The importance of understanding the true predictive value of a negative SLNB is complicated by the variations in surgical technique in practice, which could in theory alter the accuracy of the results obtained. Some groups exclusively use radiotracers transported by lymph fluid[36,46,47] or radiotracers combined with blue dye.[43,48-50] In this context, Ross and associates[43] mentioned that the false-negative rate is not significantly reduced by additional color lymphography. This team affirmed that the radioactive marking of the sentinel nodes represented the basis of sentinel lymphadenectomy in the head and neck.

In addition, application of blue dye does entail some risk of complications. Accidental injury of the lymphatics leads to an extravasation of the dye, with resulting staining of adjacent tissue and reduction in intraoperative visualization. Especially in the area of the cervical soft tissues and the oral primary site, with their numerous neural and vascular structures, assessing tissue color and texture is of great importance in oncologic surgery. Furthermore, in 1985 Longnecker and associates[51] reported a 2% incidence of anaphylaxis after subcutaneous injection of blue dye.

Intraoperative[36,46,47] or preoperative[49,50,52,53] tracer injection and intraoperative lymphatic mapping detecting several "hot" nodes within the lymphatic draining basin during elective neck dissection are performed by some groups. Intraoperative lymphatic mapping is performed after elevation of the cutaneous flaps, following mobilization and dissection of the neck dissection specimen. The latter approach to gamma probe–guided neck dissection has the disadvantage of not developing the surgeon's ability to perform the minimally invasive SLNB and cannot be considered adequate for comparative study of the two techniques.[53]

Surgical Technique: Contrast between Oral and Cutaneous Lesions

Many steps are involved in the SLNB technique for mucosal lesions.

Step 1: Patient Selection

An appropriate patient is one with a significant risk of lymphatic micrometastases who is also unlikely to have distant metastases and has a small injectable lesion. Since early oral cavity cancer has less risk of distant metastases than melanoma, the manner in which these patients are approached is a bit different from the way we approach patients with melanoma. It is very important not to miss potentially curable micrometastases and reasonable to consider using the technique for lesions that are larger and more invasive than what would be considered appropriate for a melanoma. Nonetheless, many series have confirmed that the technique is not appropriate for T3 and T4 primary tumors because of the significant volume of tissue that would need to be injected, the excessively large number of radioactive nodes generated, the greater risk that grossly positive nodes exist, the potential for false-negative results due to incomplete injection, and the technical futility of removing a large number of nodes in piecemeal fashion. On the contrary, the technique is best applied to T1 and smaller T2 lesions. If a lesion is less than 4 cm in maximal diameter but has significant tongue fixation or other manifestations of deep invasion, then this is truly a T4 lesion, and the results with SLNB are unlikely to prove accurate and useful.

If the primary tumor meets criteria, the next issue is whether the neck is grossly involved. Although the sentinel node technique is an excellent technique for detecting micrometastases, it is less useful for detecting nonpalpable but grossly involved lymph nodes. This appears to be particularly true with squamous cell carcinoma. It is postulated that when a large percentage of the lymph node is replaced by cancer, physiologic obstruction occurs, and alternative patterns of lymphatic drainage develop. Extranodal squamous cell carcinoma in the neck tissues, by definition, cannot be detected by SLNB. It is important to detect the presence of such gross disease on preoperative imaging and avoid applying this technique to that group of patients to avoid false-positives. Generally, contrast-enhanced CT and MRI (if iodine-allergic) are the imaging modalities used. These should be strictly interpreted. The role of positron emission tomography remains to be delineated, but this may ultimately also prove useful in ruling out such gross disease. It should be kept in mind that the sentinel node technology represents an excellent technique for detection of micrometastases in patients felt to have a reasonably low risk of metastases, but it is not as accurate at detecting grossly involved, nonfunctional nodes.

Step 2: Injection of the Primary Tumor

The injection is performed before the surgical procedure, generally on the morning of surgery, in the radiologic suite. Injection is also sometimes performed late on the day before surgery. Use of 500 mCi is recommended on the morning of surgery or a slightly higher dose the night before. Awake injection and imaging in radiology constitute the most commonly used technique, but as we extend this procedure to endoscopically accessible oropharyngeal, supraglottic, and hypopharyngeal lesions, it is likely that cooperative efforts with the nuclear radiologist and the use of portable cameras will allow for intraoperative endoscopic injection, with or without radiologic imaging, and gamma probe–guided sentinel node biopsy without the need for uncomfortable injections on an awake patient. Theoretical advantages of injecting under general anesthesia include better exposure of the primary tumor and prevention of patient motion related to discomfort. This may eventually further increase the reliability of this method. Taking into account that the radiolocalization of the detected hot spots does not represent the drainage of the primary tumor, but does represent the drainage of the tracer deposits, which are supposed to mimic the lymphatic drainage of the primary, the impact of a thorough and representative tracer injection becomes evident. Because of the density and direction of the head and neck lymphatics, the primary tumor may drain into several alternative lymphatic pathways, all representing the first echelon of draining sentinel lymph nodes.

Nevertheless, because of regulatory issues related to the injection of radioactive substances and the lack of widely available portable nuclear imaging, awake injection remains the most commonly used technique at present. It is important to ensure that the patient is comfortable so that an adequate preoperative injection is obtained. We use topical anesthetic, mild oral sedation, and lingual, inferior alveolar, and/or sphenopalatine nerve blocks to ensure patient comfort during manipulation and injection of the primary tumor. Direct injection of the tumor with local anesthetic should not be performed since it may affect uptake of the radionuclide and reportedly even cause it to precipitate in the tissues. The injection technique involves narrow injection with a 25-gauge needle circumferentially encompassing the leading edge of the lesion and an additional injection in the center of the lesion (Figs. 11-5 and 11-6). Five tuberculin syringes with 1-mL aliquots of ^{99m}Tc-sulfur colloid, with a total radioactiv-

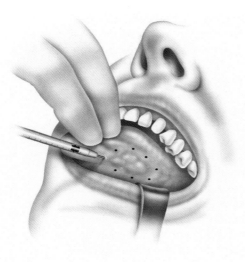

Figure 11-5. A 1.5-inch needle and tuberculin syringe are used to inject gingerly, completely encompassing the lesion. Excess force should be avoided so that nonphysiologic drainage patterns are not opened. Sedation, topical anesthetics, and nerve blocks can be used, but lidocaine should not be infiltrated into the bed of injection. Avoid injecting more widely or deeply than necessary, as the injected colloid will extravasate more widely than is apparent. (From Civantos FJ, Werner JA, and Bared A: Sentinel node biopsy in cancer of the oral cavity. Operative Techniques in Otolaryngology–Head Neck Surgery 16:275–285, 2005, Figure 1.)

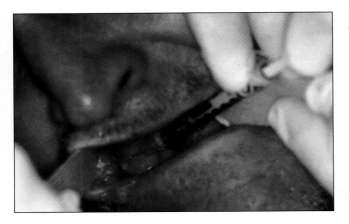

Figure 11-6. Injection of buccal mucosa tumor with radiocolloid.

ity of 500 mCi, would represent a standard dose for the morning of surgery. A slightly higher dose would be used the night before. These dosages are extrapolated from the practice for melanoma and have worked well for oral cavity cancer, but formal comparative evaluation of dosages and volumes for use in the oral cavity have yet to be performed.

To extend this technique to supraglottic and hypopharyngeal sites, arrangements must be made to handle radionuclide in the operating suite. This generally involves the participation of a nuclear medicine technician, and endoscopic injection of the primary tumor must be performed. Subsequently, adequate time must be allowed for migration of radionuclide to the lymphatic basin, and the gamma probe can be used to confirm this.

For cutaneous lesions, it is well documented that a scar from a previous excisional biopsy can be injected to allow accurate SLNB. Whether a previously excised oral lesion could undergo sentinel node excision by injection of an intraoral scar has yet to be determined. It is important to inject narrowly and not to inject the deep tissues. The radionuclide extravasates more widely in the oral cavity around the site of injection than occurs in the skin and will usually go to the neck more quickly. There is no benefit in trying to inject a margin around the tumor, since this leads to an unmanageable excess of radioactive nodes. However, injection must be just peripheral to the tumor in normal-appearing tissue and not within the gross cancer to allow migration into normal lymphatic channels. We prefer to use unfiltered ^{99m}Tc-sulfur colloid. The presence of larger particles allows for retention of radioactivity in the proximal lymphatics. Retained particles at the site of primary injection are not a major issue since we recommend removal of the primary tumor first. However, it is also possible to obtain good results using filtered ^{99m}Tc-sulfur colloid, and if there is a strong preference for addressing the lymphatics first, then this may be preferable since there is a better clearance of background radioactivity from the primary site. The more rapid migration of the filtered agent may also make it advantageous if injections of radionuclide are performed on the operating room table at the start of the procedure rather than before the surgical procedure.

As previously discussed, blue dye used concurrently with ^{99m}Tc-sulfur colloid has become popular in SLNB for melanoma. This is a reasonable technique for skin and certainly can help during the learning phase of the procedure, because the subtle blue-dyed lymphatic vessels can be traced toward the sentinel node. Furthermore, reinjection of the blue dye is performed in the operating room under anesthesia and can provide a measure of security against inadequacy of preoperative injection due to patient discomfort. The most common approach, however, for the reasons previously mentioned, is to use the radionuclide alone for mucosal lesions. We prefer to remove the primary tumor first to eliminate radioactive background at the primary site. When the technique is performed in this sequence, the blue dye has usually run through to the distal lymphatics by the time the oral resection is completed and margins are sent, making the dye less useful. The concept of injecting a second agent within the operating room for better accuracy is reasonable, however; currently, a contrast agent, Sonazoid (GE Healthcare, Oslo, Norway), which does not color the tissues but can be identified by intraoperative ultrasound, is undergoing clinical trials.[54] Sonazoid is a lipid-stabilized suspension of 2.4 to 3.5 microns of perfluorobutane microbubbles. This may someday provide an alternative to blue dye for those who desire a second tracer injection for increased accuracy.

Step 3: Nuclear Lymphatic Mapping

After injection, nuclear imaging of the lymphatics is obtained. SPECT technology, though not absolutely necessary, may eventually provide even better three-

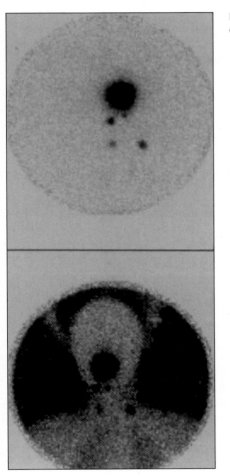

Figure 11-7. Lymphoscintigrams may show unexpected contralateral drainage.

dimensional localization of the sentinel node. The availability of both anteroposterior and lateral imaging will generally be adequate, however, to guide the surgeon. A dynamic phase should be acquired with serial images for 1 hour after injection. These images should be acquired for 1 minute each. Transmission images should be acquired for 1 to 2 minutes in each new movement of the camera. Although it is possible to perform SLNB with the intraoperative gamma probe alone, the radiologic image can be useful in providing a rough guide to the location of the sentinel node. It may provide for a more complete informed consent process by predicting unexpected drainage to the contralateral neck or other areas that were not expected to be involved (Fig. 11-7).

Step 4: Removal of the Primary Tumor

We prefer to resect the primary tumor transorally first. If the injection field is sufficiently narrow, this usually eliminates or greatly reduces background radioactivity at the primary site, or "shine-through," which can confound the sentinel node identification. The usual appropriate surgical margins with frozen-section control should be obtained. In some situations, it may be necessary to perform the nodal biopsy before primary resection. Removal of the primary tumor first is less important when the lymphatic basin is distant from the primary tumor and is often less of an issue for skin lesions (i.e., auricular scalp or nasal lesions). However, this can be important for lesions of the neck or preauricular skin, where the lymphatics are immediately deep to the primary tumor. Removal of the primary tumor is especially important for floor-of-mouth tumors because of the immediate proximity of the submandibular lymphatics.

Step 5: Gamma Probe–Guided Sentinel Lymph Node Biopsy

The hand-held gamma probe is now used to confirm the location of the sentinel lymph node(s), which previously were identified during lymphoscintigraphy (Fig. 11-8). The skin is again marked with the location of the nodes. If the patient is to undergo SLNB alone, with neck dissection planned only for positive findings intraoperatively or on permanent histopathology, the incision can be drawn narrowly over the node. However, the incision must be consistent with the possibility of subsequent neck dissection, and the planned incision for the formal lymphadenectomy should be considered. Alternatively, the incision can be drawn in the line of that to be used for neck dissection, though shorter in length, and flaps can be elevated. This latter approach is used when immediate gamma probe–guided neck dissection is the plan. After the incision is made, subplatysmal flaps are elevated sufficiently to provide access to the hot area. The neck should first be carefully palpated to identify palpable gross lymphatic disease that may not be physiologically functional, and hence may not take up radioactivity. The finding of gross cancer involvement would, of course, contraindicate SLNB and mandate formal lymphadenectomy.

If no gross disease is identified, the surgeon now localizes the sentinel node(s). Use of the probe to locate the nodes is not intuitive and is best learned through instruction by a surgeon with experience in the technique. Initial readings are taken of the precordium and back table to assess the level of hematogenous radioactivity (Fig. 11-9). Readings are also obtained from the resected tumor specimen and the bed of resection to assess the level of anticipated background activity. The probe is slowly passed over the neck at a steady rate, assessing the auditory input for radioactivity generated by the gamma probe. Care is taken to aim away from the primary resection bed. Since the probe measures radioactivity over time, rapid or unsteady movement leads to higher readings and louder auditory input and should be avoided. Using steady constant motion, the probe is moved radially across each hot spot allowing the surgeon to determine the direction in which to proceed, in three dimensions, to locate the sentinel node (Fig. 11-10). Using a fine hemostat or McCabe nerve dissector, the surgeon bluntly dissects toward the sentinel node (Fig. 11-11). Bipolar

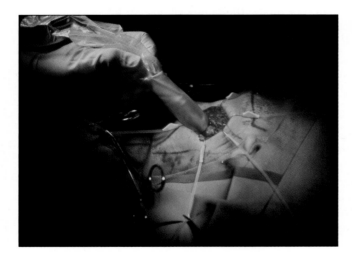

Figure 11-8. The gamma probe is used to direct dissection toward the sentinel node.

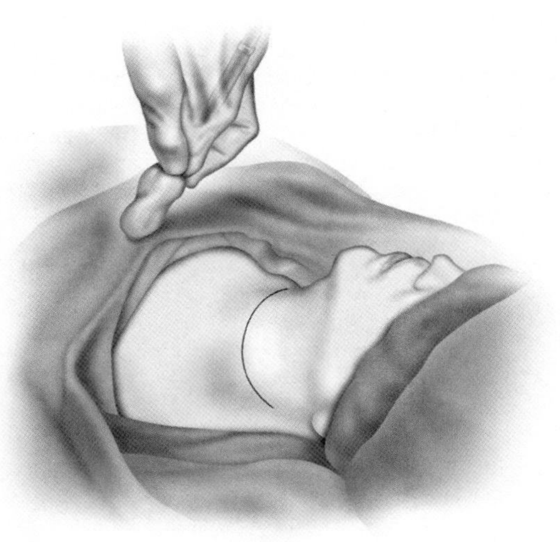

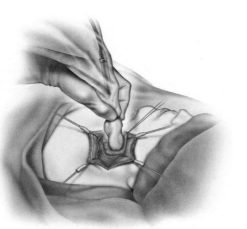

Figure 11-9. Background reading is taken at the precordium. (From Civantos FJ, Werner JA, and Bared A: Sentinel node biopsy in cancer of the oral cavity. Operative Techniques in Otolaryngology–Head Neck Surgery 16:275–285, 2005, Figure 3.)

Figure 11-10. Blunt dissection towards the "hot spot" is followed by reinsertion of the sentinel node into the path of dissection and angulation in various directions seeking the hot lymph node. (From Civantos FJ, Werner JA, and Bared A: Sentinel node biopsy in cancer of the oral cavity. Operative Techniques in Otolaryngology–Head Neck Surgery 16:275–285, 2005, Figure 6.)

cautery can be used to divide the tissues to provide wider exposure. Use of paralytics and monopolar cautery should be avoided.

After the dissection cavity is opened, the gamma probe is introduced into this space along the plane of dissection and angled in various directions to guide the surgeon to the sentinel node. The sentinel node is bluntly excised. Probe readings (counts per minute) are recorded for initial readings taken while the node is in the patient, as well as for ex vivo readings of the extracted node, away from the patient (Fig. 11-12). Repeat readings of the resection bed are taken to ensure that there are no adjacent hot nodes that also need to be removed (Fig. 11-13). Any lymph node exhibiting 10% or more of the radioactivity of the most radioactive node in the same anatomic area is considered an additional sentinel lymph node and is harvested separately. A large number of very radioactive nodes (i.e., more than six) essentially represents a failure of the technique, and piecemeal removal of a large number of nodes is not recommended. The surgeon should proceed to selective neck dissection if indicated. With a very hot sentinel node in a specific area, there may be a relatively hot node in a completely separate anatomic region (i.e., submental region versus level II jugular region) that does not reach 10% of the radioactivity of the hottest node.

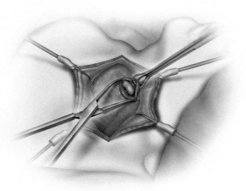

Figure 11-11. The sentinel node is excised using a combination of blunt dissection and division of tissue by means of bipolar cautery. Unipolar cautery should be avoided when the proximity of neurovascular structures is not known. (From Civantos FJ, Werner JA, and Bared A: Sentinel node biopsy in cancer of the oral cavity. Operative Techniques in Otolaryngology–Head Neck Surgery 16:275–285, 2005, Figure 7.)

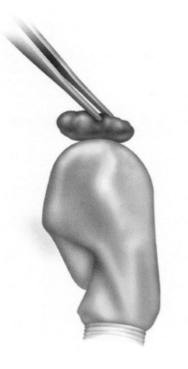

Figure 11-12. Ex vivo readings pointing away from the patient should confirm whether this is the radioactive node. (From Civantos FJ, Werner JA, and Bared A: Sentinel node biopsy in cancer of the oral cavity. Operative Techniques in Otolaryngology–Head Neck Surgery 16:275–285, 2005, Figure 8.)

If this second node is truly in a separate area and is significantly greater than background (two or more times background readings), it should still be harvested as a sentinel node because it may represent a separate drainage pattern from a different portion of the tumor (Fig. 11-13).

Review of the lymphoscintigraphic imaging and knowledge of basic anatomic principles allow the surgeon to judge whether such additional areas of borderline radioactivity need to be excised. When the sentinel lymph node dissections are performed before resection of the oral primary cancer or significant radioactivity persists in the bed of resection, intraoral lead shields can be used to block background activity at the primary site. The presence of a collimator on the gamma probe is also recommended, and most modern probes have fine tips with collimators. With tongue tumors, background activity can be avoided by using a transoral suture on the tongue to pull the primary bed away from the lymphatics.

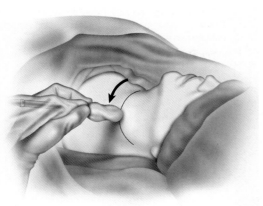

Figure 11-13. The probe is drawn slowly over the neck seeking additional hot areas. This process is repeated after the hottest node(s) are removed. (From Civantos FJ, Werner JA, and Bared A: Sentinel node biopsy in cancer of the oral cavity. Operative Techniques in Otolaryngology–Head Neck Surgery 16:275–285, 2005, Figure 5.)

The issue of dealing with background activity at the primary site is most marked for the level I nodes with floor-of-mouth tumors. In this situation, the surgeon may need to perform some initial dissection below the level of the marginal mandibular nerve, transecting the tissues down to the level of the mylohyoid muscle. In this manner, the lymph nodes are mobilized away from the oral cavity, allowing for more accurate identification of the sentinel lymph node(s) by placing the gamma probe into the tunnel thus created and directing the probe inferiorly away from the background radioactivity at the floor-of-mouth injection site. Each sentinel lymph node is labeled, measured, described, and recorded separately as to location and total ex vivo counts per second.

It is particularly important to tag the tissue adjacent to any identified marginal mandibular or spinal accessory nerve branches with permanent suture to facilitate identification during a subsequent procedure if the sentinel node is positive.

Step 6: Histopathologic Assessment of the Sentinel Node

SLNB for cutaneous lesions is gaining wide acceptance, particularly for melanoma, for which formal elective lymphadenectomy is not standard. Minimally invasive T1 oral lesions represent an emerging group in which the option of SLNB might be considered. However, in any situation in which SLNB alone is performed, exhaustive histopathologic evaluation of the sentinel node with fine sectioning and sampling at thin intervals (some have advocated as thin as 150 micron intervals) and concurrent immunohistochemistry should be performed to rule out microscopic foci of cancer and allow for therapeutic neck dissection or radiation. If such an evaluation remains negative, close follow-up and consideration of serial radiologic imaging (CT, MRI, or serial ultrasound) should be considered.

Risks of SLNB

The theoretical risk of injury to the facial nerve and spinal accessory nerve during blunt dissection through narrow exposure is one concern with SLNB in the head and neck region (Fig. 11-14). The relatively few publications addressing this issue to date have reported incidences of complications of less than 1%.[42,55] Theoretically in the hands of an inexperienced operator, the risk of injury to the facial or spinal accessory nerves may be greater with SLNB than with formal parotidectomy and selective neck dissection. Since the presence of sentinel node micrometastases may be recognized postoperatively, the potential risk of nerve injury related to re-exploration of an inflamed, recently operated wound needs to be considered. For this reason, important

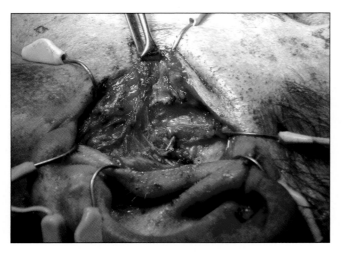

Figure 11-14. Sentinel node biopsy in the parotid region may require identification of distal facial nerve branches.

structures are tagged, and pathologic analysis is done promptly to allow for early re-exploration.

Conclusions

SLNB can be used safely and with technical success for accessible head and neck squamous cell carcinomas. It offers the potential for more anatomically accurate surgery based on each patient's unique lymphatic drainage pattern. However, selective neck dissection remains the standard approach for most oral cancers, particularly for larger T2, T3, and T4 lesions. SLNB can be advocated as a reasonable alternative to selective neck dissection for very early oral cancers. Unlike melanoma, in which the presence of lymphatic metastasis portends an extremely poor prognosis, squamous cell carcinoma with early lymphatic metastases remains curable. Thus, there is much more to lose by understaging patients or missing involved lymph nodes.

The sentinel node concept is discarded by some based on the misconception that selective neck dissection has no significant morbidity. Coming from a tradition of more radical neck procedures, the selective neck dissection is generally viewed as an intervention with negligible morbidity by many head and neck surgeons. In fact, although the morbidity of selective neck dissection is significantly less than that of modified radical and radical dissections, there is measurable morbidity in a variable percentage of patients, including issues with shoulder function secondary to temporary trapezius weakness followed by adhesive capsulitis of the shoulder, pain syndromes, contour changes, and lower lip mobility. This has been demonstrated in numerous quality-of-life studies and at least two objective functional assessments.[56-58] This moderate morbidity has led some to suggest watchful waiting as an alternative for patients of lower risk. SLNB has developed as an intermediate option in response to this controversy. All these complications are observed much less frequently with SLNB, although formal quality-of-life assessments have not yet been performed.

The sentinel node procedure would be more widely applicable if we developed the ability to immediately diagnose positive sentinel nodes. Frozen section, even with multiple sections, is not sufficiently accurate and may destroy valuable specimen material.[28] Thus, for the patient with the micrometastasis in the sentinel node, we are potentially dealing with issues of re-exploration and dissection of functionally important nerves in a recently operated wound. Ultimately, rapid reverse transcriptase-polymerase chain reaction assessment of nodes may provide immediate information regarding the status of the sentinel node.[59] As future studies are designed to safely evaluate the SLNB technique, the opportunity should be taken to plan correlative studies to validate the role of these new technologies in tumor assessment.

SLNB ultimately may have a role in the management of oral cancer, given that there are lesions and situations in which the "wait and see" approach continues to be advocated. It may provide an intermediate approach for small but invasive T1 or smaller T2 lesions for which watchful waiting is the major alternative. It appears unlikely that this technique will ever replace selective neck dissection for larger T2 and T3N0 lesions.

Equally important is the evaluation for the significant unpredictability of lymphatic pathways observed for both cutaneous and oral lesions. In fact for lesions not involving the midline but within a few centimeters of it, lymphoscintigraphy and gamma probe–guided surgery may provide the solution in these patients, for whom we often struggle with the decision regarding contralateral neck management. Increased accuracy in the identification of micrometastases will lead to more accurate staging.

The sentinel node technique is likely to have an increasing role in the management of head and neck cancer in the future. Surgeons can gain experience in the use of this technique for cutaneous malignancies, superficial oral cancers, and, with gamma probe–guided neck dissection, for invasive cancers, preferably in the context of a clinical trial. Pilot data on the use of this technique in the pharynx and larynx will continue to emerge. It is hoped that this chapter will provide a guide to surgeons as they consider the developing role of lymphoscintigraphy and sentinel node biopsy in detecting microscopic lymphatic metastases.

References

1. Morton DL, Wen D-R, Wong JH, et al: Technical details of intraoperative lymphatic mapping for early stage melanoma. Arch Surg 127:392–399, 1992.
2. Morton DL, Wen D-R, Foshag LJ, et al: Intraoperative lymphatic mapping and selective cervical lymphadenectomy for early-stage melanomas of the head and neck. J Clin Oncol 11:1751–1756, 1993.
3. Leong SP: Selective sentinel lymphadenectomy for malignant melanoma. Surg Clin North Am 83:157–185, 2003.
4. Morton DL, Thompson JF, Essner R, et al: Validation of the accuracy of intraoperative lymphatic mapping and sentinel lymphadenectomy for early-stage melanoma: a multicenter trial. Multicenter Selective Lymphadenectomy Trial Group. Ann Surg 230:453–463, 1999.
5. Alex JC, Krag DN: The gamma-probe-guided resection of radio-labeled primary lymph nodes. Surg Oncol Clin N Am 5:33–41, 1996.
6. Krag DN, Meijer SJ, Weaver DL, et al: Minimal-access surgery for staging of malignant melanoma. Arch Surg 130:654–658, 1995.
7. Glass LF, Messina JL, Cruse W, et al: The use of intraoperative radiolymphoscintigraphy for sentinel node biopsy in patients with malignant melanoma. Dermatol Surg 22:715–720, 1996.
8. Albertini JJ, Cruse CW, Rapaport D, et al: Intraoperative radio-lympho-scintigraphy improves sentinel node identification for patients with melanoma. Ann Surg 223:217–224, 1996.
9. Ross MI, Reintgen D, Balch CM: Selective lymphadenectomy: emerging role for lymphatic mapping and sentinel node biopsy in the management of early stage melanoma. Semin Surg Oncol 9:219–223, 1993.
10. O'Brien CJ, Uren RF, Thompson JF, et al: Prediction of potential metastatic sites in cutaneous head and neck melanoma using lymphoscintigraphy. Am J Surg 170:461–466, 1995.
11. Pijpers R, Collet GJ, Meijer S, Hoekstra OS: The impact of dynamic lymphoscintigraphy and gamma probe guidance on sentinel node biopsy in melanoma. Eur J Nucl Med 22:1238–1241, 1995.
12. Jesse RH, Ballantyne AJ, Larson D: Radical or modified neck dissection: a therapeutic dilemma. Am J Surg 136:516–519, 1978.
13. Spiro RH, Strong EW: Epidermoid carcinoma of the mobile tongue. Treatment by partial glossectomy alone. Am J Surg 122:707–710, 1971.
14. Spiro RH, Strong EW: Epidermoid carcinoma of the oral cavity and oropharynx. Elective versus therapeutic radical neck dissection as treatment. Arch Surg 107:382–384, 1973.
15. Vandenbrouck C, Sancho-Garnier H, Chassagne D, et al: Elective versus therapeutic radical neck dissection in epidermoid carcinoma of the oral cavity. Results of a randomized clinical trial. Cancer 46:386–390, 1980.
16. McGuirt WF, Jr, Johnson JT, Myers EN, et al: Floor of mouth carcinoma. The management of the clinically negative neck. Arch Otolaryngol Head Neck Surg 121:278–282, 1995.
17. Shah JP, Andersen PE: Evolving role of modifications in neck dissection for oral squamous carcinoma. Br J Oral Maxillofac Surg 33:3–8, 1995.
18. Kligerman J, Lima RA, Soares JR, et al: Supraomohyoid neck dissection in the treatment of T1/T2 squamous cell carcinoma of oral cavity. Am J Surg 168:391–394, 1994.
19. Martínez-Gimeno C, Rodríguez EM, Vila CN, Varela CL: Squamous cell carcinoma of the oral cavity: a clinicopathologic scoring system for evaluating risk of cervical lymph node metastasis. Laryngoscope 105:728–733, 1995.
20. Ho CM, Lam KH, Wei WI, et al: Occult lymph node metastasis in small oral tongue cancers. Head Neck 14:359–363, 1992.
21. Urist MM, O'Brien CJ, Soong SJ, et al: Squamous cell carcinoma of the buccal mucosa: analysis of prognostic factors. Am J Surg 154:411–414, 1987.
22. Mohit-Tabatabai MA, Sobel HJ, Rush BF, Mashberg A: Relation of thickness of floor of mouth stage I and II cancers to regional metastasis. Am J Surg 152:351–353, 1986.
23. Brown B, Barnes L, Mazariegos J, et al: Prognostic factors in mobile tongue and floor of mouth carcinoma. Cancer 64:1195–1202, 1989.

24. Spiro RH, Huvos AG, Wong GY, et al: Predictive value of tumor thickness in squamous carcinoma confined to the tongue and floor of the mouth. Am J Surg 152:345–350, 1986.

25. Rassekh CH, Johnson JT, Myers EN: Accuracy of intraoperative staging of the N0 neck in squamous cell carcinoma. Laryngoscope 105:1334–1336, 1995.

26. Ross G, Shoaib T, Soutar DS, et al: The use of sentinel node biopsy to upstage the clinically N0 neck in head and neck cancer. Arch Otolaryngol Head Neck Surg 128:1287–1291, 2002.

27. Shoaib T, Soutar DS, MacDonald DG, et al: The accuracy of head and neck carcinoma sentinel lymph node biopsy in the clinically N0 neck. Cancer 91:2077–2083, 2001.

28. Civantos FJ, Gomez C, Duque C, et al: Sentinel node biopsy in oral cavity cancer: correlation with PET scan and immunohistochemistry. Head Neck 25:1–9, 2003.

29. Taylor RJ, Wahl RL, Sharma PK, et al: Sentinel node localization in oral cavity and oropharynx squamous cell cancer. Arch Otolaryngol Head Neck Surg 127:970–974, 2001.

30. Alex JC, Sasaki CT, Krag DN, et al: Sentinel lymph node radiolocalization in head and neck squamous cell carcinoma. Laryngoscope 110:198–203, 2000.

31. Stoeckli SJ, Steinert H, Pfaltz M, Schmid S: Sentinel lymph node evaluation in squamous cell carcinoma of the head and neck. Otolaryngol Head Neck Surg 125:221–226, 2001.

32. Zitsch RP III, Todd DW, Renner GJ, Singh A: Intraoperative radiolymphoscintigraphy for detection of occult nodal metastasis in patients with head and neck squamous cell carcinoma. Otolaryngol Head Neck Surg 122:662–666, 2000.

33. Ross GL, Soutar DS, MacDonald D, et al: Sentinel node biopsy in head and neck cancer: preliminary results of a multicenter trial. Ann Surg Oncol 11:690–696, 2004.

34. Stoeckli SJ, Pfaltz M, Ross GL, et al: The Second International Conference on Sentinel Node Biopsy in Mucosal Head and Neck Cancer. Ann Surg Oncol 12:919–924, 2005.

35. Paleri V, Rees G, Arullendran P, et al: Sentinel node biopsy in squamous cell cancer of the oral cavity and oral pharynx: a diagnostic meta-analysis. Head Neck 27:739–747, 2005.

36. Werner JA, Dünne AA, Ramaswamy A, et al: Sentinel node detection in N0 cancer of the pharynx and larynx. Br J Cancer 87:711–715, 2002.

37. Messina JL, Reintgen DS, Cruse CW, et al: Selective lymphadenectomy in patients with Merkel cell (cutaneous neuroendocrine) carcinoma. Ann Surg Oncol 4:389–395, 1997.

38. Altinyollar H, Berberoglu U, Celen O: Lymphatic mapping and sentinel lymph node biopsy in squamous cell carcinoma of the lower lip. Eur J Surg Oncol 28:72–74, 2002.

39. Reschly MJ, Messina J, Zaulyanov LL, et al: Utility of sentinel lymphadenectomy in the management of patients with high-risk cutaneous squamous cell carcinoma. Dermatol Surg 29:135–140, 2003.

40. Nouri K, Rivas MP, Pedroso F, et al: Sentinel lymph node biopsy for high-risk cutaneous squamous cell carcinoma of the head and neck. Arch Dermatol 140:1284, 2004.

41. Devaney KO, Rinaldo A, Rodrigo JP, Ferlito A: Sentinel node biopsy in head and neck tumors—where do we stand today? Head Neck 28:1122–1131, 2006.

42. Civantos FJ, Moffat FL, Goodwin WJ: Lymphatic mapping and sentinel lymphadenectomy for 106 head and neck lesions: contrasts between oral cavity and cutaneous malignancy. Laryngoscope 112(Suppl 109):S1–S15, 2006.

43. Ross GL, Soutar DS, Shoaib T, et al: The ability of lymphoscintigraphy to direct sentinel node biopsy in the clinically N0 neck for patients with head and neck squamous cell carcinoma. Br J Radiol 75:950–958, 2002.

44. Alvi A, Johnson JT: Extracapsular spread in the clinically negative neck (N0): implications outcome. Otolaryngol Head Neck Surg 114:65–70, 1996.

45. Civantos FJ, Zitsch R, Schuller D, et al: Sentinel node biopsy for oral cancer: a multi-center validation trial. Arch Otolaryngol Head Neck Surg; 132: Abstract (Presentation to the American Head and Neck Society), 2006.

46. Barzan L, Sulfaro S, Alberti F, et al: Gamma probe accuracy in detecting the sentinel lymph node in clinically N0 squamous cell carcinoma of the head and neck. Ann Otol Rhinol Laryngol 111:794–798, 2002.

47. Werner JA, Dünne AA, Ramaswamy A, et al: Number and location of radiolabeled, intraoperatively identified sentinel nodes in 48 head and neck cancer patients with clinically staged N0 and N1 neck. Eur Arch Otorhinolaryngol 259:91–96, 2002.

48. Chiesa F, Mauri S, Grana C, et al: Is there a role for sentinel node biopsy in early N0 tongue tumors? Surgery 128:16–21, 2000.

49. Chiesa F, Tradati N, Calabrese L: Sentinel node biopsy, lymphatic pattern and selective neck dissection in oral cancer. Oral Dis 7:317–318, 2007.

50. Hyde NC, Prvulovich E, Newman L, et al: A new approach to pre-treatment assessment of the N0 neck in oral squamous cell carcinoma: the role of sentinel node biopsy and positron emission tomography. Oral Oncol 39:350–360, 2003.

51. Longnecker SM, Guzzardo MM, Van Voris LP: Life-threatening anaphylaxis following subcutaneous administration of isosulfan blue 1%. Clin Pharm 4:219–221, 1985.

52. Ionna F, Chiesa F, Longo F, et al: Prognostic value of sentinel node in oral cancer. Tumori 88:S18–S19, 2002.

53. Mozzillo N, Chiesa F, Botti G, et al: Sentinel node biopsy in head and neck cancer. Ann Surg Oncol 8(9 Suppl):S103–S105, 2001.

54. Curry JM, Bloedon E, Malloy KM, et al: Ultrasound-guided contrast-enhanced sentinel node biopsy of the head and neck in a porcine model. Otolaryngol Head Neck Surg 137:735–741, 2007.

55. Chao C, Wong SL, Edwards MJ, et al: Sentinel lymph node biopsy for head and neck melanomas. Ann Surg Oncol 10:21–26, 2003.

56. Chepeha DB, Taylor RJ, Chepeha JC, et al: Functional assessment using Constant's Shoulder Scale after modified radical and selective neck dissection. Head Neck 24:432–436, 2002.

57. Kuntz AL, Weymuller EA, Jr: Impact of neck dissection on quality of life. Laryngoscope 109:1334–1338, 1999.

58. Rogers SN, Ferlito A, Pelliteri PK, et al: Quality of life following neck dissections. Acta Otolaryngol 124:231–236, 2004.

59. Becker MT, Shores CG, Yu KK, Yarbrough WG: Molecular assay to detect metastatic head and neck squamous cell carcinoma. Arch Otolaryngol Head Neck Surg 130:21–27, 2004.

Solitary Thyroid Nodule

12

Emad H. Kandil, Martha A. Zeiger, and Ralph P. Tufano

KEY POINTS

- High-resolution ultrasonography (US) has led to the identification of nonpalpable thyroid incidentalomas during nonthyroidal US examination of the neck in 19% to 67% of randomly selected individuals.
- Incidentalomas detected by US have a cancer risk of approximately 10% to 15% (0%–29%).
- The majority of patients presenting with a solitary thyroid nodule most likely have a benign lesion; however, thyroid cancer is a definite possibility in all patients.
- Most nodules are asymptomatic; however, physical findings may suggest possible malignancy.
- US provides considerably more anatomic detail than thyroid scintigraphy or CT scannings.
- The sonographic appearances of normal lymph nodes differ from those of abnormal nodes.
- The incidence of occult nodal metastasis in well-differentiated thyroid cancer is high, with the highest probability of nodal disease occurring in levels II–IV.
- FNA biopsy is the most cost effective and direct way to determine whether a thyroid nodule is a carcinoma.
- Laryngoscopic examination should be considered for all patients undergoing thyroid surgery.
- Thyroid cancer is the most common endocrine malignancy, accounting for over 90% of all endocrine cancers. The disease kills approximately 1300 people in the United States annually.
- Papillary cancer is the most common thyroid malignancy, accounting for 70% to 80% of all newly diagnosed thyroid cancers in the United States.
- The primary mode of therapy for patients with differentiated papillary thyroid cancer (PTC) is surgery.
- Lymph node "berry picking" is discouraged in management of PTC. Central lymph node dissection may reduce the risk for nodal recurrence and improve survival.
- Patients with an FNA that is interpreted as a follicular neoplasm should undergo a lobectomy and isthmusectomy.
- Patients with medullary thyroid carcinoma can be cured only by surgical intervention. These tumors are not amenable to radioiodine therapy.

Epidemiology

Although thyroid nodules are a common clinical problem, their prevalence depends to a considerable extent on the method of screening and the population being evaluated. Earlier epidemiologic studies have shown the prevalence of palpable thyroid nodules to be approximately 5% in women and 1% in men living in iodine-sufficient parts of the world.[1] In North America, the incidence of thyroid nodules detected by palpation is estimated to be 0.1% per year, with a prevalence between 4% and 7% in the general population.[2]

The prevalence of thyroid incidentalomas estimated from autopsy studies ranges from 30% to 60%.[3-5] Simple palpation, even by experienced physicians, is the least sensitive of all screening methods. In contrast, the increasing use of sensitive high-resolution ultrasonography has led to the identification of nonpalpable thyroid nodules during nonthyroidal ultrasonographic examination of the neck in 19% to 67% of randomly selected individuals, with higher frequencies in women and the elderly.[6,7]

Nodules are 10 times more common when the thyroid is examined at autopsy, intraoperatively, or by ultrasonography; half the glands studied have nodules, most of which are benign.[8]

Evaluation of a Clinically or Incidentally Discovered Thyroid Nodule

Most patients presenting with a solitary thyroid nodule most likely have a benign lesion; however, thyroid cancer is a definite possibility in all patients (Fig. 12-1). Management has evolved from surgical removal of all solitary nodules to a conservative approach; however, deciding between conservative management or surgical therapy relies on the careful analysis of the presentation, image assessment, and interventional diagnostic methods[9,10] (Fig. 12-2). In making this distinction, several

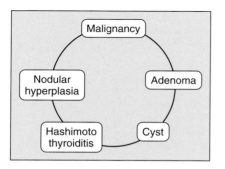

Figure 12-1. Differential diagnosis of thyroid nodule.

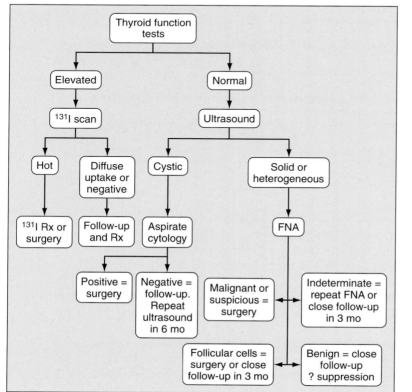

Figure 12-2. Algorithm for thyroid nodule workup.

clinical features must be considered, including patient age, sex, status of thyroid function, history of exposure to irradiation, family history, and preexisting thyroid disorders. However, none of these factors is sufficiently reliable in predicting whether a specific nodule will harbor malignant disease.

History

Nodules occurring at the extremes of age, particularly in men, are especially likely to be cancerous. Symptoms of local invasion and rapid tumor growth increase the likelihood of cancer. It is important to ask whether a patient has had external irradiation to the head, neck, and chest, since exposure to external irradiation raises the probability of malignant nodules. The chance that a thyroid nodule is malignant is higher when there is a history of childhood radiation exposure.[11]

Radiation-induced thyroid cancer may be diminishing in frequency, but radiation remains an important cause of cancer even though such a history is more commonly associated with benign thyroid abnormalities.[12,13] A family history of medullary or papillary thyroid cancer increases the likelihood that a thyroid nodule is cancerous.[14]

Physical Examination

Most nodules are asymptomatic; however, physical findings suggesting possible malignancy include fixation of the nodule to surrounding tissues, a very firm or hard nodule, vocal cord paralysis, obstructive symptoms, and cervical lymphadenopathy[15,16] (Table 12-1).

Laboratory Examination

Serum Thyroid-Stimulating Hormone

Low serum thyroid-stimulating hormone (TSH) concentration indicates overt or subclinical hyperthyroidism, increasing the possibility that the nodule is hot, and thus thyroid scintigraphy should be obtained to document whether the nodule is hyperfunctioning, isofunctioning, or nonfunctioning. However, the risk of malignancy in a thyroid nodule increases with serum thyroid-stimulating hormone concentrations within the normal range.[14]

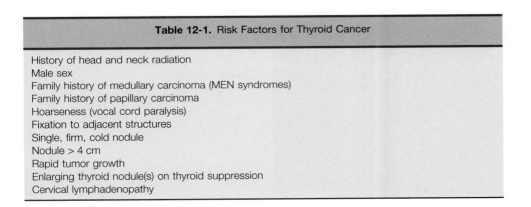

Table 12-1. Risk Factors for Thyroid Cancer

History of head and neck radiation
Male sex
Family history of medullary carcinoma (MEN syndromes)
Family history of papillary carcinoma
Hoarseness (vocal cord paralysis)
Fixation to adjacent structures
Single, firm, cold nodule
Nodule > 4 cm
Rapid tumor growth
Enlarging thyroid nodule(s) on thyroid suppression
Cervical lymphadenopathy

Serum Calcitonin

Unstimulated serum calcitonin greater than 100 pg/mL is likely to be associated with medullary cancer. Several series of prospective, nonrandomized studies have suggested that serum calcitonin should be measured routinely in patients with nodular thyroid disease in order to detect C-cell hyperplasia and medullary thyroid cancer (MTC) at an earlier stage. However, controversy remains regarding the routine use of serum calcitonin measurements because of the high false-positive rate (59%), cost-effectiveness, and unresolved issues of assay performance.[17]

Radiologic Evaluation

Neck Ultrasound

Routine screening of a population of individuals at low risk for thyroid cancer does not seem to be cost-effective. However, a recent report of ultrasonographic mass screening for thyroid carcinoma in women who require breast examinations was considered effective for the detection of subclinical thyroid carcinoma.[18]

A nodule not discovered clinically but detected by ultrasonography (such as with carotid Doppler scans) is considered an *incidentaloma.* Incidentalomas detected by ultrasound have a cancer risk of approximately 10% to 15% (0% to 29%).[19-21]

Thyroid ultrasonography is helpful in determining the volume of a nodule, its multicentricity, and whether it is solid or cystic. In addition, ultrasound is extremely useful in patients who are managed conservatively for follow-up of possible increased volume of a suspicious lesion. Ultrasound provides considerably more anatomic detail than thyroid scintigraphy or computed tomography (CT) scans, and it is being increasingly used as an extension of the physical examination.

For the patient with a thyroid nodule and normal thyroid function tests, an ultrasound should be performed. Ultrasound has proved highly effective in determining the location and characteristics (cystic versus solid) of nodules, but it is unable to accurately predict the diagnosis of solid nodules (Fig. 12-3). The finding of a cystic lesion may be reassuring, but these represent only 1% to 5% of thyroid nodules. In addition, up to 25% of well-differentiated thyroid cancers had cystic components. Patients with recurrent cysts should be considered surgical candidates.

Most nodules with apparent microcalcifications are benign, since colloid may have an appearance on ultrasound similar to that of microcalcifications associated with thyroid cancer (Table 12-2; Fig. 12-4).

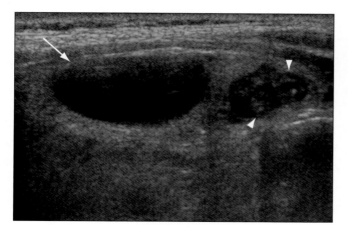

Figure 12-3. Cystic thyroid nodules (colloid cyst).   Sagittal sonogram of the left thyroid lobe shows two cystic nodules. The largest (*arrow*) is for a simple cyst (anechoic); the smaller inferior nodule (*arrowheads*) shows a lace-like pattern of multiple small cysts, which is also characteristic of colloid nodules.

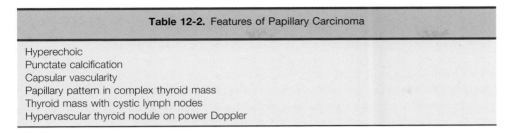

Table 12-2. Features of Papillary Carcinoma

Hyperechoic
Punctate calcification
Capsular vascularity
Papillary pattern in complex thyroid mass
Thyroid mass with cystic lymph nodes
Hypervascular thyroid nodule on power Doppler

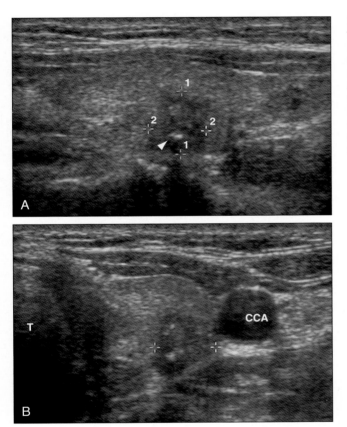

Figure 12-4. Incidentaloma with papillary thyroid cancer. A 57-year-old woman with history of low-grade lymphoma and incidentally noted FDG ([18]fluorodeoxyglucose)-avid thyroid nodule on positron emission tomography scan. **A,** Sagittal sonogram of the left thyroid lobe shows a hypoechoic mass with irregular borders (between calipers) and small foci of microcalcifications (arrowhead). **B,** Transverse sonogram confirms the presence of the 7-mm mass. CCA, common carotid artery; T, trachea.

The sonographic appearances of normal nodes differ from those of abnormal nodes. Abnormal nodes have sonographic features that include round shape, absent hilus, calcification, intranodal necrosis, reticulation, matting, soft tissue edema, and peripheral vascularity. However, many nodal metastases demonstrate a wide variety of nondiagnostic features.[22]

The incidence of occult nodal metastasis in well-differentiated thyroid cancer is high, with the highest probability of nodal disease in levels II-IV. In a recent study from the Mayo Clinic, preoperative ultrasound detected metastatic nonpalpable lymph nodes in 32.9% of patients with papillary thyroid cancer, thus altering surgical planning. In addition, in patients with palpable lymphadenopathy, ultrasound can guide the extent of lymphadenectomy.[23]

Thyroid Scan

A thyroid scan can help to determine whether a nodule is autonomously functioning or is nonfunctional. Nodules that do not take up radioactive iodine are called cold and have a 5% risk of being malignant. Generally, 95% of nodules are cold. The use of radionuclide scanning has decreased as fine-needle aspiration (FNA) has improved. The determination of increased or poor uptake in a thyroid nodule does not have acceptable accuracy to warrant its exclusive use for diagnostic decision making.

Fine-Needle Aspiration Biopsy

Fine-needle aspiration (FNA) biopsy has resulted in substantial improvements in diagnostic accuracy and a higher malignancy yield at time of surgery. FNA technique was first used in Sweden in the 1960s. FNA biopsy is the most cost-effective and direct way to determine whether a thyroid nodule is a carcinoma. Every patient with a palpable thyroid nodule is a candidate for FNA. Before a decision is made to perform FNA, a complete history should be obtained; a directed physical examination to the thyroid gland and cervical lymph nodes should be performed; and thyroid function tests and thyroid ultrasound should be obtained. Ultrasonography can enhance the efficiency of this technique (Fig. 12-5).

Contraindications to thyroid FNA are few: a severe bleeding disorder and an uncooperative patient. Medical consultation should be obtained prior to the FNA. Intrathyroidal hemorrhage with acute upper airway obstruction is an extremely rare complication, limited to a few case reports.[24]

Four major categories of results can be obtained from FNA (Fig. 12-1): (1) non-diagnostic; (2) benign: colloid, adenomas, Hashimoto's, or subacute thyroiditis; (3) indeterminate (suspicious): microfollicular or cellular adenomas (follicular neoplasm); and (4) malignant: papillary cancer, medullary cancer, thyroid lymphoma, anaplastic cancer, or metastatic cancer.

Benign nodules diagnosed by FNA should be followed sequentially with ultrasound to make sure the characteristics do not change.

All thyroid biopsy techniques are limited by their inability to distinguish differentiated follicular cancer from microfollicular or cellular adenomas. As a result, approxi-

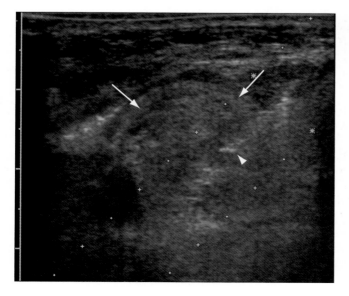

Figure 12-5. Fine-needle aspiration (FNA) biopsy under ultrasound guidance. Transverse sonogram of FNA of right thyroid nodule shows the echogenic tip of the needle (*arrowhead*) within the nodule (*arrow*).

Table 12-3. Indications for Diagnostic Ipsilateral Thyroid Lobectomy

Thyroid nodule
  Suspicious cytology
  Indeterminate cytology
  Enlarging nodule
  Associated compressive symptoms
  Nondiagnostic FNA biopsy ×2
Thyroid cysts
  >4 cm
  Compound solid/cystic lesions
  >3 recurrences of the cyst

FNA, fine-needle aspiration.

mately 20% of all biopsies are classified as indeterminate or suspicious. If FNA leads to a diagnosis that is "suspicious but not confirmatory," an aggressive workup should continue designed to look for a possible malignancy. If an FNA is indeterminate, a repeat aspiration might be considered. Patients who are male, have solid nodules, are older than 40 years, or have a history of radiation exposure have an increased likelihood of having a malignancy in a thyroid nodule. These patients should be counseled to consider a surgical option (Table 12-3).

FNA cannot confirm follicular cancer, nor can it confirm a benign adenoma. Patients with follicular cells seen on FNA have up to a 20% incidence of malignancy. Therefore, older male patients with a history of radiation should be considered for surgical intervention.

There is no agreement regarding whether thyroid suppression is superior to observation in patients with colloid nodules. However, thyroid hormone should not be used in patients with suppressed serum thyroid-stimulating hormone levels so that toxic symptoms can be avoided. Thyroid suppression is often unsuccessful and has the potential for untoward effects from exogenous hyperthyroidism. If the decision is made to use thyroid suppression, it must be carefully monitored, particularly in postmenopausal women because of the significant risk of osteoporosis.[25]

Cystic nodules should be reevaluated with ultrasound every 6 months to establish stability of nodule size. Increase in nodule size should be an indication for surgical intervention.

Preoperative Laryngoscopy in Patients Undergoing Thyroidectomy

Vocal cord paralysis is usually associated with extrathyroidal invasive malignancy. Voice change is associated with vocal cord paralysis in only one third of patients. Preoperative radiographic evaluation with CT scans is positive for vocal cord paralysis in only 25% of patients with vocal cord paralysis. Laryngoscopic examination should be considered for all patients undergoing thyroid surgery.[26,27]

Preoperative recognition of thyroid cancer extent allows for appropriate operative planning, and helps in counseling patients appropriately about the risks of surgery while minimizing the medicolegal ramifications of iatrogenic recurrent laryngeal nerve injury.

Thyroid Cancer

Thyroid cancer is an uncommon tumor, with an annual incidence in the United States of about 30,000 cases (1.5% of all cancers); 74% of newly diagnosed patients are women, making thyroid cancer the seventh most commonly diagnosed malignancy

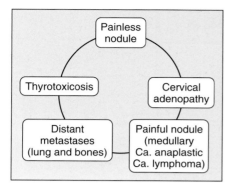

Figure 12-6. Clinical presentation of thyroid cancer.

Table 12-4. Pathologic Classification of Thyroid Cancers

Tumors of Follicular Cell Origin	Occurrence (%)
Differentiated	
Papillary	75
Follicular	10
Hürthle cell	5
Undifferentiated	
Anaplastic	1.6
Tumors of Parafollicular or C-cell Origin	
Medullary	5–10
Other	
Lymphoma	<1
Squamous cell carcinoma, secondary tumors	<1

in women.[28] It is the most common endocrine malignancy, accounting for over 90% of all endocrine cancers, and kills approximately 1300 people annually.[29] Most patients present with a thyroid nodule, but a few present with cervical lymphadenopathy or distant metastases (Fig. 12-6).

Ninety to ninety-five percent of thyroid cancer cases are categorized as well-differentiated tumors arising from follicular cell origin (papillary, follicular, and Hürthle cell carcinomas). Medullary thyroid cancer is responsible for about 5% to 10% of thyroid malignancies. Anaplastic carcinoma accounts for 1.6% of thyroid carcinomas and accounts for more than half the deaths from thyroid cancer in the United States (Table 12-4). Primary squamous cell carcinoma and metastatic disease to the thyroid gland are rare. This diagnosis can be made by FNA.

Papillary Thyroid Cancer

Papillary cancer is the most common thyroid malignancy, accounting for about 70% to 80% of all newly diagnosed thyroid cancers in the United States.

Pathology

Histologically, papillary thyroid cancer has characteristic features including psammoma bodies (calcified clumps of cells from sloughed papillary projections), cyto-

Table 12-5. Histologic Variants of Papillary Carcinoma
Pure papillary
Follicular variant
Tall-cell variant
Columnar cell variant
Oxyphilic cell variant
Diffuse sclerosing variant
Encapsulated variant

plasmic inclusions, and intranuclear grooves. The finding of psammoma bodies is diagnostic of papillary cancer. Nucleoli are prominent and have holes due to intranuclear cytoplasmic inclusions (Orphan Annie eyes). Papillary carcinoma consists of the following histologic subtypes (Table 12-5):

Pure papillary variant
Follicular variant (10%): In the past, these were mistakenly called follicular adenomas or carcinomas because of the near total absence of papillae. The pathologic and clinical behavior is comparable to that of pure papillary variant.[30]
Other variants: The following papillary cancers are rare and tend to be relatively radioiodine-resistant, more aggressive, and associated with a poorer prognosis:

Tall cell variant (1%)
Insular variant
Columnar cell variant
Hürthle (oxyphilic) cell variant
Diffuse sclerosing variant

Clinical Presentation

Papillary cancer occurs two times more often in women than in men, and the mean age at presentation ranges from 38 to 45 years. Patients usually present with a solitary mass or masses that are painless and firm. Occasionally, a painless mass is seen in the lateral neck, and an FNA biopsy helps to confirm a metastatic papillary thyroid carcinoma, even in the case of a normal thyroid examination. Papillary cancer may be found incidentally in a thyroidectomy specimen resected for a benign process. These masses are usually less than 5 mm in size.

Papillary thyroid carcinoma accounts for 90% of radiation-induced thyroid malignancy. The use of external-beam radiation in the 1950s and 1960s for tonsillitis and acne in the juvenile and adolescent population has been shown to result in an increased incidence of well-differentiated thyroid malignancy at any time, usually 5 years after exposure. Approximately 30% to 35% of patients who have received external-beam radiation for soft tissue malignancy have an increased incidence of thyroid nodules and cancer.[31] Areas near known nuclear fallout contamination, such as Chernobyl in the former Soviet Union, have increased incidence rates of well-differentiated thyroid carcinoma.[32] Radiation exposure is associated with the development of thyroid nodules. Risk of thyroid cancer is high in atomic bomb survivors with solid thyroid nodules, suggesting the need for careful observation of irradiated persons with such nodules.[33] Familial variant accounts for 3% of patients with papillary thyroid carcinoma.

Surgery

The primary mode of therapy for patients with differentiated papillary thyroid cancer is surgery. Controversy exists regarding the use of lobectomy versus total thyroidectomy in young patients with a 1- to 2-cm papillary thyroid carcinoma. We recommend total thyroidectomy in the following conditions:

- Primary tumor is more than 1 cm
- Contralateral thyroid nodules
- Regional or distant metastases
- History of head and neck radiation therapy
- Age > 45 years
- First-degree family history of differentiated thyroid cancer

Total thyroidectomy decreased the recurrence of papillary thyroid carcinoma in both low-risk and high-risk patients and death and recurrence rates in high-risk patients.[23] Unilateral lobectomy for low-risk papillary thyroid carcinoma resulted in an 11% recurrence rate, and 33% of these patients subsequently died of thyroid carcinoma.[34]

Multiple studies documented improved survival in addition to decreased recurrence when patients were treated with total thyroidectomy and postoperative iodine therapy.[35,36] The benefits of total thyroidectomy include the following:

- Effective radioiodine ablative therapy after removal of thyroid tissue
- Usage of serum thyroglobulin levels for detecting recurrent or persistent disease
- Removal of multicentric thyroid cancer, which is present in up to 80% of patients
- Elimination of the risk of transformation of a well-differentiated papillary thyroid cancer to an undifferentiated one.

Recurrence in regional lymph nodes after initial surgery should be treated with completion thyroidectomy if residual thyroid exists, in addition to comprehensive regional lymph node dissection. Radioiodine therapy should still be used as adjunctive therapy.

Lymph Node Dissection

The role of lymph node dissection is also debated. Metastatic regional lymph nodes are present in 20% to 90% of patients at the time of diagnosis.[37-39] On preoperative ultrasonography, suspicious lymph nodes in the central and lateral neck should undergo FNA. For positive findings in the central neck, a central neck dissection should be performed. For positive findings in the lateral neck, a lateral neck dissection should be undertaken. Lymph node "berry picking" is discouraged. Central lymph node dissection may reduce the risk of nodal recurrence and improve survival.[40,41]

Prognostic Features

Most patients with papillary carcinoma do not die of their disease and can expect an excellent prognosis (95% 10-year survival rate for well-differentiated stages). Certain clinical and pathologic features have been identified that portend a higher risk of tumor recurrence and cancer-related mortality. The most important clinical and pathologic prognostic factors include age at diagnosis, size of the primary tumor, and the presence of soft tissue invasion or distant metastases[35,42-44] (Table 12-6).

Table 12-6. Prognostic Scoring Systems for Well-Differentiated Thyroid Carcinoma

AGES	AMES	DAMES	SAG	MACIS
Age	Age	DNA	Size	Metastasis (distant)
Grade	Metastasis (distant)	Age	Age	Age
				Completeness of resection
				Invasion
Extent	Extent	Metastasis (Distant)	Grade	Size

Failure to take up radioiodine, aneuploid DNA content, *N-ras* mutations, and *p53* oncogene expression are associated with a poorer prognosis. Patients with *BRAF* mutation are more likely to have extrathyroidal invasion, lymph node metastases, and tumor recurrence.[45]

Follicular Thyroid Cancer

Follicular thyroid cancer (FTC) is the second most common type of thyroid cancer after papillary thyroid cancer, accounting for approximately 10% of all thyroid cancer.

Pathology

Histologically, follicular thyroid cancer is characterized by follicle formation and the absence of any papillary elements in the tumor. A follicular adenoma is distinguished from a carcinoma based on the presence of capsular or vascular invasion on permanent section of the thyroid. FNA biopsy or frozen section cannot distinguish between follicular adenomas and carcinomas. Distant metastases occur in 10% to 15% of patients, even in those with small primary tumors. Common sites of distant metastases are bone (lytic lesions) and lung.[46]

There are two patterns of growth that relate to capsular invasion: (1) minimally invasive (encapsulated) follicular carcinoma (MIFC); and (2) widely invasive follicular carcinoma (WIFC), which invades the tumor capsule and adjacent thyroid parenchyma. Recently, the term "angioinvasive" has been used and may be associated with distant metastases.[47]

Clinical Presentation

The mean age at presentation of follicular thyroid cancer is 50 years and predominantly affects women. The female-to-male ratio is 3 : 1. It usually presents as a painless thyroid mass. The mass is typically uninodular, and the coexistence of cervical lymphadenopathy is rare, occurring in less than 5% of patients. Follicular thyroid malignancy is very rarely associated with a hyperfunctioning or hypofunctioning thyroid.

Treatment

Surgical intervention is the primary treatment for follicular thyroid cancer. Patients with an FNA biopsy that is interpreted as a follicular neoplasm should undergo a lobectomy and isthmusectomy. A completion thyroidectomy should be performed when the permanent section shows a clinically significant follicular cancer. Lymph node dissection is performed only for evident metastatic disease.

Radioiodine therapy is most efficacious in patients who have undergone total thyroidectomy. Higher doses of iodine-131 are needed for remnant ablation in patients who have undergone subtotal thyroidectomy.

Medullary Thyroid Cancer

Medullary thyroid carcinoma is a neuroendocrine tumor of the parafollicular (C cells) of the thyroid gland. It accounts for approximately 5% of thyroid carcinomas.

Clinical Presentation

Most medullary thyroid carcinomas are sporadic (80% of all cases). The mean age of presentation is 50 years, and there may be a slight female preponderance.[39] Patients with sporadic medullary thyroid carcinoma usually present with a solitary thyroid nodule (75% to 95%). The cancer generally is confined to one lobe in sporadic cases, whereas in hereditary cases both lobes are usually involved.

In most patients, the disease has already metastasized at the time of diagnosis. Systemic symptoms may occur as a result of hormonal secretion by the tumor. Calcitonin secretion can cause diarrhea or facial flushing in patients with advanced disease. In addition, medullary thyroid tumors occasionally secrete corticotropin (ACTH), causing Cushing's syndrome.

Multiple endocrine neoplasia (MEN) type IIA usually has a more favorable long-term outcome than MEN IIB or sporadic medullary carcinoma.[48]

Medullary thyroid cancer is a component comprising two well-defined syndromes (Table 12-7):

MEN IIA, which may be associated with pheo.chromocytoma and/or hyperparathyroidism;
MEN IIB, which occurs early and is accompanied by developmental abnormalities.

All patients who inherit the MEN type II syndrome develop medullary thyroid cancer. MENIIB patients with medullary thyroid cancer present at an extremely early age, and this disease is considered the most aggressive form of hereditary medullary thyroid cancer. Once it manifests clinically, it is rarely curable.[49]

Table 12-7. Multiple Endocrine Neoplasias (MEN)

Sporadic MTC
No associated endocrinopathies

MEN IIA
Medullary thyroid carcinoma
Pheochromocytoma
Hyperparathyroidism
Lichen planus amyloidosis
Hirschsprung's disease

MEN IIB
Medullary thyroid carcinoma
Pheochromocytoma
Marfanoid body habitus
Mucosal neuromas
Ganglioneuromatosis of the gastrointestinal tract

Familial medullary thyroid cancer (FMTC)
No associated endocrinopathies

The *RET* proto-oncogene is the causative gene of the MEN II syndromes and mutations in this gene are found in over 90% of inherited cases, allowing a reliable family screening. Sporadic and familial medullary thyroid cancers (FMTC) are not associated with any endocrinopathy. Medullary thyroid cancer spreads to the perithyroidal and paratracheal lymph nodes (central compartment, level VI lymph nodes).

A characteristic feature of this tumor is the production of calcitonin. Although plasma calcitonin serum level is a specific and sensitive marker of medullary thyroid cancer, in the United States, measurement of serum calcitonin has not been a part of the routine evaluation of thyroid nodules. Patients with thyroid nodules had a high serum calcitonin of up to 3%. However, only 40% of patients with high serum calcitonin values proved to have medullary thyroid cancer.[50,51]

As mentioned earlier in this chapter, controversy remains concerning the routine use of serum calcitonin measurements because of the high false-positive rate (59%), cost-effectiveness, and unresolved issues of assay performance.[14] Patients with higher preoperative serum calcitonin concentrations have larger tumors and are less likely to have normal serum concentrations postoperatively than those with lower preoperative values.[52]

Treatment

Patients with medullary thyroid carcinoma can be cured only by surgical intervention, which, at least, consists of a total thyroidectomy with central lymph node dissection. These tumors are not amenable to radioiodine therapy.

Central lymph node compartment (level VI lymph nodes) dissection allows appropriate staging of this disease. Lateral neck dissection should be performed for any palpable lymph nodes in the lateral compartments. Postoperatively, serum calcitonin level should be checked. Documentation of an elevated postoperative serum calcitonin level should prompt a search for locally resectable disease as well as metastatic disease. Serum calcitonin concentration falls slowly in some patients, with the nadir not being reached for several months. Metastatic medullary thyroid cancer is most commonly found in the liver, lungs, and bones. Ultrasound of the neck is the most sensitive study to identify residual disease.

References

1. Vander JB, Gaston EA, Dawber TR: The significance of nontoxic thyroid nodules. Final report of a 15-year study of the incidence of thyroid malignancy. Ann Intern Med 69(3):537–640, 1968.
2. Rojeski MT, Gharib H: Nodular thyroid disease. Evaluation and management. N Engl J Med 313(7):428–436, 1985.
3. Mortensen JD, Woolner LB, Bennett WA: Gross and microscopic findings in clinically normal thyroid glands. J Clin Endocrinol Metab 15(10):1270–1280, 1955.
4. Hermanson L, Gargill SL, Lesses MF: The treatment of nodular goiter. J Clin Endocrinol Metab 12(1):112–129, 1952.
5. Furmanchuk AW, Roussak N, Ruchti C: Occult thyroid carcinomas in the region of Minsk, Belarus. An autopsy study of 215 patients. Histopathology 23(4):319–325, 1993.
6. Tan GH, Gharib H: Thyroid incidentalomas: management approaches to nonpalpable nodules discovered incidentally on thyroid imaging. Ann Intern Med 126(3):226–231, 1997.
7. Solbiati L, Volterrani L, Rizzatto G, et al: The thyroid gland with low uptake lesions: evaluation by ultrasound. Radiology 155(1):187–191, 1985.
8. Mazzaferri EL: Management of a solitary thyroid nodule. N Engl J Med 328(8):553–559, 1993.
9. Wong CK, Wheeler MH: Thyroid nodules: rational management. World J Surg 24(8):934–941, 2000.
10. Castro MR, Gharib H: Thyroid fine-needle aspiration biopsy: progress, practice, and pitfalls. Endocr Pract 9(2):128–136, 2003.
11. Mihailescu DV, Schneider AB: Size, number, and distribution of thyroid nodules and the risk of malignancy in radiation-exposed patients who underwent surgery. J Clin Endocrinol Metab 93(6):2188–2193, 2008.
12. Fogelfeld L, Wiviott MB, Shore-Freedman E, et al: Recurrence of thyroid nodules after surgical removal in patients irradiated in childhood for benign conditions. N Engl J Med 320(13):835–840, 1989.
13. Hrafnkelsson J, Tulinius H, Jonasson JG, et al: Papillary thyroid carcinoma in Iceland. A study of the occurrence in families and the coexistence of other primary tumours. Acta Oncol 28(6):785–788, 1989.
14. Boelaert K, Horacek J, Holder RL, et al: Serum thyrotropin concentration as a novel predictor of malignancy in thyroid nodules investigated by fine-needle aspiration. J Clin Endocrinol Metab 91(11):4295–4301, 2006.
15. Hegedus L: The thyroid nodule. N Engl J Med 351:1764–1771, 2004.
16. Alexander EK, Hurwitz S, Heering JP, et al: Natural history of benign solid and cystic thyroid nodules. Ann Intern Med 138:315–318, 2003.

17. Castro MR, Gharib H: Continuing controversies in the management of thyroid nodules. Ann Intern Med 142(11):926–931, 2005.

18. Chung WY, Chang HS, Kim EK, Park CS: Ultrasonographic mass screening for thyroid carcinoma: a study in women scheduled to undergo a breast examination. Surg Today 31(9):763–767, 2001.

19. Cooper DS, Doherty GM, Haugen BR, et al: Management guidelines for patients with thyroid nodules and differentiated thyroid cancer. Thyroid 16:109–142, 2006.

20. Liebeskind A, Sikora AG, Komisar A, et al: Rates of malignancy in incidentally discovered thyroid nodules evaluated with sonography and fine-needle aspiration. J Ultrasound Med 24:629–634, 2005.

21. Nan-Goong IS, Kim HY, Gong G, et al: Ultrasonography-guided fine-needle aspiration of thyroid incidentaloma: correlation with pathological findings. Clin Endocrinol 60:21–28, 2004.

22. Ahuja AT, Ying M: Sonographic evaluation of cervical lymph nodes. AJR Am J Roentgenol 184(5):1691–1699, 2005.

23. Stulak JM, Grant CS, Farley DR, et al: Value of preoperative ultrasonography in the surgical management of initial and reoperative papillary thyroid cancer. Arch Surg 141(5):489–494; discussion 494–496, 2006.

24. Roh JL: Intrathyroid hemorrhage and acute upper airway obstruction after fine needle aspiration of the thyroid gland. Laryngoscope 116:154–156, 2006.

25. Hurley DL, Gharib H: Evaluation and management of multinodular goiter. Otolaryngol Clin North Am 29(4):527–540, 1996.

26. Farrag TY, Lin FR, Cummings CW, et al: Importance of routine evaluation of the thyroid gland prior to open partial laryngectomy. Arch Otolaryngol Head Neck Surg 132(10):1047–1051, 2006.

27. Randolph GW, Kamani D: The importance of preoperative laryngoscopy in patients undergoing thyroidectomy: voice, vocal cord function, and the preoperative detection of invasive thyroid malignancy. Surgery 139(3):357–362, 2006.

28. Jemal A, Siegel R, Ward E, et al: Cancer statistics, 2006. CA Cancer J Clin 56(2):106–130, 2006.

29. Boring CC, Squires TS, Tong T, Montgomery S: Cancer statistics, 1994. CA Cancer J Clin 44(1):7–26, 1994.

30. Zidan J, Karen D, Stein M, et al: Pure versus follicular variant of papillary thyroid carcinoma: clinical features, prognostic factors, treatment, and survival. Cancer 97(5):1181–1185, 2003.

31. Fraker DL: Radiation exposure and other factors that predispose to human thyroid neoplasia. Surg Clin North Am 75(3):365–375, 1975.

32. Pacini F, Vorontsova T, Demidchik EP, et al: Post-Chernobyl thyroid carcinoma in Belarus children and adolescents: comparison with naturally occurring thyroid carcinoma in Italy and France. J Clin Endocrinol Metab 82(11):3563–3569, 1997.

33. Imaizumi M, Usa T, Tominaga T, et al: Long-term prognosis of thyroid nodule cases compared with nodule-free controls in atomic bomb survivors. J Clin Endocrinol Metab 90(9):5009–5014, 2005.

34. Cady B, Sedgwick CE, Meissner WA, et al: Risk factor analysis in differentiated thyroid cancer. Cancer 43(3):810–820, 1979.

35. Mazzaferri EL, Jhiang SM: Long-term impact of initial surgical and medical therapy on papillary and follicular thyroid cancer. Am J Med 97(5):418–428, 1994.

36. Loh KC, Greenspan FS, Gee L, et al: Pathological tumor-node-metastasis (pTNM) staging for papillary and follicular thyroid carcinomas: a retrospective analysis of 700 patients. J Clin Endocrinol Metab 82(11):3553–3562, 1997.

37. Grebe SK, Hay ID: Prognostic factors and management in thyroid cancer–consensus or controversy? West J Med 165(3):156–157, 1996.

38. Grebe SK, Hay ID: Thyroid cancer nodal metastases: biologic significance and therapeutic considerations. Surg Oncol Clin N Am 5(1):43–63, 1996.

39. Kouvaraki MA, Shapiro SE, Fornage BD, et al: Role of preoperative ultrasonography in the surgical management of patients with thyroid cancer. Surgery 134(6):946–954; discussion 954–945, 2003.

40. Tisell LE, Nilsson B, Molne J, et al: Improved survival of patients with papillary thyroid cancer after surgical microdissection. World J Surg 20(7):854–859, 1996.

41. Scheumann GF, Gimm O, Wegener G, et al: Prognostic significance and surgical management of locoregional lymph node metastases in papillary thyroid cancer. World J Surg 18(4):559–567; discussion 567–568, 1994.

42. Eustatia-Rutten CF, Corssmit EP, Biermasz NR, et al: Survival and death causes in differentiated thyroid carcinoma. J Clin Endocrinol Metab 91(1):313–319, 2006.

43. Voutilainen PE, Multanen MM, Leppaniemi AK, et al: Prognosis after lymph node recurrence in papillary thyroid carcinoma depends on age. Thyroid 11(10):953–957, 2001.

44. Xing M, Westra WH, Tufano RP, et al: BRAF mutation predicts a poorer clinical prognosis for papillary thyroid cancer. J Clin Endocrinol Metab 90(12):6373–6379, 2005.

45. Grebe SK, Hay ID: Follicular thyroid cancer. Endocrinol Metab Clin North Am 24(4):761–801, 1995.

46. Baloch ZW, LiVolsi VA: Prognostic factors in well-differentiated follicular-derived carcinoma and medullary thyroid carcinoma. Thyroid 11(7):637–645, 2001.

47. Roman S, Lin R, Sosa JA: Prognosis of medullary thyroid carcinoma: demographic, clinical, and pathologic predictors of survival in 1252 cases. Cancer 107(9):2134–2142, 2006.

48. You YN, Lakhani V, Wells SA, Jr, Moley JF: Medullary thyroid cancer. Surg Oncol Clin N Am 15(3):639–660, 2006.

49. O'Riordain DS, O'Brien T, Crotty TB, et al: Multiple endocrine neoplasia type 2B: more than an endocrine disorder. Surgery 118(6):936–942, 1995.

50. Pacini F, Fontanelli M, Fugazzola L, et al: Routine measurement of serum calcitonin in nodular thyroid diseases allows the preoperative diagnosis of unsuspected sporadic medullary thyroid carcinoma. J Clin Endocrinol Metab 78(4):826–829, 1994.

51. Niccoli P, Wion-Barbot N, Caron P, et al: Interest of routine measurement of serum calcitonin: study in a large series of thyroidectomized patients. The French Medullary Study Group. J Clin Endocrinol Metab 82(2):338–341, 1997.

52. Cohen R, Campos JM, Salaun C, et al: Preoperative calcitonin levels are predictive of tumor size and postoperative calcitonin normalization in medullary thyroid carcinoma. Groupe d'Etudes des Tumeurs a Calcitonine (GETC). J Clin Endocrinol Metab 85(2):919–922, 2000.

13 Conclusion: Impediments to Finding and Using an Effective Tool in Early Detection

Wayne M. Koch and Rachel A. Koch

Importance of an Early Detection Tool

Early detection of cancer is a highly prized goal. Indeed, the very reason for this book is that early detection of head and neck cancer (head and neck squamous cell carcinoma [HNSCC]) is widely viewed as a prime opportunity to improve the management of this disease in the population at large. This notion is based on the fact that most clinical reports indicate that the success of treatment varies directly with the stage at diagnosis. The hypothesis at play, therefore, is that cancers of the mouth and throat are more successfully treated if discovered before signs and symptoms are sufficient to arouse clinical attention leading to detection. Statistics show up to a 44% reduction in the rate of mortality in breast cancer associated with screening mammography.[1] No analogous data are available for HNSCC. This is probably because there is no effective means of screening for HNSCC that is easily accomplished on a mass scale throughout the country. Furthermore, the rate of HNSCC is much lower than that of breast, colon, and prostate cancers, making it more difficult to derive meaningful statistical data from this demographic group. But with little other hope of improved outcomes after several decades of improved reconstruction, combined chemotherapy and radiation, or even a decade of biologic treatments arising from the molecular biology revolution, early detection remains perhaps the best possibility for progress against HNSCC.

It is not known how much reduction in morbidity and mortality would accompany the development and implementation of an effective HNSCC early detection tool. Preclinical studies indicate marked variation in the growth rate of HNSCC in tissue culture and mice implants.[2] It could be that most cancers amenable to early detection by any means are of a slower-growing phenotype that lingers at an early stage over a longer time, whereas fast-growing tumors offer only a brief duration of time between development of a diagnosable lesion and achieving late-stage criteria. In addition, these lesions of more aggressive phenotype would convey a poorer prognosis. Therefore, it might not follow that early detection of lesions with a more aggressive genotype would have the same benefit in terms of outcome as would the discovery of indolent lesions at a low stage.

Specific Challenges

Some HNSCC metastasizes to neck nodes, and perhaps even to distant sites before the clinical appearance of the primary site. This not uncommon phenomenon is termed "unknown primary." In some cases, the primary site may be detected using radiographic testing or expert examination; in a few others, it may be identified by directed biopsy of typical sites in which cancer is likely to lie hidden. However, in a minority of cases, the primary site is not detected even with these steps taken, perhaps being identified years later and perhaps being sterilized by an effective local immune response or by radiation therapy applied to at-risk regions.[3] This well-known phenomenon illustrates the challenge of early detection efforts. Molecular analysis of directed biopsy tissues may help; identification of tumor-specific alterations identified in the metastatic implant in histologically normal tissue is strong evidence of the site of origin of the cancer.[4]

There are other impediments to effective clinical application of an early detection method. Delivering the test to those at risk requires mass communication to health care providers and patients as to (1) availability and appropriate application of the technology; (2) motivation and facilitation of health care systems and providers to make the test available; (3) distribution of necessary equipment, technical expertise, and reagents to perform the test; (4) overcoming of barriers that exist within society for individuals to seek out or accept screening; (5) an effective method for follow-up of positive results, including appropriate referral to specialist providers; (6) accurate localization of the clinical manifestation of disease underlying the positive test signal; and (7) availability of effective treatment options to halt early lesions (Box 13-1). Each of these must be in place; otherwise, the mere existence of a screening test is meaningless.

An ideal early detection test must be robust and reproducible with reliable results and must have high sensitivity and specificity. It must be inexpensive, minimally invasive, and simple to perform, permitting widespread distribution of equipment and reagents needed. When sensitivity is low, a false sense of security may derive from a negative result. This has been seen with mammography in that some breast cancers are not visualized well on mammogram. Magnetic resonance imaging (MRI)

Box 13-1. Challenges Facing Early Detection of HNSCC

Tumor Related

Molecular change precedes physical change

Field cancer effect

Variable aggressiveness/timing of metastasis

Host Related

Variable topography of mucosal sites—crypts, folds, crevices

Provider Related

Availability of equipment and expertise to examine upper aerodigestive tract

Population

Low incidence

Variable inherited risk profile

Variable exposure/lifestyle profile

Psychosocial

Avoidance of screening by at-risk individuals

Economic/Policy

Communicate availability of screening technology

Level of evidence required to win support

Access to care restrictions among indigent at-risk and remote populations

---

HNSCC, head and neck squamous cell carcinoma.

scanning and digital mammography are being tested as a means of enhancing sensitivity.[5] On the other hand, false-positive results from cancer screening tests have several untoward ramifications: time and expense must be allotted for follow-up examination(s), and patients incorrectly labeled as having cancer suffer mental anxiety and could lose insurance coverage or be otherwise stigmatized. The acceptance of a test by society at large is dependent on the perception of its accuracy.

One way to enhance the cost-effectiveness of a screening approach is to accurately identify those at risk for the disease. HNSCC presents a challenge in this regard. Unlike some breast, thyroid, and colon cancers, there is no known inherited tendency to develop HNSCC. Efforts to identify genotypic features associated with risk have been of marginal success and no clinical usefulness to date. A recent example is a case-control study consisting of 147 patients with premalignant oral or oropharyngeal lesions and 147 matched controls, who were evaluated for the associations of 10 genetic variants in 9 genes of the double-strand break (DSB) DNA repair pathway with an oral premalignant lesion (OPL) risk. The most notable finding was an intronic polymorphism (A17893G) of the XRCC3 gene in which the GG variant had one fifth the risk of cancer development of the AA form.[6] Demographic and lifestyle features associated with risk, though distinctive with regard to risk of smoking and excessive alcohol use, have been made more complicated by the advent of human papillomavirus (HPV)-related HNSCC with its distinctively different risk profile. Although HPV infection with seroconversion may indicate exposure sufficient to risk cancer development, most individuals with antibody response to HPV do not develop HNSCC.[7] The risk of developing cancer declines after smoking cessation, but only gradually. In recent years, as the rate of cigarette smoking declines in America, proportionally more ex-smokers are presenting with HNSCC many years after quitting regular tobacco use. This observation indicates the difficulty in defining who is at risk for HNSCC and therefore should be subjected to new detection approaches.

Oral Screening

Dental providers are encouraged to perform oral screening through training programs and the American Dental Association. If every dentist had proper training and motivation to provide this screening and identify visible lesions and if most persons regularly visited a dentist, a policy of oral screening would go a long way toward effective early detection of cancers of the visible oral tissues. A variety of products designed to enhance this visual screening by dentists are being developed and marketed. Most of these products require some degree of expertise and render many equivocal calls that require referral to more highly trained specialists for further workup and confirmation. This is useful for those discovered to have HNSCC who would be otherwise unaware of their disease for many months, but it also identifies many who must pursue further expensive, invasive, anxiety-inducing, and often painful medical evaluation including biopsy—all to learn that no cancer is present. Moreover, cancers that arise elsewhere in the upper aerodigestive tract (UADT) from tonsil arch and circumvallate papillae and beyond into the pharynx would still not be detected. Unfortunately, many people do not visit the dentist regularly for a variety of reasons: only a small subset of Americans has dental insurance through their employee benefits programs, and often these are the very individuals with the lowest risk for cancer. Persons with poor oral hygiene, who are most at risk for cancer, shun dental care, and in many cases have been rendered edentulous at an early age. Primary care physicians, who see a somewhat broader cross-section of Americans, are able to examine the oral cavity using a hand-held flashlight, but have little training in identifying lesions. Together with the rarity of HNSCC, this means that most physicians do nothing to screen for this disease.

Screening programs offered free of charge are gaining in popularity through the efforts of organizations such as the Yul Brynner Society Oral Cancer Awareness events held annually in April nationwide. However, these programs tend to attract people who are concerned and careful about their oral health, not the smoker-drinker population at risk. Indeed, a screening event held at a veterans' convention several years ago by the senior author and colleagues was attended primarily by nonsmoking spouses of at-risk veterans who remained in adjacent smoke-filled recreational facilities during screening hours despite vigorous public announcement and encouragement. Similar problems are noted in other screening endeavors. Even the highly recognized value of screening mammography has recently been met with a decline in compliance among at-risk women.[8] Patient navigators are being field tested in urban populations with the goal of increasing compliance among indigent patients with colonoscopy screening.[9] Similar organized efforts to encourage oral screening are nonexistent.

Imaging and Other Methods of Screening

Radiographic imaging is limited in its ability to detect early HNSCC lesions. These surface cancers typically are often not detectable by any currently available radiographic method. Even positron emission tomography (PET) scanning requires a substantial concentration of tumor cells—each with high metabolic activity clustered together to produce a signal that would draw attention. Slow-growing clonal populations of a precancerous nature do not take up enough radiolabeled glucose. Transformed cells that spread across the mucosa producing a field of premalignancy are too thin to produce adequate signal. T1 lesions only a few millimeters thick will not appear as a mass on computed tomography (CT) or MRI scans. On the other hand, PET and CT/MRI scanning frequently produces findings that ultimately prove to be false-positives, necessitating extensive further workup to investigate and rule out cancer. Inflammation may yield enough metabolic activity to produce suspicious regions in the mucosa or regional lymph nodes on PET scanning. For this reason, most third party payers do not support PET scans as screening tools for cancer.

In addition to expense and procedural risk, screening programs have a psychological impact on patients. A recent report indicates that that impact may not be all negative in a population of women receiving false-positive reports from screening mammography. In this report, a trend to conduct more frequent self-examination was seen along with a higher, but not pathologic, elevation in levels of distress and thoughts about cancer.[10] However, these patients need high-quality educational information appropriate to their degree of education and interest. The additional expense involved in providing that information is critical to the success of early detection programs.

To date, no commercially viable blood or saliva test has emerged for early detection of HNSCC. In large part, this may be attributed to the expense and time required for detection of the few highly tumor-specific molecular targets (such as *p53* mutation), and the decreased specificity of protein and mRNA markers that may be overexpressed but are also present to a lesser degree in normal tissues.

The best example of an available cancer blood test is prostate-specific antigen (PSA). Though widely used for prostate cancer screening in men over age 40 to 50, this approach is not without consternation and controversy (including the age at which testing should begin). The Center for Primary Care, Prevention, and Clinical Partnerships of the Agency for Healthcare Research and Quality recently concluded: "Prostate-specific antigen screening is associated with psychological harms, and its potential benefits remain uncertain."[11] This conclusion is based on lack of evidence of a reduction in prostate cancer mortality and morbidity rates since the introduction of PSA screening and on evidence that false-positive results cause adverse psychological effects for up to 1 year after the test. Observations such as this may serve to dampen enthusiasm for searching for blood and saliva screening targets for other cancers.

Even if a blood or saliva test did exist, positive results would still require careful physical evaluation to discover the location of the offending tissue. Small areas of dysplasia, perhaps deep within crypts in the tonsil, or mucosal folds in hypopharynx or larynx would not be easily identified, even by expert examiners. Given the potential for false-positive results, invasive measures such as tonsillectomy, direct laryngoscopy with directed biopsy of tongue base and pyriform, or empiric delivery of radiation or chemotherapy would seem not to be indicated unless the positive predictive value of the test is very high indeed. Expensive radiologic evaluations such as PET scanning have an unsatisfactory lower level of sensitivity with a lack of specificity, thus rendering PET more likely to produce a false-positive than a true-positive result when applied to a population of only limited risk.

Cost of Oral Screening

The economics of HNSCC cancer screening reflects technical imperfections. Dental visits are expensive and therefore shunned by those most at risk. Enhancing technology for dental visual examination is an additional expense passed on to the patient. Oral rinse or blood tests, when available, may be covered by health insurance, but it is unclear whether the entire population of Americans should be screened using expensive technology, when it becomes available, for detecting the 45,000 persons who will develop HNSCC each year. When a test turns positive, referral to a specialist would be required at minimum, with subsequent fiberoptic laryngoscopy, examination under anesthesia, surgical biopsy, or radiographic imaging adding to the price tag. Although early detection with its promise of simpler, more effective treatment should be a substantial cost savings for those who are identified with early cancer, the extent of that economic advantage might be modest for a large population. However, note that many women are screened annually by Pap smear for cervical cancer, which affects only 10,000 individuals annually and yet is well accepted by the public and third party payers. Indeed, regular screening is coincident with a dramatic decline in the incidence of cervical cancer (due perhaps to effective discovery and treatment of precancerous lesions).[12]

Identifying Precancerous Lesions

To intensify the dilemma, molecular alterations may predate morphologic cellular change, making clinical identification of precancerous clonal populations even more difficult, if not impossible. The field effect surrounding a known cancerous lesion may have some telltale clinical features (leukoplakia, erythroplakia), and histologic alterations (atypia, dysplasia), but these do not necessarily coexist (areas of carcinoma in situ may even be clinically unapparent), and tissues that have normal gross and histologic appearance can harbor molecular changes that predispose toward tumor recurrence and second primary development.[13]

At present, no effective measures are available for treating precancerous lesions let alone completely occult clonal populations of cells with malignant potential in an effort to prevent progression. Hence, once early detection is pressed below the threshold in which available therapeutic interventions are rationally applied, only enhanced surveillance and elevated efforts to avoid further carcinogen exposure (i.e., smoking cessation) can be prescribed in the effort to improve the clinical outcome of at-risk individuals. Chemopreventive agents effective in disrupting the tumor-progression pathway of transforming epithelial cells have long been sought with disappointing results (see Chapter 6). Awareness of being at high risk for developing cancer may help some persons to stop tobacco use. However, most smokers are well aware that their habit has negative health implications. Adoption of a diet rich in antioxidants and nutrients thought to enhance immune function seems to be a commonsense precaution available to at-risk individuals. However, consumption of leafy dark-green vegetables and purple berries is expensive and is atypical of persons with heavy smoking and alcohol use unless some epiphany has already occurred, such as a cancer diagnosis.

The Future of Early Detection of HNSCC

What is needed for enhancement of early detection efforts that would yield real clinical benefit (Box 13-2)? First, improved identification of individuals at risk would help limit the use of expensive testing and increase the specificity of results. This goal will likely be achieved through a combination of refinement of information of genetic risk profiles and cofactors that may influence known risk-inducing exposures. Very little data exist about inheritable risk for HNSCC, in part because of the rarity of the disease, together with the fact that exposure profiles related to lifestyle habits are often similar among family members. The sheer number of genes that have been studied because of a suggested link to cancer risk is daunting and growing. DNA repair and carcinogen metabolism functions intuitively make sense as potential risk profile candidates. The mapping of the human genome and ever-improving methods of high-throughput screening of thousands of genes may be helpful, but properly designed case-control studies are expensive and time-consuming.

Cofactors may contribute to simple paradigms of risk. For example, preliminary evidence suggests that marijuana use may contribute to the development of oropharyngeal cancer in patients with HPV exposure.[14] Cigarette smoking, though not increasing the risk of developing HPV-related oropharyngeal cancer, may be associated with increased metastatic potential once cancer does arise. Declining social stigma regarding discussion of sexual activity has permitted the collection of compelling data linking HPV-related cancer with sexual contact history. These issues are now common knowledge, opening the door to routine inclusion of sexual history in clinical workup of cancer patients, as well as in primary care risk assessment. Persons with a history of multiple oral sex partners should be watched more closely for HPV-related oropharyngeal cancer and should be among the first to be tested with new molecular approaches targeting the HPV genome.

The fact that HPV-related cancer of the oropharynx has been shown to have a distinctive clinical and molecular profile illustrates another problem challenging the

---

Box 13-2. Future Requirements for Effective Early Detection and Treatment

High-quality molecular markers (high sensitivity and specificity)

Noninvasive methods for specimen procurement

Economical, high-throughput, robust platform for testing

Societal recognition of need

Economic support of testing

Availability of expert diagnosticians

Availability of effective treatment for early but diffuse disease

Availability of effective preventive measures for precancerous lesions

development of an early detection schema for HNSCC: diversity within the disease at large. Nasopharyngeal carcinoma is another well-documented example of a particular disease entity distinct from mucosal epithelial carcinoma and arising in other areas of the upper aerodigestive tract. Cancers of the lateral tongue in young non-smokers is also a distinctive clinical entity within HNSCC (though less well understood) that may have its own unique features amenable to some screening methods while eluding others. HNSCC that develops in the extremes of age (under 25/over 75) also is probably associated with unique features that may be missed when screening for more typical HNSCC.

It is often suggested that prophylactic tonsillectomy might be considered to prevent HPV-related tonsil cancer. However, the palatine tonsils that are removed at standard tonsillectomy are only about half of the volume of at-risk tissue, since lingual tonsils that cover the tongue base are also frequently the site of HPV-related cancer development. These lymphoepithelial inclusions are less accessible and anatomically less well defined, making prophylactic extirpation of all tonsil tissue a much more dubious endeavor. Indeed, no effective surgical treatment exists to prevent HNSCC in high-risk situations. Some women submit to bilateral mastectomy in the setting of a very high familial risk for cancer, and some care providers have advocated total thyroidectomy for individuals with a strong family history of medullary thyroid carcinoma.[15] These other cancers benefit from the availability of specific genetic profiling, sufficient clinical data to confirm the high risk of individuals carrying the affected genes, and well-defined surgical procedures that can reduce risk by complete removal of at-risk tissue with manageable sequelae. For example, risk-reducing mastectomy has been shown to reduce the risk of breast cancer by 90% in *BRCA*-mutation carriers.[16]

Some slow-growing preclinical cancers arising in elderly patients may not require any treatment at all. This has been recognized in prostate cancer, resulting in proposals not to screen PSA after age 75.[17] In addition, well-differentiated microscopic thyroid cancers discovered incidentally at thyroidectomy performed for goiter, or at autopsy, are of no substantial clinical significance.[18] There is no obvious corresponding HNSCC entity that might go untreated throughout the natural life-span of even elderly patients. Because lesions of the upper aerodigestive tract quickly create pain and functional difficulty and because most lesions grow to increase symptom production within months, some treatment is generally contemplated, even if associated with substantial morbidity, in all patients except those already in active decline from another disease process.

Molecular testing for HNSCC is the focus of intense research activity at several major research centers worldwide. Laboratory testing for cancer awaits the discovery of markers (alone or in combination) that provide adequate sensitivity and specificity to permit an economical application of screening, whereas the throughput platform must be economical and robust. Again, sequencing of the entire HNSCC genome may be useful[19] through the discovery of new markers, whereas endeavors to enhance panels targeting epigenetic events such as methylation, and mitochondrial mutations may contribute.

Finally, public policy must make provision for the development of screening procedures for HNSCC. National health insurance coverage focused on health maintenance should embrace effective screening methods and make them available to persons at risk. Governmental endorsement of efforts to raise awareness regarding HNSCC would enhance the application of early detection tests. Continued support of research for the development and testing of screening methods by the National Institutes of Health (NIH) and industry partners is vital to the establishment of effective methods. Health and life insurance policies that penalize cancer survivors and cancer risk must also be addressed to remove a real source of fear that may prevent a person from wanting to know the truth about possible cancer.

Novel therapeutic tools are needed to reverse or block early steps in tumorigenesis in order to capitalize on early detection. Chemoprotective agents might be provided to persons at highest risk for exposure-driven carcinogenesis. One of the earliest alterations in HNSCC appears to affect the cell cycle (loss of *p16* through 9p heterozygous deletion or promoter methylation), making restoration of cell-cycle control a prime target for reversal of foundational events in tumorigenesis. Use of the anti-EGFR (epidermal growth factor receptor) antibody cetuximab for persons with premalignant lesions is being tested in clinical trial, another example of this line of reasoning.

Concluding Remarks

Despite numerous real and anticipated impediments, efforts at early detection of HNSCC must continue. This remains one of the best approaches to manage an otherwise deadly and devastating disease. Activity must progress in several arenas at once to bring to the public effective screening programs. Cooperation among the small society of HNSCC care providers, researchers, policy makers, and cancer providers is needed to achieve meaningful results.

References

1. Brem RF: Mammography screening of women in their forties: the impact of changes in screening guidelines. [Editorial]. Cancer 112(3):456–460, 2008.
2. Meck RA, Ingram M, Meck JM, et al: Establishment and cell cycle kinetics of a human squamous cell carcinoma in nude mice and in vitro. Cancer Res 41(3):1076–1085, 1981.
3. McQuone SJ, Eisele DW, Lee DJ, et al: Occult tonsillar carcinoma in the unknown primary. Laryngoscope 108:1605–1610, 1998.
4. Bedi GC, Westra WH, Gabrielson E, et al: Multiple head and neck tumors: evidence for a common clonal origin. Cancer Res 56:2484–2487, 1996.
5. Robson M, Offit K: Management of an inherited predisposition to breast cancer. N Engl J Med 357(2): 154–162, 2007.
6. Yang H, Lippman SM, Huang M, et al: Genetic polymorphisms in double-strand break DNA repair genes associated with risk of oral premalignant lesions. Eur J Cancer 44(11):1603–1611.
7. D'Souza G, Kreimer AR, Viscidi R, et al: Case-control study of human papillomavirus and oropharyngeal cancer. N Engl J Med 356;19:1944–1956, 2007.
8. Breen N, Cronin K, Meissner HI, et al: Reported drop in mammography: is this cause for concern? Cancer 109:2405–2409, 2007.
9. Chen LA, Santos S, Jandorf L, et al: A program to enhance completion of screening colonoscopy among urban minorities. Clin Gastroenterol Hepatol 6(4):443–450, 2008.
10. Brewer NT, Salz T, Lillie SE: Systematic review: the long-term effects of false-positive mammograms. Ann Intern Med 146(7): 502–510, 2007.
11. Lin K, Lipsitz R, Miller T, Janakiraman S, U.S. Preventive Services Task Force: Benefits and harms of prostate-specific antigen screening for prostate cancer: an evidence update for the U.S. Preventive Services Task Force. Ann Intern Med 149(3):192–199, 2008.
12. Milbourne A: Access, access, access: cervical cancer screening and management practices among providers in the National Breast and Cervical Cancer Early Detection Program (NBCCEDP). Cancer 110(5):941–942, 2007.
13. Califano J, Westra WH, Meininger G, et al: Genetic progression and clonal relationship of recurrent premalignant head and neck lesions. Clin Cancer Res 6:347–352, 2000.
14. Gillison ML, D'Souza G, Westra W, et al: Distinct risk factor profiles for human papillomavirus type 16-positive and human papillomavirus type 16-negative head and neck cancers. J Natl Cancer Inst 100(6):407–420, 2008.
15. Sakorafas GH, Friess H, Peros G: The genetic basis of hereditary medullary thyroid cancer: clinical implications for the surgeon, with a particular emphasis on the role of prophylactic thyroidectomy. Endocr Relat Cancer 15(4):871–884, 2008.
16. Rebbeck TR, Friebel T, Lynch HT, et al: Bilateral prophylactic mastectomy reduces breast cancer risk in BRCA1 and BRCA2 mutation carriers: the PROSE Study Group. J Clin Oncol 22:1055–1062, 2004.
17. Twombly R: Preventive Services Task Force recommends against PSA screening after age 75. J Natl Cancer Inst 100(22):1571–1573, 2008.
18. Solares CA, Penalonzo MA, Xu M, Orellana E: Occult papillary thyroid carcinoma in postmortem species: prevalence at autopsy. Am J Otolaryngol 26(2):87–90, 2005.
19. Leary RJ, Lin JC, Cummins J, et al: Integrated analysis of homozygous deletions, focal amplifications, and sequence alterations in breast and colorectal cancers. Proc Natl Acad Sci U S A 105(42):16224–16229, 2008.

Index

Note: Page numbers followed by f indicate figures; those followed by t indicate tables; and those followed by b indicate boxed material.